AF559742

A Handbook for Veterinary Physician

A Handbook for Veterinary Physician

Kurra Venkata Gopaiah

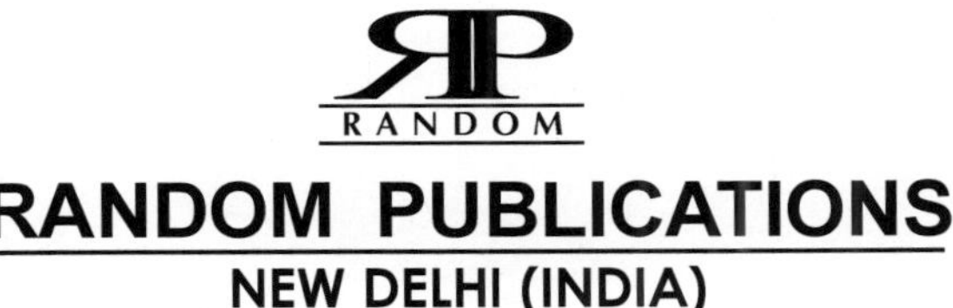

RANDOM PUBLICATIONS
NEW DELHI (INDIA)

A Handbook for Veterinary Physician

ISBN 978-93-5111-782-7

Published in 2016 in India by

RANDOM PUBLICATIONS

4376-A/4B, Gali Murari Lal, Ansari Road
New Delhi-110 002
Phone : +9111-43580356, 011-23289044, 011-43142548
e-mail: sales@randompublications.com,
info@randompublications.com, randomexports@gmail.com

Reprinted 2024

Type Setting by : Friends Media, Delhi-110089
Digitally Printed at: Replika Press Pvt. Ltd.

Preface

A veterinary physician, colloquially called a vet, shortened from veterinarian or veterinary surgeon, is a professional who practices veterinary medicine by treating disease, disorder, and injury in non-human animals.

In many countries, the local nomenclature for a veterinarian is a regulated and protected term, meaning that members of the public without the prerequisite qualifications and/or licensure are not able to use the title. In many cases, the activities that may be undertaken by a veterinarian (such as treatment of illness or surgery in animals) are restricted only to those professionals who are registered as a veterinarian. For instance, in the United Kingdom, as in other jurisdictions, animal treatment may only be performed by registered veterinary physicians (with a few designated exceptions, such as paraveterinary workers), and it is illegal for any person who is not registered to call themselves a veterinarian or prescribe any treatment.

Most veterinary physicians work in clinical settings, treating animals directly. These veterinarians may be involved in a general practice, treating animals of all types; they may be specialized in a specific group of animals such as companion animals, livestock, zoo animals or equines; or may specialize in a narrow medical discipline such as surgery, dermatology or internal medicine. As with other healthcare professionals, veterinarians face ethical decisions about the care of their patients. Current debates within the profession include the ethics of certain procedures believed to be purely cosmetic or unnecessary for behavioral issues, such as declawing of cats, docking of tails, cropping of ears and debarking on dogs.

The book shall also be useful for the neo-vets and budding veterinarians, practicing veterinary clinicians, livestock development officers, animal health workers, Pranibandhu and progressive livestock farmers in India and other tropical countries.

– Author

Contents

1

Introduction

A veterinarian is a medical professional who protects the health and well-being of both animals and people. They diagnose and control animal diseases and treat sick and injured animals. They also advise owners on proper care of their pets and livestock. Veterinarians provide a wide range of services in private practice, teaching, research, government service, public health, military service, private industry, and other areas.

When taking the veterinarian's oath, a doctor solemnly swears to use his or her scientific knowledge and skills "for the benefit of society, through the protection of animal health, the relief of animal suffering, the conservation of animal resources, the promotion of public health, and the advancement of medical knowledge."

A Veterinarian is a specialized type of Doctor.

FIND YOUR COMPATIBILITY

Would you make a good veterinarian? Sokanu's free assessment reveals your exact compatibility with this career, your strengths, and any unique areas of interest.

WHAT DOES A VETERINARIAN DO

A Veterinarian:

- Diagnoses animal health problems
- Vaccinates against diseases, such as distemper and rabies
- Medicates animals suffering from infections or illnesses
- Treats and dresses wounds
- Sets fractures
- Performs minor to complex surgery, depending on training
- Advises owners about animal feeding, behaviour and breeding
- Euthanizes animals when necessary
- Provides preventive care to maintain the health of livestock
- Performs diagnostic tests such as X-ray, EKG, ultrasound, blood, urine, and faeces

In many respects a veterinarian is similar to a pediatrician. Animals cannot talk like human beings, and much of the clinical history is obtained from the owner or client, as a pediatrician would obtain from a child's parents. Excellent people skills and communication skills are required. What cannot be obtained from the clinical history is acquired with the fingers, eyes, and smell. The ability to listen with a stethoscope and palpate with the fingers and hands will reveal much of the physical findings. The sense of smell is also important in detecting the fruity odour of the ketotic cow's breath, or the urea from the breath of a cat in renal failure.

What cannot be revealed by the history and exam is further supported by diagnostic tests like blood work, urinalysis, and fecal exams. Veterinarians are well trained in laboratory medicine and parasitology.

The general practice veterinarian spends one third to one half of his or her time in surgery. Animal neutering operations are done in most veterinarians' offices. Many veterinarians also perform orthopedic procedures, bone setting, dentistry, and trauma surgery. Surgery requires good hand and eye coordination, and fine motor skills. A veterinarian's job is similar to that of a human doctor.

When health problems arise, veterinarians diagnose the problem and treat the animal. Accurate diagnosis frequently requires laboratory tests, radiography, and specialized equipment. Treatments may involve a number of different procedures including emergency lifesaving techniques, prescribing medication, setting fractures, birthing, performing surgery, or advising an owner on feeding and care of the animal. To prevent the introduction of foreign diseases, veterinarians employed by government agencies quarantine and inspect animals brought into the country from other countries. They supervise shipments of animals, test for the presence of diseases, and manage campaigns to prevent and eradicate many diseases such as tuberculosis, brucellosis and rabies, which threaten animal and human health.

A veterinarian in research looks for better ways to prevent and solve animal and human health problems. Many problems, such as cancer and heart disease, are studied through the use of laboratory animals, which are carefully bred, raised, and maintained under the supervision of veterinarians.

There are many veterinarians that are professors, teaching at schools and universities of veterinary medicine. In addition to teaching, veterinary school faculty members conduct basic and clinical research, contribute to scientific publications, and develop continuing education programmes to help graduate veterinarians acquire new knowledge and skills.

Veterinarians also work in the area of public health. They help to prevent and control animal and human diseases and promote good health. As epidemiologists they investigate animal and human disease outbreaks such as food-borne illness, influenza, plague, rabies, AIDS, and encephalitis. They evaluate the safety of food processing plants, restaurants, and water supplies. Veterinarians in environmental health programmes study and evaluate the effects of various pesticides, industrial pollutants, and other contaminants on people as well as on animals.

As opposed to human medicine, general practice veterinarians greatly outnumber veterinary specialists. Most veterinary specialists work at a veterinary school, or at a referral centre in large cities. As opposed to human medicine, where each organ system has its own medical and surgical specialties, veterinarians often combine both the surgical and medical aspect of an organ system into one field. The specialties in veterinary medicine often encompass several medical and surgical specialties that are found in human medicine. Within each veterinary specialty, one will often find a separation of large animal medicine from small animal medicine. Some veterinary specialties are evolving, some are limited only in the teaching universities, and some are practiced only in the field.

LABORATORY ANIMAL SOURCES

Animals used by laboratories for testing purposes are largely supplied by dealers who specialize in selling them to universities, medical and veterinary schools, and companies that provide contract animal-testing services. It is comparatively rare that animals are procured from sources other than specialized dealers, as this poses the threat of introducing disease into a colony and confounding any data collected. However, suppliers of laboratory animals may include breeders who supply purpose-bred animals, businesses that trade in wild animals, and dealers who supply animals sourced from pounds, auctions, and newspaper ads. Animal shelters may also supply the laboratories directly. Some animal dealers, termed Class B dealers, have been reported to engage in kidnapping pets from residences or illegally trapping strays, a practice dubbed as bunching.

DEALERS IN THE UNITED STATES

All laboratories using vertebrate lab animals in the United States are required by law to have a licensed veterinarian on staff and to adhere to the NIH Guide for the Use and Care of Laboratory Animals, which further stipulates that all protocols, including the sources for obtaining the animals, must be reviewed by an independent committee.

Class A Dealers

Class A breeders are licensed by the U.S. Department of Agriculture (USDA) to sell animals bred specifically for research. In July 2004, there were 4,117 licensed Class A dealers in the United States.

Class B Dealers

Class B dealers are licensed by the USDA to buy animals from "random sources". This refers to animals who were not purpose-bred or raised on the dealers' property.Animals from "random sources" come from auctions, pounds, newspaper ads (including "free-to-home" ads), and some may be stolen pets or illegally trapped strays. As of February 2013, there were only seven active Class B dealers remaining in the United States. However, these sources round up "thousands" of cats and dogs each year for sale.

Animal Shelters

Animals are also sold directly to laboratories by shelters. According to the American Society for the Prevention of Cruelty to Animals (ASPCA), Iowa, Minnesota, Oklahoma, South Dakota, and Utah require publicly funded shelters to surrender animals to any Class B dealer who asks for them. Fourteen states prohibit the practice, and the remainder either have no relevant legislation, or permit the practice in certain circumstances.

Bunching

According to a paper presented to the American Society of Criminology in 2006, an illegal economy in the theft of pets, mostly dogs, has emerged in the U.S. in recent years, with the thieves known as "bunchers". The bunchers sell the animals to Class B animal dealers, who pay $25 per animal. The dealers then sell the animals to universities, medical and veterinary schools, and companies providing animal-testing services. Lawrence Salinger and Patricia Teddlie of Arkansas State University told the conference that these institutions pay up to $500 for a stolen animal, who is often accompanied by forged documents and fake health certificates. Salinger and Teddlie argue that the stolen animals may affect research results, because they come from unknown backgrounds and have an uncertain health profile. Conversely the Foundation for Biomedical Research claim that pets being stolen for animal research is largely an urban myth and that the majority of stolen dogs are most likely used for dog fighting. The largest Class B dealer in dogs in the U.S. was investigated for bunching by the U.S. Department of Agriculture (USDA) in 2005.

Chester C. Baird, of Martin Creek Kennels and Pat's Pine Tree Farms in Willifore, Arkansas, lost his licence after being convicted of 100 counts of animal abuse and neglect, and of stealing pets for laboratories and forging documentation. The criminal charges were filed after an eight-year investigation by an animal protection group, Last Chance for Animals. The group filmed over 72 hours of undercover video at Martin Creek Kennels, which included footage of dogs being shot. In 2006, HBO produced Dealing Dogs, a documentary film based on this footage. Baird's customers included the University of Missouri, University of Colorado Health Sciences Centre, and Oregon State University. According to the Humane Society of the United States, Missouri was experiencing such a high rate of pet theft that animal protection groups had dubbed it the "Steal Me State". Last Chance for Animals estimates that around two million pets are stolen in the U.S. each year.

DEALERS IN THE EUROPEAN UNION

Animal dealers in the European Union (EU) are governed by Council Directive 86/609/EEC. This directive sets forth specific requirements regulating the supply and breeding of animals intended for use by testing facilities within the EU. The directive defines 'breeding establishment' as a facility engaged in breeding animals for their use in experiments, and 'supplying establishment' as a facility other than a breeding establishment, which supplies animals for experiments.

Article 15 of the directive requires supplying establishments to obtain animals only from approved breeding or other supplying establishments, "unless the animal has been lawfully imported and is not a feral or stray animal." Nonetheless, the directive allows exemptions from this sourcing requirement "under arrangements determined by the authority."

Animal rights supporters have raised concerns that these rules allow strays and pets to be used for experimentation, either by exemptions or by importing animals from non-EU countries, where the rules may be more lax.

In 2010, a new EU directive was published on the protection of animals used for scientific purposes, repealing the old directive 86/609/EEC on January 1, 2013, with the exception of Article 13 (statistical information on the use of animals in experiments) which shall be repealed on May 10, 2013.

VETERINARY SCIENCE

Veterinary science is the study, diagnosis, treatment and prevention of disease in animals both as individuals and as groups. There is also a key role for members of the profession as guardians of human health in the context of disease transmission from animal or animal products to man.

HISTORICAL AND CURRENT PERSPECTIVE

Once early man had moved from hunting to herding he had an interest in the health and husbandry of his stock. By the time of the ancient civilisations there is evidence of close interaction between man and animals in contexts which are still familiar today including the use of animals for production, draught and war and, increasingly, as human companions. The first book of the modern era devoted to veterinary medicine, 'Artis Veterinariae', was produced by Publius Vegetius Renatus in the second half of the 5th century.

The 'veterinarii' were the animal doctors of ancient Rome, and the word came back into use in the 17th and 18th centuries as the veterinary profession emerged from its origins amongst the farriers. By the 18th century several veterinary texts had been published and the first veterinary school in Europe was established at Lyon in 1762. The first to be established in the United Kingdom was the Royal Veterinary College in 1792. Although the term 'veterinary surgeon' is widely used within the UK, the term 'veterinarian' is employed here. The veterinary workplace has changed in the last century with less emphasis on the horse (especially as a draught animal), an increasing emphasis on companion animals kept for pleasure, and greater veterinary involvement in production animals, public health and food hygiene. The role of the profession in protecting the health and welfare of more diverse species groups such as laboratory animals, zoological collections, wildlife and, indeed, the contribution to conservation of endangered species, continues to grow.

There is also an increasing body of specialists, both in individual species and in disciplines which cut across species groups, as opportunities for training and the demand for specialist services have grown. The comparative approach of veterinary science will continue to provide insight and support for basic scientists and contribute to the understanding of human disease. The beginning of the 21st century finds the veterinary profession and its work held in high esteem by the general public and a source of considerable interest, with unprecedented exposure of veterinary matters in the popular media. Veterinarians are regarded as guardians of animal health and welfare, and the veterinary schools have a responsibility to continue to produce graduates in whom the public will have confidence.

The sustained public appeal of veterinary work has led to a level of demand for places on veterinary courses which far exceed supply. This demand enables the schools to select strongly motivated, high achievers with entry qualifications among the highest in UK university courses. Most applicants are attracted in the first instance by the prospect of veterinary clinical practice with its unique combination of science, art, practical skills, human-animal and interpersonal interaction. However, an increasing number follow other career paths as they become aware of the diverse opportunities provided by a veterinary degree.

ANALYTICAL EPIDEMIOLOGY

The major aims of epidemiology are to *describe* the health status of populations, to *explain* the aetiology of diseases, to *predict* disease occurrence and to *control* the distribution of disease. An understanding of causal relationships is the basis of the last three objectives.

Such associations between causes and disease occurrence can be discovered through individual *case studies*, by experimental *laboratory studies* and by *field studies*. *Case studies* focusing on individual sick animals have long been at the centre of clinical knowledge. They are based on direct personal observations relating to anatomical structure and physiological function, which can be quantified and are systematic but still largely qualitative. While these observations can be extremely intensive and detailed their disadvantage is their subjectivity and the possibly extreme variation between cases. In the *laboratory experiment* - the classic experiment- great precision in measurements and optimal control of influencing variables can be achieved resulting in sound inferences.

The disadvantage is that it is usually not possible to represent the myriad of factors affecting disease occurrence in the natural environment of the animal and it may be difficult to work with sufficient numbers of animals to represent true variation between animals in the natural population. A *field study* is conducted in the natural environment of the animals and measurements are made on sick as well as healthy animals. The differences between sick and healthy animals can be described with respect to the frequency of presence or absence of potential risk factors. With this type of study, animals are exposed to all the known and unknown environmental factors present in their natural environment.

Field research is *empirical* and involves measurement of variables, estimation of population parameters and statistical testing of hypotheses. It is of a *probabilistic nature* in that as a result of a population study it will not be possible to predict with certainty which animal will develop a particular disease given the presence of certain risk factors. But it will be possible to predict how many cases of the disease will occur in the population in the future. Field research involves comparisons among groups in order to estimate the magnitude of an *association* between a putatively causal factor and a disease. The objective is to assess if there is the potential of a cause-effect relationship between a single or multiple risk factors and the disease.

The interrelatedness of phenomena within a biological system complicates the situation for an investigator who will always have to select a segment of the system for the investigation. Attempting to isolate the segment from the rest of the system can result in an outcome which does not represent the real situation in the system anymore.

Analytical epidemiology is aimed at determining the *strength*, *importance* and *statistical significance* of epidemiological associations. The process typically begins with data collection and eventually leads to data analysis and interpretation. The data collection can be based on a *survey* or a *study*. Both terms are often used interchangeably. A *survey* typically involves *counting* members of an aggregate of units and *measuring* their characteristics. In contrast, a *study* is aimed at comparison of different groups and investigation of cause-effect relationships.

Both designs can be based on a *census* where all members of the population are included thus allowing exact measurement of variables of interest, or alternatively on a *sample* where a subset of the population is included, thereby providing only estimates of the variables of interest.

EPIDEMIOLOGICAL STUDIES

Epidemiological studies are broadly categorised into *non-observational* (or *experimental* studies) and *observational* studies. The first group includes clinical trials or intervention studies and the basic principle is that the design of the study involves deliberately changing population parameters and assessing the effect. With this type of study an attempt is made to simplify observation by *creating* suitable conditions for the study. The second group assumes that the study does not interfere with the population characteristics.

Here, the investigator is only allowed to *select* suitable conditions for the study. *Observational studies* can be further categorised into *prospective cohort* studies and *retrospective* studies as well as *cross-sectional* studies. *Retrospective studies* include case-control and retrospective cohort studies. Another type of observational study is the *longitudinal* study which is a mix between prospective cohort and repeated cross-sectional studies. Within the group of observational studies mixtures of study designs are common, such as for example the case-cohort study. The *case series* is a separate group of studies and frequently used in a clinical context.

This type of study typically involves dividing a group of animals into a subgroup which is being *treated* and another subgroup which is being left *untreated* and acts as a control. The decision to treat an animal or leave it untreated is typically based on random allocation - *randomisation*. After a period of time the status with respect to a response variable (e.g. disease status) is assessed for each animal.

Summary measures of the response are then compared between both subgroups. Differences in the summary values suggest the presence of an effect of the *treatment* on the response variable. Non-observational or experimental studies can be conducted as *laboratory experiments* or as *field studies* such as *clinical trials*. The latter are usually used to evaluate therapeutic or preventive effects of particular interventions, but are also useful to investigate etiologic relationships.

The *non-observational study* provides the researcher with effective control over the study situation. If the sample size is large enough a well-designed experiment will limit the effect of unwanted factors even if they are not measurable. Control of factors other than the treatment which are likely to have an effect on disease can be achieved by using them to define homogeneous subgroups with respect to the status of these variables - *blocking* or *matching*- within which treatment is then allocated randomly.

The possibility to have excessive control over the study situation can become a weakness of the non-observational approach as it may not be representative of the real situation in the biological system anymore. *Clinical trials* are considered the method of choice for investigation of causal hypotheses about the effectiveness of preventive measures, and compared with the other types of field studies they can provide the strongest evidence about causality.

There is less opportunity for systematic error compared with the observational studies. Amongst their disadvantages are the following characteristics. They require large groups, are costly, bias may be introduced through selection error and the required duration can be long if disease incidence is low.

SAMPLING OF ANIMAL POPULATIONS

The main objectives of sampling are to provide data which will allows making inferences in relation about a larger population on the basis of examining a sample in relation to for example presence/absence of animal disease or other parameters of interest. Inferences might relate to proving that disease is not present, to detecting presence of disease or establishing the level of disease occurrence. The objective could also be to describe levels of milk production in a population of dairy cattle or more generally provide a descriptive analysis of an animal production system for example in an African country.

DATA SOURCES

Any *data sources* for epidemiological analyses have to be evaluated with respect to their *completeness*, *validity* and *representativeness*. The data can be collected as part of *routine data collection* which includes laboratory submissions, disease surveillance programmes, industry- or farm/ bureau based data recording systems and abattoirs.

More recently, *structured data collection* has been found to provide a more effective way for regular monitoring of disease / production. And finally, data can be collected as part of *epidemiological studies*. Data which is based on *laboratory submissions* is useful for detecting disease.

It can become the basis of case series and case control studies. It does not provide sufficient data to allow prevalence estimation, because the enumerator and denominator are likely to both be biased. In isolation, laboratory submissions do not provide information about causation !!!! They are also not useful for evaluation of therapies or economic effects.

The data collection process can include the whole population of interest (=*census*) or it can be restricted to a *sample*. The latter has the advantage over the *census* that results can be obtained more quickly. A sample is less expensive to collect, and sample results may be more accurate as it is possible to make more efficient use of resources. In addition, *probability samples* result in probability estimates which allow inferences to be used for other populations.

Heterogeneity in the results can be reduced by targeted sampling of particular sub-groups within the population. Involvement of the whole population such as is necessary for a census may not be possible due to logistic or administrative problems, so that sampling becomes the method of choice. The sampling process can be described using the following terminology. The *target population* represents the population at risk. The population effectively sampled is called the *study population*. Frequently, the target population is not completely accessible, so that it differs to a possibly unknown extent from the study population.

It is then necessary to use common sense judgement in order to assess the representativeness of the study population in relation to the target population. The *sampling frame* lists all sampling units in the study population, and is an essential requirement for probability sampling. *Sampling units* are the individual members of the sampling frame.

INTERPRETATION OF DIAGNOSTIC TESTS

UNCERTAINTY AND THE DIAGNOSTIC PROCESS

The duties of the veterinary profession include "to maintain and enhance the health, productivity and well-being of all animals" and "to prevent and relieve animal suffering". In order to fulfill this duty, the veterinarian has to be able to diagnose disease or production problems as well as identify possible causes.

Diagnosis is the basis for a decision, such as whether to treat (or implement a programme) or to do nothing, to further evaluate, euthanase or to wait. The tools which the veterinarian uses to come to a diagnosis include factual knowledge, experience, intuition as well as diagnostic tests. Correct use of these four mechanisms maximises the probability of a correct diagnosis. The uncertainty with regard to the effect of a treatment on a patient's health made the ancient Greeks call medicine a *stochastic art*.

Clearly, the main task of any veterinarian is to deal with the uncertainty of both, diagnosis and the outcome of treatment. It has been shown in studies of the medical profession that fear of personal inadequacy and failure in reacting to this uncertainty is a common characteristic among physicians. This has become an even more important problem as our society becomes increasingly specialized and technological, relying on science rather than religion or magic to explain uncertainties.

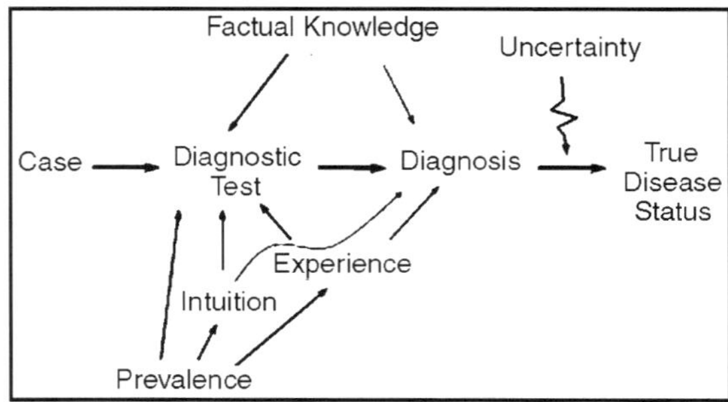

Fig. Factors Influencing Veterinary

In this context, one should be aware of two major paradigms used to explain biological processes. The *mechanistic paradigm* assumes deterministic causation, and experiments are conducted to develop rules or laws according to which nature is thought to 'work'. Obviously, the client in a diagnostic situation does prefer this kind of interpretation, as it increases confidence in the diagnostic and the therapeutic process. The *probabilistic paradigm* on the other hand assumes probabilistic causation. Diagnostic and therapeutic procedures are seen as gambles and it is recognised that the decision making process incorporates subjective judgement. The conclusion has to be though that given our incomplete understanding of biological systems and the presence of true biological variation, in veterinary diagnosis one must be content to end not in certainties, but rather statistical probabilities.

The outcome of the *diagnostic process* is a statement as to whether an animal is considered normal or not normal. This could relate to disease or infection status as well as to productive performance or quality of life from an animal welfare perspective.

DIAGNOSTIC TESTS

The diagnostic test is a more or less objective method for reducing *diagnostic uncertainty*. As the consequential decisions are typically dichotomous (treat or do not), the outcome of the diagnostic process often is interpreted as a dichotomous variable as well, such as the animal having or not having the disease. The unit of measurement of the diagnostic device can be dichotomous, such as presence or absence of bacteria, which facilitates interpretation significantly. But if the diagnostic device measures on a continuous scale, such as serum antibody levels or somatic cell counts, a *cut-off value* has to be determined so that the result can be condensed into a dichotomous scale.

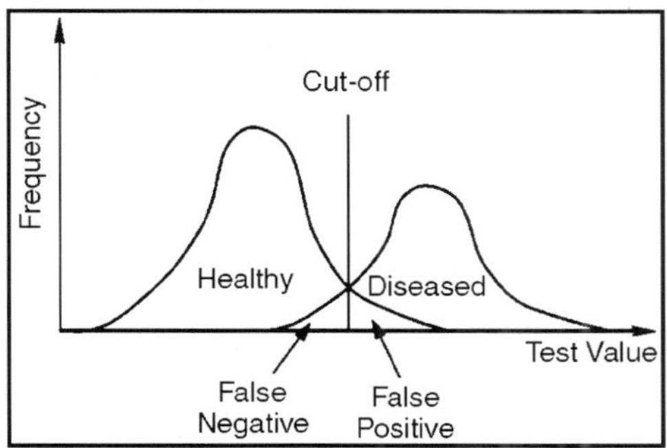

Fig. Test Result Measured on Continuous Scale

Given a clinical measurement on a continuous scale, the problem with any cut-off point is that it is likely to result in overlap between healthy and diseased individuals with regard to test results.

The consequences of this situation are that uncertainty in addition to any other potential sources of measurement error (such as operator error) is being introduced. It is desirable to quantify this relationship between diagnostic test result and "true" disease status so that the clinician can take account of this uncertainty when interpreting test results.

The performance of a diagnostic method can be described using the *accuracy* which refers to the closeness between test result and "true" clinical state, the *bias* which is a measure of the systematic deviation from "true" clinical state, and the *precision* or *repeatability* representing the degree of fluctuation of a test series around a central measurement.

Any evaluation of diagnostic tests needs a measure of the "true" condition of individuals to compare with which is usually called the *gold standard*. Most of the time it is impossible to define with 100% accuracy what the true diagnosis should be. There may also be disagreement amongst experts such as for example in the case of mastitis where the presence of the particular pathogen *or* the presence of an inflammatory response in the udder could be defined as the gold standard.

MEDICAL ETHICS

Medical ethics is primarily a field of applied ethics, the study of moral values and judgments as they apply to medicine. As a scholarly discipline, medical ethics encompasses its practical application in clinical settings as well as work on its history, philosophy, theology, and sociology.

Medical ethics tends to be understood narrowly as an applied professional ethics, whereas bioethics appears to have worked more expansive concerns, touching upon the philosophy of science and the critique of biotechnology. Still, the two fields often overlap and the distinction is more a matter of style than professional consensus. Medical ethics shares many principles with other branches of healthcare ethics, such as nursing ethics.

There are various ethical guidelines. The Declaration of Helsinki is regarded as one of the most authoritative.By the 18th and 19th centuries, medical ethics emerged as a more self-conscious discourse. For instance, authors such as Thomas Percival wrote about "medical jurisprudence" and reportedly coined the phrase "medical ethics."

Percival's guidelines related to physician consultations have been criticized as being excessively protective of the home physician's reputation. Jeffrey Berlant is one such critic who considers Percival's codes of physician consultations as being an early example of the anti-competitive, "guild"-like nature of the physician community.

In 1847, the American Medical Association adopted its first code of ethics, with this being based in large part upon Percival's work. While the secularized field borrowed largely from Catholic medical ethics, in the 20th century a distinctively liberal Protestant approach was articulated by thinkers such as Joseph Fletcher. In the 1960s and 1970s, building upon liberal theory and procedural justice, much of the discourse of medical ethics went through a dramatic shift and largely reconfigured itself into bioethics.

Since the 1970s, the growing influence of ethics in contemporary medicine can be seen in the increasing use of Institutional Review Boards to evaluate experiments on human subjects, the establishment of hospital ethics committees, the expansion of the role of clinician ethicists, and the integration of ethics into many medical school curricula.

VALUES IN MEDICAL ETHICS

In the United Kingdom, General Medical Council provides clear overall modern guidance in the form of its 'Good Medical Practice' statement. Other organisations, such as the Medical Protection Society and a number of university departments, are often consulted by British doctors regarding issues relating to ethics.

How does one ensure that appropriate ethical values are being applied within hospitals? Effective hospital accreditation requires that ethical considerations are taken into account, for example with respect to physician integrity, conflicts of interest, research ethics and organ transplantation ethics.

Autonomy

Autonomy is a general indicator of health. Many diseases are characterised by loss of autonomy, in various manners. This makes autonomy an indicator for both personal well-being, and for the well-being of the profession. This has implications for the consideration of medical ethics: "is the aim of health care to do good, and benefit from it?"; or "is the aim of health care to do good to others, and have them, and society, benefit from this?". (Ethics - by definition - tries to find a beneficial balance between the activities of the individual and its effects on a collective.)

By considering Autonomy as a gauge parameter for (self) health care, the medical and ethical perspective both benefit from the implied reference to Health.

Beneficence

James Childress and Tom Beauchamp in *Principle of Biomedical Ethics* (1978) identify beneficence as one of the core values of health care ethics. Some scholars, such as Edmund Pellegrino, argue that beneficence is the *only* fundamental principle of medical ethics. They argue that healing should be the sole purpose of medicine, and that endeavors like cosmetic surgery, contraception and euthanasia fall beyond its purview.

Non-Maleficence

In practice, however, many treatments carry some risk of harm. In some circumstances, e.g. in desperate situations where the outcome without treatment will be grave, risky treatments that stand a high chance of harming the patient will be justified, as the risk of not treating is also very likely to do harm. So the principle of *non-maleficence* is not absolute, and must be balanced against the principle of *beneficence* (doing good).

Some American physicians interpret this principle to exclude the practice of euthanasia, though not all concur. Probably the most extreme example in recent history of the violation of the non-maleficence dictum was Dr. Jack

Kevorkian, who was convicted of second-degree homicide in Michigan in 1998 after demonstrating active euthanasia on the TV news show, 60 Minutes.

In some countries euthanasia is accepted as standard medical practice. Legal regulations assign this to the medical profession. In such nations, the aim is to alleviate the suffering of patients from diseases known to be incurable by the methods known in that culture. In that sense, the "Primum no Nocere" is based on the realisation that *the inability of the medical expert to offer help, creates a known great and ongoing suffering in the patient*. "Not acting" in those cases is believed to be more damaging than actively relieving the suffering of the patient. Evidently the ability to offer help depends on the limitation of what the practitioner can do. These limitations are characteristic for each different form of healing, and the legal system of the specific culture. The aim to "not do harm" is still the same. It gives the medical practitioner a responsibility to help the patient, in the intentional and active relief of suffering, in those cases where no cure can be offered.

"Non-maleficence" is defined by its cultural context. Every culture has its own cultural collective definitions of 'good' and 'evil'. Their definitions depend on the degree to which the culture sets its cultural values apart from nature. In some cultures the terms "good" and "evil" are absent: for them these words lack meaning as their experience of nature does not set them apart from nature. Other cultures place the humans in interaction with nature, some even place humans in a position of dominance over nature. The religions are the main means of expression of these considerations.

Depending on the cultural consensus conditioning (expressed by its religious, political and legal social system) the legal definition of Non-maleficence differs. Violation of non-maleficence is the subject of medical malpractice litigation. Regulations thereof differ, over time, per nation.

Double Effect

Some interventions undertaken by physicians can create a positive outcome while foreseeably, but unintentionally, doing harm. The combination of these two circumstances is known as the "double effect". A commonly cited, but fallacious, example of this phenomenon is the use of morphine in the dying patient. Such use of morphine can ease the pain and suffering of the patient, while simultaneously hastening the demise of the patient through suppression of the respiratory drive. If correct, this would be an example of the double effect; however, no research evidence supports the claim that appropriately administered opioid drugs depress the respiratory system.

Informed Consent

Informed consent in ethics usually refers to the idea that a person must be fully-informed about and understand the potential benefits and risks of their choice of treatment. An uninformed person is at risk of mistakenly making a choice not reflective of his or her values or wishes. It does not specifically mean the process of obtaining consent, nor the specific legal requirements, which vary from place to place, for capacity to consent. Patients can elect to make their own medical decisions, or can delegate decision-making authority to another party. If the patient is incapacitated, laws around the world designate different processes for obtaining informed consent, typically by having a person appointed by the patient or their next-of-kin make decisions for them. The value of informed consent is closely related to the values of autonomy and truth telling.A correlate to "informed consent" is the concept of informed refusal.

Confidentiality

Confidentiality is commonly applied to conversations between doctors and patients. This concept is commonly known as patient-physician privilege.Legal protections prevent physicians from revealing their discussions with patients, even under oath in court.

Confidentiality is mandated in America by HIPAA laws, specifically the Privacy Rule, and various state laws, some more rigorous than HIPAA. However, numerous exceptions to the rules have been carved out over the years. For example, many states require physicians to report gunshot wounds to the police and impaired drivers to the Department of Motor Vehicles. Confidentiality is also challenged in cases involving the diagnosis of a sexually transmitted disease in a patient who refuses to reveal the diagnosis to a spouse, and in the termination of a pregnancy in an underage patient, without the knowledge of the patient's parents.

Many states in the U.S. have laws governing parental notification in underage abortion.Traditionally, medical ethics has viewed the duty of confidentiality as a relatively non-negotiable tenet of medical practice. More recently, critics like Jacob Appel have argued for a more nuanced approach to the duty that acknowledges the need for flexibility in many cases.

Criticisms of Orthodox Medical Ethics

It has been argued that mainstream medical ethics is biased by the assumption of a framework in which individuals are not simply free to contract with one another to provide whatever medical treatment is demanded, subject to the ability to pay. Because a high proportion of medical care is typically provided via the welfare state, and because there are legal restrictions on what treatment may be provided and by whom, an automatic divergence may exist between the wishes of patients and the preferences of medical practitioners and other parties. Tassano has questioned the idea that Beneficence might in some cases have priority over Autonomy. He argues that violations of Autonomy more often reflect the interests of the state or of the supplier group than those of the patient. Routine regulatory professional bodies or the courts of law are valid social recourses.

Importance of Communication

Many so-called "ethical conflicts" in medical ethics are traceable back to a lack of communication. Communication breakdowns between patients and their healthcare team, between family members, or between members of the medical community, can all lead to disagreements and strong feelings. These breakdowns should be remedied, and many apparently insurmountable "ethics" problems can be solved with open lines of communication.

Ethics Committees

Often, simple communication is not enough to resolve a conflict, and a hospital ethics committee must convene to decide a complex matter.

These bodies are composed primarily of health care professionals, but may also include philosophers, lay people, and clergy - indeed, in many parts of the world their presence is considered mandatory in order to provide balance.

With respect to the expected composition of such bodies in the USA, Europe and Australia, the following applies. U.S. recommendations suggest that Research and Ethical Boards (REBs) should have five or more members, including at least one scientist, one non-scientist and one person not affiliated with the institution. The REB should include people knowledgeable in the law and standards of practice and professional conduct. Special memberships are advocated for handicapped or disabled concerns, if required by the protocol under review. The European Forum for Good Clinical Practice (EFGCP) suggests that REBs include two practicing physicians who share experience in biomedical research and are independent from the institution where the research is conducted; one lay person; one lawyer; and one paramedical professional, e.g. nurse or pharmacist. They recommend that a quorum include both sexes from a wide age range and reflect the cultural make-up of the local community.

The 1996 Australian Health Ethics Committee recommendations were entitled, "Membership Generally of Institutional Ethics Committees". They suggest a chairperson be preferably someone not employed or otherwise connected with the institution. Members should include a person with knowledge and experience in professional care, counselling or treatment of humans; a minister of religion or equivalent, e.g. Aboriginal elder; a layman; a laywoman; a lawyer and, in the case of a hospital-based ethics committee, a nurse. The assignment of philosophers or religious clerics will reflect the importance attached by the society to the basic values involved. An example from Sweden with Torbjörn Tännsjö on a couple of such committees indicates secular trends gaining influence.

Cultural Concerns

Culture differences can create difficult medical ethics problems. Some cultures have spiritual or magical theories about the origins of disease, for example, and reconciling these beliefs with the tenets of Western medicine can be difficult.

Truth-telling

Some cultures do not place a great emphasis on informing the patient of the diagnosis, especially when cancer is the diagnosis. Even American culture did not emphasize truth-telling in a cancer case, up until the 1970s. In American medicine, the principle of informed consent takes precedence over other ethical values, and patients are usually at least asked whether they want to know the diagnosis.

Online Business Practices

The delivery of diagnosis online leads patients to believe that doctors in some parts of the country are at the direct service of drug companies. Finding diagnosis as convenient as what drug still has patent rights on it. Physicians and drug companies are found to be competing for top ten search engine ranks to lower costs of selling these drugs with little to no patient involvement

Conflicts of Interest

Physicians should not allow a conflict of interest to influence medical judgment. In some cases, conflicts are hard to avoid, and doctors have a responsibility to avoid entering such situations. Unfortunately, research has shown that conflicts of interests are very common among both academic physicians and physicians in practice. The The Pew Charitable Trusts has announced the Prescription Project for "academic medical Centres, professional medical societies and public and private payers to end conflicts of interest resulting from the $12 billion spent annually on pharmaceutical marketing".

Referral

For example, doctors who receive income from referring patients for medical tests have been shown to refer more patients for medical tests. This practice is proscribed by the American College of Physicians Ethics Manual.

Fee splitting and the payments of commissions to attract referrals of patients is considered unethical and unacceptable in most parts of the world - while it is rapidly becoming routine in other countries, like India, where many urban practitioners currently pay a per centage of office-visit charges, lab tests as well as hospital care to unaccredited "quacks", or semi-accredited "practitioners of alternative medicine", who refer the patient. It is tolerated in some areas of US medical care as well.

Vendor Relationships

Studies show that doctors can be influenced by drug company inducements, including gifts and food. Industry-sponsored Continuing Medical Education

(CME) Programmes influence prescribing patterns. Many patients surveyed in one study agreed that physician gifts from drug companies influence prescribing practices. A growing movement among physicians is attempting to diminish the influence of pharmaceutical industry marketing upon medical practice, as evidenced by Stanford University's ban on drug company-sponsored lunches and gifts. Other academic institutions that have banned pharmaceutical industry-sponsored gifts and food include the University of Pennsylvania, and Yale University.

Treatment of Family Members

Many doctors treat their family members. Doctors who do so must be vigilant not to create conflicts of interest or treat inappropriately.

Sexual Relationships

Sexual relationships between doctors and patients can create ethical conflicts, since sexual consent may conflict with the fiduciary responsibility of the physician. Doctors who enter into sexual relationships with patients face the threats of deregistration and prosecution. In the early 1990s it was estimated that 2-9 % of doctors had violated this rule. Sexual relationships between physicians and patients' relatives may also be prohibited in some jurisdictions, although this prohibition is highly controversial.

Futility

The concept of medical futility has been an important topic in discussions of medical ethics. What should be done if there is no chance that a patient will survive but the family members insist on advanced care? Previously, some articles defined futiliy as the patient having less than a one per cent chance of surviving. Some of these cases wind up in the courts. Advanced directives include living wills and durable powers of attorney for health care. In many cases, the "expressed wishes" of the patient are documented in these directives, and this provides a framework to guide family members and health care professionals in the decision making process when the patient is incapacitated. Undocumented expressed wishes can also help guide decisions in the absence of advanced directives, as in the Quinlan case in Missouri.

"Substituted judgment" is the concept that a family member can give consent for treatment if the patient is unable (or unwilling) to give consent himself. The key question for the decision making surrogate is not, "What would you like to do?", but instead, "What do you think the patient would want in this situation?".

Courts have supported family's arbitrary definitions of futility to include simple biological survival, as in the Baby K case (in which the courts ordered a child born with only a brain stem instead of a complete brain to be kept on a ventilator based on the religious belief that all life must be preserved).

A more in-depth discussion of futility is available at futile medical care. In some hospitals, medical futility is referred to as "non-beneficial care."

- Baby Doe Law establishes state protection for a disabled child's right to life, ensuring that this right is protected even over the wishes of parents or guardians in cases where they want to withhold treatment.

Critics claim that this is how the State, and perhaps the Church, through its adherents in the executive and the judiciary, interferes in order to further its own agenda at the expense of the patient's. Ronald Reagan's Americans With Disabilities Act was a direct response to the Baby K Case, in an effort to prop up "Right to Life" philosophies.

2

Laboratory and Animal Testing

ANIMAL TESTING

Animal testing, also known as animal experimentation, animal research, and in vivo testing, is the use of non-human animals in experiments. It is estimated that 50 to 100 million vertebrate animals worldwide — from zebrafish to non-human primates — are used annually. Although much larger numbers of invertebrates are used and the use of flies and worms as model organisms is very important, experiments on invertebrates are largely unregulated and not included in statistics.

Most animals are euthanized after being used in an experiment. Sources of Labouratory animals vary between countries and species; while most animals are purpose-bred, others may be caught in the wild or supplied by dealers who obtain them from auctions and pounds.

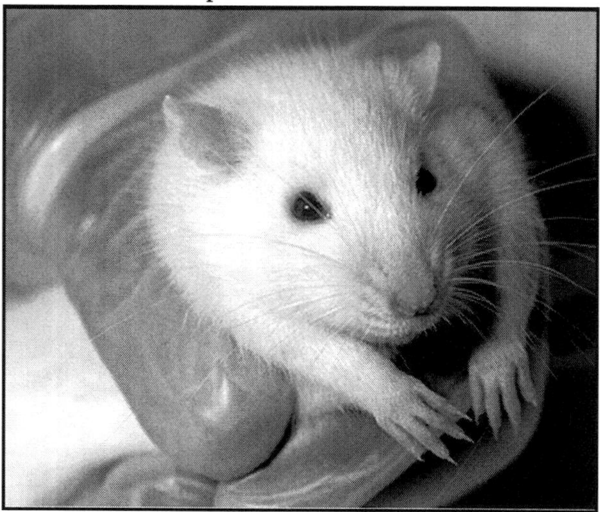

Fig. Animal Testing

The research is conducted inside universities, medical schools, pharmaceutical companies, farms, Defence establishments, and commercial facilities that provide animal-testing services to industry. It includes pure research such as genetics, developmental biology, behavioural studies, as well as applied research such as biomedical research, xenotransplantation, drug testing and toxicology tests, including cosmetics testing. Animals are also used for education, breeding, and Defence research.

Supporters of the practice, such as the British Royal Society, argue that virtually every medical achievement in the 20th century relied on the use of animals in some way, with the Institute for Labouratory Animal Research of the U.S. National Academy of Sciences arguing that even sophisticated computers are unable to model interactions between molecules, cells, tissues, organs, organisms, and the environment, making animal research necessary in many areas.

Some scientists and animal rights organizations, such as PETA and BUAV, question the legitimacy of it, arguing that it is cruel, poor scientific practice, poorly regulated, that medical progress is being held back by misleading animal models, that some of the tests are outdated, that it cannot reliably predict effects in humans, that the costs outweigh the benefits, or that animals have an intrinsic right not to be used for experimentation.

The practice of animal testing is regulated to various extents in different countries.

DEFINITIONS

The terms animal testing, animal experimentation, animal research, *in vivo* testing, and vivisection have similar denotations but different connotations. Literally, "vivisection" means the "cutting up" of a living animal, and historically referred only to experiments that involved the dissection of live animals. The term is occasionally used to refer pejoratively to any experiment using living animals; for example, the *Encyclopaedia Britannica* defines "vivisection" as: "Operation on a living animal for experimental rather than healing purposes; more broadly, all experimentation on live animals", although dictionaries point out that the broader definition is "used only by people who are opposed to such work".

The word has a negative connotation, implying torture, suffering, and death. The word "vivisection" is preferred by those opposed to this research, whereas scientists typically use the term "animal experimentation".

HISTORY OF ANIMAL TESTING

The history of animal testing goes back to the writings of the Greeks in the third and fourth centuries BCE, with Aristotle (384-322 BCE) and Erasistratus (304-258 BCE) among the first to perform experiments on living animals.

Galen, a physician in second-century Rome, dissected pigs and goats, and is known as the "father of vivisection."

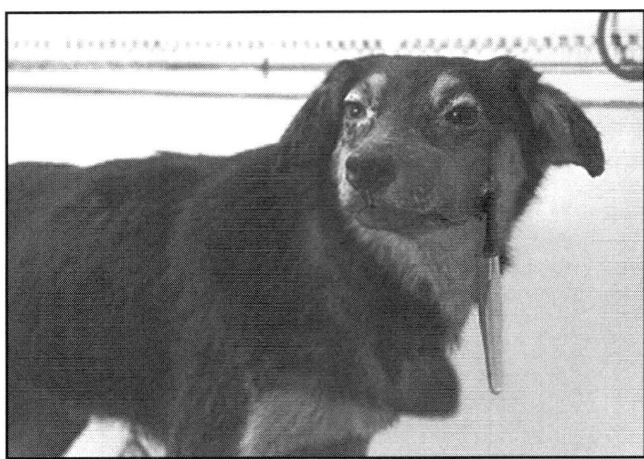

Fig. One of Pavlov's Dogs with a Saliva-catch Container and Tube Surgically Implanted in his Muzzle.

EARLY DEBATE

In 1655, physiologist Edmund O'Meara is recorded as saying that "the miserable torture of vivisection places the body in an unnatural state." O'Meara thus expressed one of the chief scientific objections to vivisection: that the pain that the subject endured would interfere with the accuracy of the results.

In 1822, the first animal protection law was enacted in the British parliament, followed by the Cruelty to Animals Act (1876), the first law specifically aimed at regulating animal testing. The legislation was promoted by Charles Darwin, who wrote to Ray Lankester in March 1871:

You ask about my opinion on vivisection. I quite agree that it is justifiable for real investigations on physiology; but not for mere damnable and detestable curiosity. It is a subject which makes me sick with horror, so I will not say another word about it, else I shall not sleep to-night."

Opposition to the use of animals in medical research arose in the United States during the 1860s, when Henry Bergh founded the American Society for the Prevention of Cruelty to Animals (ASPCA), with America's first specifically anti-vivisection organization being the American Antivivisection Society (AAVS), founded in 1883.

In the UK, an article in the *Medical Times and Gazette* on April 28, 1877, indicates that anti-vivisectionist campaigners, mainly clergymen, had prepared a number of posters entitled, "This is vivisection," "This is a living dog," and "This is a living rabbit," depicting animals in a poses that they said copied the work of Elias von Cyon in St. Petersburg, though the article says the images differ from the originals. It states that no more than 10 or a dozen men were actively involved in animal testing on living animals in the UK at that time.

Antivivisectionists of the era generally believed the spread of mercy was the great cause of civilization, and vivisection was cruel. However, in the U.S., the antivivisectionists' efforts were defeated in every legislature, overwhelmed by the superior organization and influence of the medical community. The early antivivisectionist movement in the U.S. dwindled greatly in the 1920s, potentially caused by a variety of factors including opposition of the medical community, improvement in medicine through the use of animals, and the tendency of the antivivisectionists to misrepresentation and exaggeration, and their use of inaccurate, vague and outdated references. Overall, this movement had no US legislative success until the passing of the Labouratory Animal Welfare Act, in 1966.

Basic Science Advances

In the 1600s, William Harvey described the movement of blood in mammals. In the 1700s, Antoine Lavoisier, used a guinea pig in a calorimeter to prove that respiration was a form of combustion, and Stephen Hales measured blood pressure in the horse. In the 1780s, Luigi Galvani demonstrated that electricity applied to a dead, dissected, frog's leg muscle caused it to twitch, which led to an appreciation for the relationship between electricity and animation. In the 1880s, Louis Pasteur convincingly demonstrated the germ theory of medicine by giving anthrax to sheep. In the 1890s, Ivan Pavlov famously used dogs to describe classical conditioning.

In 1921 Otto Loewi provided the first strong evidence that neuronal communication with target cells occurred via chemical synapses. He extracted two hearts from frogs and left them beating in an ionic bath. He stimulated the attached Vagus nerve of the first heart, and observed its beating slowed. When the second heart was placed in the ionic bath of the first, it also slowed.

In the 1920s, Edgar Adrian formulated the theory of neural communication that the frequency of action potentials, and not the size of the action potentials, was the basis for communicating the magnitude of the signal. His work was performed in an isolated frog nerve-muscle preparation. Adrian was awarded a Nobel Prize for his work.

In the 1960s David Hubel and Torsten Wiesel demonstrated the macrocolumnar organization of visual areas in cats and monkeys, and provided physiological evidence for the critical period for the development of disparity sensitivity in vision (ie: the main cue for depth perception), and were awarded a Nobel Prize for their work.

In 1996 Dolly the sheep was born, the first mammal to be cloned from an adult cell.

ALTERNATIVES TO ANIMAL TESTING

Scientists and governments state that animal testing should cause as little suffering to animals as possible, and that animal tests should only be performed where necessary. The "three Rs" are guiding principles for the use of animals in research in most countries:

- Reduction refers to methods that enable researchers to obtain comparable levels of information from fewer animals, or to obtain more information from the same number of animals.
- Replacement refers to the preferred use of non-animal methods over animal methods whenever it is possible to achieve the same scientific aim.
- Refinement refers to methods that alleviate or minimize potential pain, suffering or distress, and enhance animal welfare for the animals still used.

Although such principles have been welcomed as a step forwards by some animal welfare groups, they have also been criticized as both outdated by current research, and of little practical effect in improving animal welfare.

ANIMAL TESTING ON NON-HUMAN PRIMATES

Experiments involving non-human primates (NHPs) include toxicity testing for medical and non-medical substances; studies of infectious disease, such as HIV and hepatitis; neurological studies; Behaviour and cognition; reproduction; genetics; and xenotransplantation. Around 65,000-70,000 are used every year in the United States and European Union. Most are purpose-bred, while some are caught in the wild. Their use is controversial. According to the Nuffield Council on Bioethics, NHPs are used because their brains share structural and functional features with human brains, but "[w]hile this similarity has scientific advantages, it poses some difficult ethical problems, because of an increased likelihood that primates experience pain and suffering in ways that are similar to humans." Some of the most publicized attacks on animal research facilities by animal rights groups have occurred because of primate research. Some primate researchers have abandoned their studies because of threats or attacks.

In December 2006, an inquiry chaired by Sir David Weatherall, emeritus professor of medicine at Oxford University, concluded that there is a "strong scientific and moral case" for using primates in some research. The British Union for the Abolition of Vivisection argues that the Weatherall report failed to address "the welfare needs and moral case for subjecting these sensitive, intelligent creatures to a lifetime of suffering in UK labs.

LEGAL STATUS

Human beings are recognized as persons and protected in law by the United Nations Universal Declaration of Human Rights and by all governments to varying degrees. Non-human primates are not classified as persons, which largely means their individual interests have no formal recognition or protection. The status of non-human primates has generated much debate, particularly through the Great Ape Project (GAP), which argues that great apes (gorillas, orangutans, chimpanzees, bonobos) be given limited legal status and the protection of three basic interests: the right to live, the protection of individual liberty, and the prohibition of torture. On June 25, 2008, Spain became the first country to announce that it will extend rights to the great apes in accordance with GAP's proposals. An all-party parliamentary group advised the government to write legislation giving chimpanzees, bonobos, gorillas, and orangutans the right to life, to liberty, and the right not to be used in experiments. *The New York Times* reported that the legislation will make it illegal to kill apes, except in self-Defence. "Torture," which will include medical experiments, will be allowed, as will arbitrary imprisonment, such as for circuses or films.

An increasing number of other governments are enacting bans. As of 2006, Austria, New Zealand, the Netherlands, Sweden, and the UK had introduced either *de jure* or *de facto* bans. The ban in Sweden does not extend to non-invasive Behavioural studies, and graduate work on Great Ape cognition in Sweden continues to be carried out on zoo gorillas, and supplemented by studies of chimpanzees held in the U.s. Sweden's legislation also bans invasive experiments on gibbons.

In December 2005, Austria outlawed experiments on any apes, unless it is conducted in the interests of the individual animal. In 2002, Belgium announced that it was working toward a ban on all primate use, and in the UK, 103 MPs signed an Early Day Motion calling for an end to primate experiments, arguing that they cause suffering and are unreliable. No licenses have been issued in the UK since 1998. The Boyd Group, a British group comprising animal researchers, philosophers, primatologists, and animal advocates, has recommended a global prohibition on the use of great apes.

Species and Numbers Used

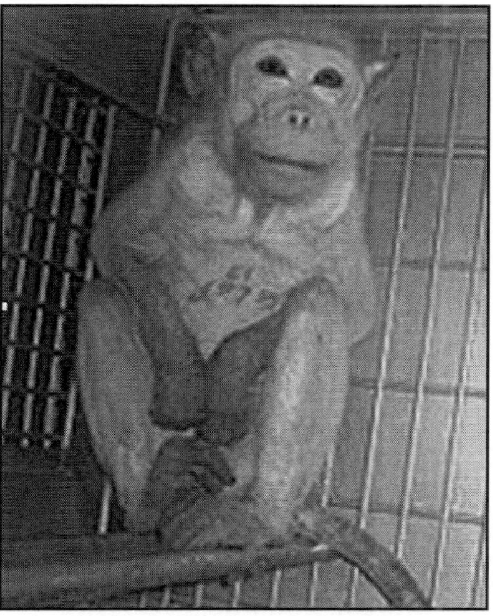

Fig. Covance Primate-Testing Lab.

Most of the NHPs used are one of three species of macaques, accounting for 79 per cent of all primates used in research in the UK, and 63 per cent of all federally funded research grants for projects using primates in the U.S. Lesser numbers of marmosets, tamarins, spider monkeys, owl monkeys, vervet monkeys, squirrel monkeys, and baboons are used in the UK and the U.S. Licenses approving the use of great apes, such as gorillas, chimpanzees, and orangutans, are not currently being issued in Britain, though their use has not been outlawed, but chimpanzees are used in the U.S., with 1,133 in research Labouratories as of October 2006.

In the United States, nearly 55,000 NHPs were used in 2004, an annual figure that has held steady since 1973, and 10,000 in the European Union in 2002. Just over 4,000 were used in the UK in 2004.

In 1996, the British Animal Procedures Committee recommended new measures for dealing with NHPs. The use of wild-caught primates was banned, except where "exceptional and specific justification can be established"; specific justification must be made for the use of old world primates (but not for the use of new world primates); approval for the acquisition of primates from overseas is conditional upon their breeding or supply Centre being acceptable to the Home Office; and each batch of primates acquired from overseas must be separately authorized.

Prevalence

There are indications that NHP use is on the rise, in part because biomedical research funds in the U.S. have more than doubled since the 1990s. In 2000, the NIH published a report recommending that the Regional Primate Research Centre System be renamed the National Primate Research Centre System and calling for an increase in the number of NHPs available to researchers, and stated that "nonhuman primates are crucial for certain types of biomedical and Behavioural research." This assertion has been challenged. In the U.S., the Oregon and California National Primate Research Centres and New Iberia Research Centre have expanded their facilities. In 2000 the National Institutes of Health (NIH) invited applications for the establishment of new breeding specific pathogen free colonies; and a new breeding colony projected to house 3,000 NHPs has been set up in Florida.

The NIH's National Centre for Research Resources claimed a need to increase the number of breeding colonies in its 2004-2008 strategic plan, as well as to set up a database, using information provided through a network of National Primate Research Centres, to allow researchers to locate NHPs with particular characteristics. China is also increasing its NHP use, and is regarded as attractive to Western companies because of the low cost of research, the relatively lax regulations and the increase in animal-rights activism in the West.

In 2005, British Home Office figures show that the number of primates used in the UK rose by 11 per cent in 2005 to 4,650 procedures, 440 more than in 2004. In 2004, the government had reported a long-term downward trend in the use of new world primates (for example, marmosets, tamarins, squirrel, owl, spider and capuchin monkeys), but stated that the use of old world primates (for example, baboons and macaques) fluctuates and is more difficult to determine. Crab-eating macaques and rhesus macaques are the most commonly used species in the UK.

Sources

The American Society of Primatologists writes that most NHPs in Labouratories in the United States are bred domestically. Between 12,000-15,000 are imported each year, specifically rhesus macaque monkeys, cynomolgus (crab-eating) macaque monkeys, squirrel monkeys, owl monkeys, and baboons. Monkeys are imported from the China, Mauritius, Israel, the Philippines, and Peru.China exported over 12,000 macaques for research in 2001 (4,500 to the U.S.), all from self-sustaining purpose-bred colonies.

The second largest source is Mauritius, from which 3,440 purpose-bred cynomolgous macaques were exported to the U.S. in 2001.In Europe, an estimated 70 per cent of research primates are imported, and the rest are purpose-bred in Europe. Around 74 per cent of these imports come from China, with most of the rest coming from Mauritius and Israel.

USE

General

NHPs are used in research into HIV, neurology, Behaviour, cognition, reproduction, Parkinson's disease, stroke, malaria, respiratory viruses, infectious disease, genetics, xenotransplantation, drug abuse, and also in vaccine and drug testing.

According to The Humane Society of the United States, chimpanzees are most often used in hepatitis research, and monkeys in SIV research. Animals used in hepatitis and SIV studies are often caged alone.

Eighty-two per cent of primate procedures in the UK in 2006 were in applied studies, which the Home Office defines as research conducted for the purpose of developing or testing commercial products. Toxicology testing is the largest use, which includes legislatively required testing of drugs. The second largest category of research using primates is "protection of man, animals, or environment", accounting for 8.9 per cent of all procedures in 2006. The third largest category is "fundamental biological research,", accounting for 4.9 per cent of all UK primate procedures in 2006. This includes neuroscientific study of the visual system, cognition, and diseases such as Parkinson's, involving techniques such as inserting electrodes to record from or stimulate the brain, and temporary or permanent inactivation of areas of tissue.

Primates are the species most likely to be re-used in experiments. The Research Defence Society writes that re-use is allowed if the animals have been used in mild procedures with no lasting side-effects. This is contradicted by Dr. Gill Langley of the British Union for the Abolition of Vivisection, who gives as an example of re-use the licence granted to Cambridge University to conduct brain experiments on marmosets. The protocol sheet stated that the animals would receive "multiple interventions as part of the whole lesion/graft repair procedure."

Under the protocol, a marmoset could be given acute brain lesions under general anaesthetic, followed by tissue implantation under a second general anaesthetic, followed again central cannula implantation under a third. The re-use is allowable when required to meet scientific goals, such as this case in which some procedures are required as preparatory for others.

METHODS OF RESTRAINT

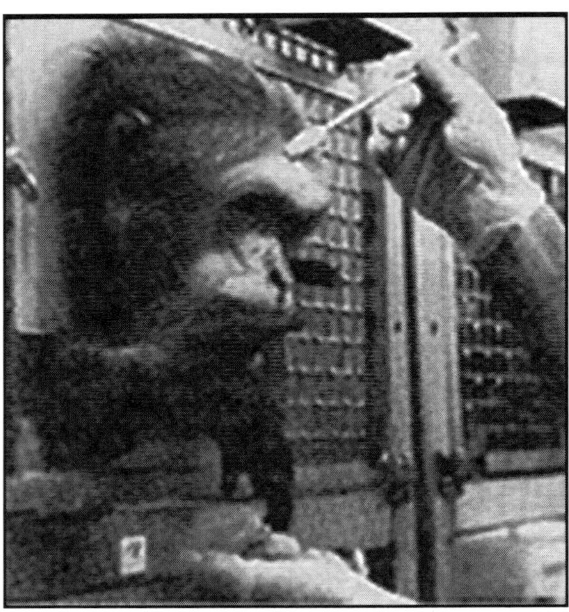

Fig. The Holes are Placed in Such a Way as to Allow the Primate to Reach for Food While Presenting his Head for the Experiment.

One of the disadvantages of using NHPs is that they can be difficult to handle, and various methods of physical restraint have to be used. Viktor Reinhardt of the Wisconsin Regional Primate Research Centre writes that scientists may be unaware of the way in which their research animals are handled, and therefore fail to take into account the effect the handling may have had on the animals' health, and thereby on any data collected. Reinhardt writes that primatologists have long recognized that restraint methods may introduce an "uncontrolled methodological variable", by producing resistance and fear in the animal. "Numerous reports have been published demonstrating that non-human primates can readily be trained to cooperate rather than resist during common handling procedures such as capture, venipuncture, injection and veterinary examination. Cooperative animals fail to show behavioural and physiological signs of distress."

Reinhardt lists common restraint methods as: squeeze-back cages, manual restraint, restraint boards, restraint chairs, restraint chutes, tethering, and nets. Alternatives include:

- Chemical restraint; for example, ketamine, a sedative, may be given to the animal before a restraint procedure, reducing stress-hormone production;
- Psychological support, in which an animal under restraint has visual and auditory contact with the animal's cage-mate. Blood pressure and heart rate responses to restraint have been measurably reduced using psychological support.
- Training animals to cooperate with restraint. Such methods have been used and resulted in unmeasurable stress hormone responses to venipuncture, and no notable distress to being captured in a transport box.

Chimpanzees in the U.S.

There are around 1133 chimpanzees in research Labouratories in the United State as of October 2006, and this number has been monotonically decreasing since the breeding ban of 1996. Many have been used in hepatitis research, often caged alone because of the design of the research protocol. Chimps routinely live 30 years in captivity, and can reach 60 years of age.

Most of the labs either conduct or make the chimps available for invasive research, defined as "inoculation with an infectious agent, surgery or biopsy conducted for the sake of research and not for the sake of the chimpanzee, and/or drug testing." Two federally funded Labouratories use chimps: Yerkes National Primate Research Centre at Emory University in Atlanta, Georgia, and the Southwest National Primate Centre in San Antonio, Texas. Five hundred chimps have been retired from Labouratory use in the U.S. and live in sanctuaries in the U.S. or Canada.

Their importation from the wild was banned in 1973. From then until 1996, chimpanzees in U.S. facilities were bred domestically. Some others were transferred from the entertainment industry to animal testing facilities as recently as 1983, although it is not known if any animals that were transferred from the entertainment industry are still in testing Centres. Animal sanctuaries were not an option until the first North American sanctuary that would accept chimps opened in 1976. In 1986, to prepare for research on AIDS, the U.S. bred them aggressively, with 315 breeding chimpanzees used to produce 400 offspring. By 1996, it was clear that SIV/HIV-2/SHIV in macaque monkeys was a preferred scientific AIDS model to the chimps, which meant there was a surplus. A five-year moratorium on breeding was therefore imposed by the U.S. National Institutes of Health (NIH) that year, and it has been extended annually since 2001. As of October 2006, the chimp population in US Labouratories had declined to 1133 from a peak of 1500 in 1996.

Chimpanzees tend to be used repeatedly over decades, rather than used and killed as with most Labouratory animals. Some individual chimps currently in U.S. Labouratories have been used in experiments for over 40 years. The oldest known chimp in a U.S. lab is Wenka, who was born in a Labouratory in Florida on May 21, 1954. She was removed from her mother on the day of birth to be used in a vision experiment that lasted 17 months, then sold as a pet to a family in North Carolina. She was returned to the Yerkes National Primate Research Centre in 1957 when she became too big to handle. Since then, she has given birth six times, and has been used in research into alcohol use, oral contraceptives, aging, and cognitive studies.

With the publication of the chimpanzee genome, there are reportedly plans to increase the use of chimps in labs, with scientists arguing that the federal moratorium on breeding chimps for research should be lifted. Other researchers argue that chimps are unique animals and should either not be used in research, or should be treated differently. Pascal Gagneux, an evolutionary biologist and primate expert at the University of California, San Diego, argues that, given chimpanzees' sense of self, tool use, and genetic similarity to human beings, studies using chimps should follow the ethical guidelines that are used for human subjects unable to give consent. Stuart Zola, director of the Yerkes National Primate Research Labouratory, disagrees. He told *National Geographic*: "I don't think we should make a distinction between our obligation to treat humanely any species, whether it's a rat or a monkey or a chimpanzee. No matter how much we may wish it, chimps are not human."

A list of facilities holding chimpanzees and the numbers:

- Alamogordo Primate Facility (affiliated with the National Institutes of Health and Charles River Labouratories) at Holloman Airforce base (245)
- M.D. Anderson Cancer Centre, affiliated with the University of Texas (133)
- New Iberia Research Centre, affiliated with the University of Louisiana (342)
- Primate Foundation of Arizona (a holding facility), affiliated with M.D. Anderson/University of Texas (73)
- Southwest National Primate Research Centre, affiliated with the Southwest Foundation for Biomedical Research (236)
- Yerkes National Primate Research Centre, affiliated with Emory University and Georgia State University (109 held); BIOQUAL, Inc. (15)

- Language Research Centre, Georgia State University (4)
- Centres for Disease Control and Prevention (18)
- Food & Drug Administration (11 held) National Institutes of Health (11).

NOTABLE STUDIES

Polio

In the 1940s, Jonas Salk used Rhesus monkey cross-contamination studies to isolate the three forms of the polio virus that crippled hundreds of thousands of people yearly across the world at the time. Salk's team created a vaccine against the strains of polio in cell cultures of Green monkey kidney cells. The vaccine was made publicly available in 1955, and reduced the incidence of polio 15-fold in the USA over the following five years. Albert Sabin made a superior "live" vaccine by passing the polio virus through animal hosts, including monkeys. The vaccine was produced for mass consumption in 1963 and is still in use today. It had virtually eradicated polio in the USA by 1965. It has been estimated that 100,000 monkeys were killed in the course of developing the polio vaccines, and 65 doses of vaccine were produced for each monkey.

Split-Brain Experiments

In the 1950s, Roger Sperry developed split-brain preparations in non-human primates that emphasized the importance of information transfer that occurred in these neocortical connections. For example, learning on simple tasks, if restricted in sensory input and motor output to one hemisphere of a split-brain animal, would not transfer to the other hemisphere. The right brain has no idea what the left brain is up to, if these specific connections are cut.

Those experiments were followed by tests on human beings with epilepsy who had undergone split-brain surgery, which established that the neocortical connections between hemispheres are the principal route for cognition to transfer from one side of the brain to another. These experiments also formed the modern basis for lateralization of function in the human brain.

Vision Experiments

In the 1960s, David Hubel and Torsten Wiesel demonstrated the macrocolumnar organization of visual areas in cats and monkeys, and provided physiological evidence for the critical period for the development of disparity sensitivity in vision (ie: the main cue for depth perception). They were awarded a Nobel Prize for their work.

Deep-Brain Stimulation

In 1983, designer drug users took MPTP, which created a Parkinsonian syndrome. Later that same year, researchers reproduced the effect in non-human primates. Over the next seven years, the brain areas that were over- and under-active in Parkinson's were mapped out in normal and MPTP-treated macaque monkeys using metabolic labelling and microelectrode studies. In 1990, deep brain lesions were shown to treat Parkinsonian symptoms in macaque monkeys treated with MPTP, and these were followed by pallidotomy operations in humans with similar efficacy. By 1993, it was shown that deep brain stimulation could effect the same treatment without causing a permanent lesion of the same magnitude. Deep brain stimulation has largely replaced pallidotomy for treatment of Parkinson's patients that require neurosurgical intervention. Current estimates are that 20,000 Parkinson's patients have received this treatment.

AIDS

The non-human primate models of AIDS, using HIV-2, SHIV, and SIV in macaques, have been used as a complement to ongoing research efforts against the virus. The drug tenofovir has had its efficacy and toxicology evaluated in macaques, and found longterm-highdose treatments had adverse effects not found using shortterm-highdose treatment followed by longterm-lowdose treatment. This finding in macaques was translated into human dosing regimens. Prophylactic treatment with anti-virals has been evaluated in macaques, because introduction of the virus can only be controlled in an animal model. The finding that prophylaxis can be effective at blocking infection has altered the treatment for occupational exposures, such as needle exposures. Such exposures are now followed rapidly with anti-HIV drugs, and this practice has resulted in measurable transient virus infection similar to the NHP model. Similarly, the mother-to-fetus transmission, and its fetal prophylaxis with antivirals such as tenofovir and AZT, has been evaluated in controlled testing in macaques not possible in humans, and this knowledge has guided antiviral treatment in pregnant mothers with HIV. "The comparison and correlation of results obtained in monkey and human studies is leading to a growing validation and recognition of the relevance of the animal model. Although each animal model has its limitations, carefully designed drug studies in nonhuman primates can continue to advance our scientific knowledge and guide future clinical trials."

ALLEGATIONS

Many of the best-known allegations of abuse made by animal protection or animal rights groups against animal-testing facilities involve NHPs.

University of Wisconsin–Madison

The so-called "pit of despair" was used in experiments conducted on rhesus macaque monkeys during the 1970s by American comparative psychologist Harry Harlow at the University of Wisconsin–Madison. The aim of the research was to produce clinical depression. The vertical chamber was a stainless-steel bin with slippery sides that sloped to a rounded bottom. A 3/8 in. wire mesh floor 1 in. above the bottom of the chamber allowed waste material to drop out of holes.

The chamber had a food box and a water-bottle holder, and was covered with a pyramid top so that the monkeys were unable to escape. Harlow placed baby monkeys in the chamber alone for up to six weeks. Within a few days, they stopped moving about and remained huddled in a corner. The monkeys generally exhibited marked social impairment and peer hostility when removed from the chamber; most did not recover.

University of California

On April 21, 1985, activists of the Animal Liberation Front (ALF) broke into the UC Riverside Labouratories and removed hundreds of animals. According to Vicky Miller of PETA, who reported the raid to newswire services, UC-Riverside "has been using animals in experiments on sight deprivation and isolation for the last two years and has recently received a grant, paid for with our tax dollars, to continue torturing and killing animals." According to UCR officials, the ALF claims of animal mistreatment were "absolutely false," and the raid would result in long-term damage to some of the research projects, including those aimed at developing devices and treatment for blindness. UCR officials also reported the raid also included smashing equipment and resulted in several hundred thousand dollars of damage.

In Germany in 2004, journalist Friedrich Mülln took undercover footage of staff in Covance in Münster, Europe's largest primate-testing Centre. Staff were filmed handling monkeys roughly, screaming at them, and making them dance to blaring music. The monkeys were shown isolated in small wire cages with little or no natural light, no environmental enrichment, and subjected to high noise levels from staff shouting and playing the radio. Primatologist Jane Goodall described their living conditions as "horrendous."

A veterinary toxicologist employed as a study director at Covance in Vienna, Virginia from 2002 to 2004, told city officials in Chandler, Arizona, that Covance was dissecting monkeys while the animals were still alive and able to feel pain. The employee approached the city with her concerns when she learned that Covance planned to build a new Labouratory in Chandler.

She alleged that three monkeys in the Vienna Labouratory had pushed themselves up on their elbows and had gasped for breath after their eyes had been removed, and while their intestines were being removed during necropsies (autopsy). When she expressed concern at the next study directors' meeting, she says she was told that it was just a reflex. She told city officials that she believed such movements were not reflexes but suggested "botched euthanasia performed by inadequately trained personnel." She alleged that she was ridiculed and subjected to thinly veiled threats when she contacted her supervisors about the issue.

In the UK, after an undercover investigation in 1998, the British Union for the Abolition of Vivisection (BUAV), a lobby group, reported that researchers in Cambridge University's primate-testing labs were sawing the tops off marmosets' heads, inducing strokes, then leaving them overnight without veterinarian care, because staff worked only nine to five. The experiments used marmosets that were first trained to perform certain Behavioural and cognitive tasks, then re-tested after brain damage to determine how the damage had affected their skills. The monkeys were deprived of food and water to encourage them to perform the tasks, with water being withheld for 22 out of every 24 hours.

The Research Defence Society defended Cambridge's research. The RDS wrote that the monkeys were fully anaesthetised, and appropriate pain killers were given after the surgery. "On recovery from the anaesthesia, the monkeys were kept in an incubator, offered food and water and monitored at regular intervals until the early evening. They were then allowed to sleep in the incubators until the next morning. No monkeys died unattended during the night after stroke surgery." A court rejected BUAV's application for a judicial review. BUAV has appealed and a decision is expected in 2006. In 2003, CNN reported that a post-doctoral veterinarian at Columbia University complained to the university's Institutional Animal Care and Use Committee about experiments being conducted on baboons by E. Sander Connolly, an assistant professor of neurosurgery.

Connolly was mimicking strokes by removing the baboons' left eyeballs and using the empty sockets to reach and clamp a particular blood vessel in their brains. He would then test a neuroprotective drug on the baboon. The baboons were kept alive after the surgery for observation for three to ten days in a state of "profound disability" which would have been "terrifying," according to neurologist Robert Hoffman. Connolly's published animal model states that animals were kept alive for three days, and that animals that were successfully self-caring were kept alive for 10 days. People for the Ethical Treatment of Animals published the description of one experiment:

On September 19, 2001, baboon B777's left eye was removed, and a stroke was induced. The next morning, it was noted that the animal could not sit up, that he was leaning over, and that he could not eat. That evening, the baboon was still slouched over and was offered food but couldn't chew. On September 21, 2001, the record shows that the baboon was 'awake, but no movement, can't eat (chew), vomited in the a.m.' With no further notation about consulting with a veterinarian, the record reads, 'At 1:30 p.m. the animal died in the cage.'"

An investigation by the U.S. Department of Agriculture found "no indication that the experiments.violated federal guidelines." The Dean of Research at Columbia's School of Medicine said that Connolly had stopped the experiments because of threats from animal rights activists, but still believed his work was humane and potentially valuable.

MEDICAL ADVANCES OF ANIMAL TESTING

In the 1880s and 1890s, Emil von Behring isolated the diphtheria toxin and demonstrated its effects in guinea pigs. He went on to demonstrate immunity against diphtheria in animals in 1898 by injecting a mix of toxin and antitoxin. This work constituted in part the rationale for awarding von Behring the 1901 Nobel Prize in Physiology and Medicine. Roughly 15 years later, Behring announced such a mix suitable for human immunity which largely banished the diphtheria from the scourges of mankind. The antitoxin is famously commemorated each year in the Iditarod race, which is modeled after the delivery of diphtheria antitoxin to Nome in the 1925 serum run to Nome. The success of the animal studies in producing the diphtheria antitoxin are attributed by some as a cause in the decline of the early 1900s antivivisectionist movement in the USA.

In 1921, Frederick Banting tied up the pancreatic ducts of dogs, and discovered that the isolates of pancreatic secretion could be used to keep dogs with diabetes alive. He followed up these experiments with chemical isolation of insulin in 1922 with John Macleod. These experiments used bovine sources instead of dogs to improve the supply. The first person treated was Leonard Thompson, a 14 year old diabetic who only weighed 65 pounds and was about to slip into a coma and die. After the first dose, the formulation had to be re-worked, a process that took 12 days. The second dose was effective. These two won the Nobel Prize in Physiology or Medicine in 1923 for their discovery of insulin and its treatment of diabetes mellitus. Thompson lived 13 more years taking insulin. Before insulin's clinical use, a diagnosis of diabetes mellitus meant death; Thompson had been diagnosed in 1919.

In the 1943, Selman Waksman's Labouratory discovered streptomycin using a series of screens to find antibacterial substances from the soil. Waksman coined the term antibiotic with regards to these substances. Waksman would win the Nobel Prize in Medicine in 1952 for his discoveries in antibiotics. Corwin Hinshaw and William Feldman took the streptomycin samples and cured tuberculosis in four guinea pigs with it. Hinshaw followed these studies with human trials that provided a dramatic advance in the ability to stop and reverse the progression of tuberculosis.

Mortality from tuberculosis in the UK has diminished from the early 20th century due to better hygiene and improved living standards, but from the moment antibiotics were introduced, the fall became much steeper, so that by the 1980s mortality in developed countries was effectively zero.

In the 1940s, Jonas Salk used Rhesus monkey cross-contamination studies to isolate the three forms of the polio virus that affected hundreds of thousands yearly. Salk's team created a vaccine against the strains of polio in cell cultures of Rhesus monkey kidney cells. The vaccine was made publicly available in 1955, and reduced the incidence of polio 15-fold in the USA over the following five years. Albert Sabin made a superior "live" vaccine by passing the polio virus through animal hosts, including monkeys. The vaccine was produced for mass consumption in 1963 and is still in use today. It had virtually eradicated polio in the USA by 1965. It has been estimated that 100,000 Rhesus monkeys were killed in the course of developing the polio vaccines, and 65 doses of vaccine were produced for each monkey.

Also in the 1940s, John Cade tested lithium salts in guinea pigs in a search for pharmaceuticals with anticonvulsant properties. The animals seemed calmer in their mood. He then tested lithium on himself, before using it to treat recurrent mania. The introduction of lithium revolutionized the treatment of manic-depressives by the 1970s. Prior to Cade's animal testing, manic-depressives were treated with lobotomy or electro-convulsive therapy.

In the 1950s the first safer, non-volatile anaesthetic halothane was developed through studies on rodents, rabbits, dogs, cats and monkeys. This paved the way for a whole new generation of modern general anaesthetics - also developed by animal studies - without which modern, complex surgical operations would be virtually impossible.

In 1960, Albert Starr pioneered heart valve replacement surgery in humans after a series of surgical advances in dogs. He received the Lasker Medical Award in 2007 for his efforts, along with Alain Carpentier. In 1968 Carpentier made heart valve replacements from the heart valves of pigs, which are pre-treated with gluteraldehyde to blunt immune response. Over 300,000 people receive heart valve replacements derived from Starr and Carpentier's designs annually. Carpentier said of Starr's initial advances "Before his prosthetic, patients with valvular disease would die".

In the 1970s, leprosy multi-drug antibiotic treatments were refined using leprosy bacteria grown in armadillos, and were then tested in human clinical trials. Today, the nine-banded armadillo is still used to culture the bacteria that causes leprosy, for studies of the proteomics and genomics (the genome was completed in 1998) of the bacteria, for the purposes of improving therapy and developing vaccines. Leprosy is still prevalent in Brazil, Madagascar, Mozambique, Tanzania, India and Nepal, with over 400,000 cases at the beginning of 2004. Throughout the twentieth century, research that used live animals has led to many other medical advances and treatments for human diseases, such as: organ transplant techniques and anti-transplant rejection medications, the heart-lung machine, antibiotics like penicillin, and whooping cough vaccine.Presently, animal experimentation continues to be used in research that aims to solve medical problems from Alzheimer's disease, multiple sclerosis spinal cord injury, and many more conditions in which there is no useful *in vitro* model system available.

The earliest references to animal testing are found in the writings of the Greeks in the second and fourth centuries BCE. Aristotle (384-322 BCE) and Erasistratus (304-258 BCE) were among the first to perform experiments on living animals. Galen, a physician in second-century Rome, dissected pigs and goats, and is known as the "father of vivisection."

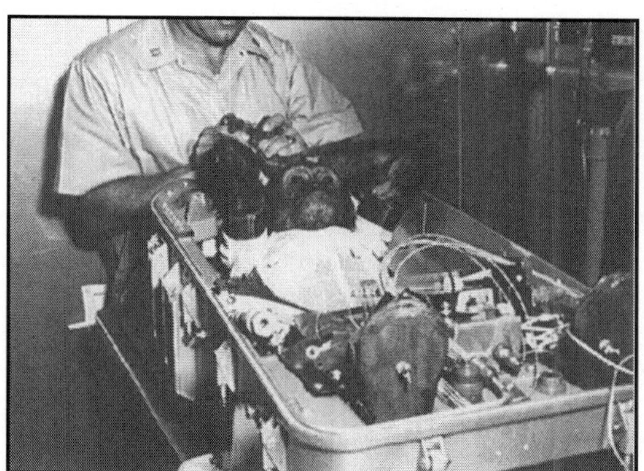

Fig. Enos the Space Chimp Before Insertion into the Mercury-Atlas 5 capsule in 1961.

Animals have been used throughout the history of scientific research. In the 1880s, Louis Pasteur convincingly demonstrated the germ theory of medicine by inducing anthrax in sheep. In the 1890s, Ivan Pavlov famously used dogs to describe classical conditioning.

Insulin was first isolated from dogs in 1922, and revolutionized the treatment of diabetes. On November 3, 1957, a Russian dog, Laika, became the first of many animals to orbit the earth. In the 1970s, antibiotic treatments and vaccines for leprosy were developed using armadillos, then given to humans. The ability of humans to change the genetics of animals took a large step forwards in 1974 when Rudolf Jaenisch was able to produce the first transgenic mammal, by integrating DNA from the SV40 virus into the genome of mice. This genetic research progressed rapidly and, in 1996, Dolly the sheep was born, the first mammal to be cloned from an adult cell.

Toxicology testing became important in the 20th century. In the 19th century, laws regulating drugs were more relaxed. For example, in the U.S., the government could only ban a drug after a company had been prosecuted for selling products that harmed customers.

However, in response to a tragedy in 1937 where a drug labeled "Elixir of Sulfanilamide" killed more than 100 people, the U.S. congress passed laws that required safety testing of drugs on animals before they could be marketed. Other countries enacted similar legislation. In the 1960s, in reaction to the Thalidomide tragedy, further laws were passed requiring safety testing on pregnant animals before a drug can be sold.

The controversy surrounding animal testing dates back to the 17th century. In 1655, the advocate of Galenic physiology Edmund O'Meara said that "the miserable torture of vivisection places the body in an unnatural state." O'Meara and others argued that animal physiology could be affected by pain during vivisection, rendering results unreliable. There were also objections on an ethical basis, contending that the benefit to humans did not justify the harm to animals. Early objections to animal testing also came from another angle — many people believed that animals were inferior to humans and so different that results from animals could not be applied to humans.

On the other side of the debate, those in Favour of animal testing held that experiments on animals were necessary to advance medical and biological knowledge. Claude Bernard, known as the "prince of vivisectors" and the father of physiology — whose wife, Marie Françoise Martin, founded the first anti-vivisection society in France in 1883 — famously wrote in 1865 that "the science of life is a superb and dazzlingly lighted hall which may be reached only by passing through a long and ghastly kitchen". Arguing that "experiments on animals. are entirely conclusive for the toxicology and hygiene of man.the effects of these substances are the same on man as on animals, save for differences in degree," Bernard established animal experimentation as part of the standard scientific method.

In 1896, the physiologist and physician Dr. Walter B. Cannon said "The antivivisectionists are the second of the two types Theodore Roosevelt described when he said, 'Common sense without conscience may lead to crime, but conscience without common sense may lead to folly, which is the handmaiden of crime.' " These divisions between pro- and anti- animal testing groups first came to public attention during the brown dog affair in the early 1900s, when hundreds of medical students clashed with anti-vivisectionists and police over a memorial to a vivisected dog.

In 1822, the first animal protection law was enacted in the British parliament, followed by the Cruelty to Animals Act (1876), the first law specifically aimed at regulating animal testing. The legislation was promoted by Charles Darwin, who wrote to Ray Lankester in March 1871: "You ask about my opinion on vivisection. I quite agree that it is justifiable for real investigations on physiology; but not for mere damnable and detestable curiosity. It is a subject which makes me sick with horror, so I will not say another word about it, else I shall not sleep to-night."

Opposition to the use of animals in medical research first arose in the United States during the 1860s, when Henry Bergh founded the American Society for the Prevention of Cruelty to Animals (ASPCA), with America's first specifically anti-vivisection organization being the American Antivivisection Society (AAVS), founded in 1883. Antivivisectionists of the era generally believed the spread of mercy was the great cause of civilization, and vivisection was cruel. However, in the USA the antivivisectionists' efforts were defeated in every legislature, overwhelmed by the superior organization and influence of the medical community. Overall, this movement had little legislative success until the passing of the Labouratory Animal Welfare Act, in 1966.

CARE AND USE OF ANIMALS

REGULATIONS

The regulations that apply to animals in Labouratories vary across species. In the U.S., under the provisions of the Animal Welfare Act and the *Guide for the Care and Use of Labouratory Animals* (the *Guide*), published by the National Academy of Sciences, any procedure can be performed on an animal if it can be successfully argued that it is scientifically justified. In general, researchers are required to consult with the institution's veterinarian and its Institutional Animal Care and Use Committee (IACUC), which every research facility is obliged to maintain.

The IACUC must ensure that alternatives, including non-animal alternatives, have been considered, that the experiments are not unnecessarily duplicative, and that pain relief is given unless it would interfere with the study.

Larry Carbone, a Labouratory animal veterinarian, writes that, in his experience, IACUCs take their work very seriously regardless of the species involved, though the use of non-human primates always raises what he calls a "red flag of special concern." However, a study published in Science magazine on July 27, 2001 confirmed the low reliability of IACUC reviews of animal experiments. Funded by the National Science Foundation, the three-year study found that animal use committees that do not know the specifics of the university and personnel do not make the same approval decisions as those made by animal use committees that do know the university and personnel.

Specifically, blinded committees more often ask for more information rather than approving studies.The IACUCs regulate all vertebrates in testing at institutions receiving federal funds in the USA. Although the provisions of the Animal Welfare Act do not include purpose-bred rodents and birds, these species are equally regulated under Public Health Service policies that govern the IACUCs. Animal Welfare Act regulations are enforced by the USDA, whereas Public Health Service regulations are enforced by OLAW and in many cases by AAALAC.

Numbers

Accurate global figures for animal testing are difficult to obtain. The British Union for the Abolition of Vivisection (BUAV) estimates that 100 million vertebrates are experimented on around the world every year, 10–11 million of them in the European Union. The Nuffield Council on Bioethics reports that global annual estimates range from 50 to 100 million animals. None of the figures, including those given in this article, include invertebrates, such as shrimp and fruit flies. Animals bred for research then killed as surplus, animals used for breeding purposes, and animals not yet weaned (which most Labouratories do not count) are also not included in the figures.

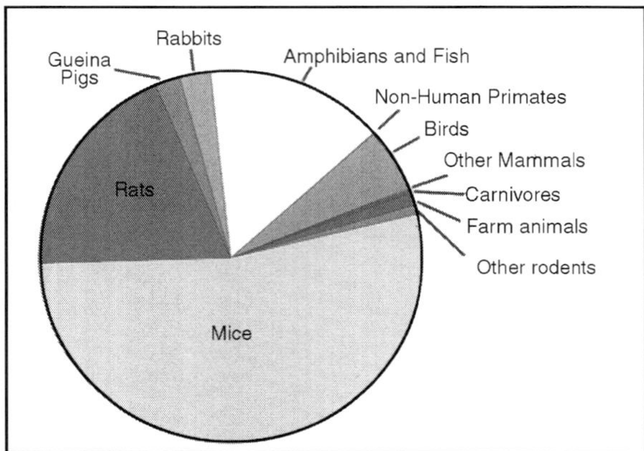

According to the U.S. Department of Agriculture (USDA), the total number of animals used in that country in 2005 was almost 1.2 million, but this does not include rats and mice, which make up about 90 per cent of research animals. In 1995, researchers at Tufts University Centre for Animals and Public Policy estimated that 14-21 million animals were used in American Labouratories in 1992, a reduction from a high of 50 million used in 1970. In 1986, the U.S. Congress Office of Technology Assessment reported that estimates of the animals used in the U.S. range from 10 million to upwards of 100 million each year, and that their own best estimate was at least 17 million to 22 million.

In the UK, Home Office figures show that nearly three million procedures were carried out in 2004 on just under the same number of animals. It is the third consecutive annual rise and the highest figure since 1992. Most animals are used in only one procedure: animals either die because of the experiment or are euthanized afterwards. A "procedure" refers to an experiment that might last minutes, several months, or years.

SPECIES

Invertebrates

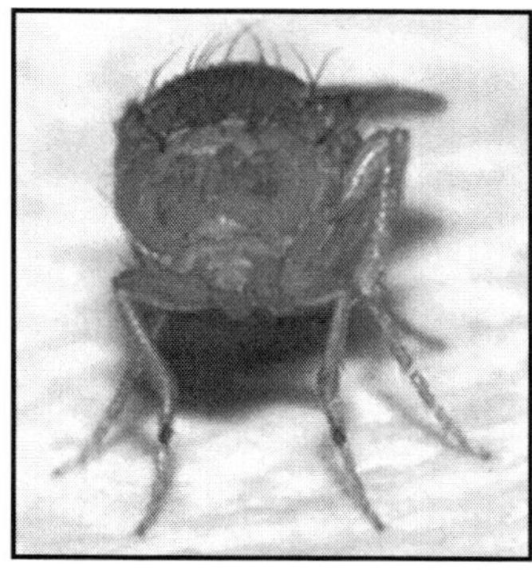

Fig. Drosophila Melanogaster is Commonly Used for Animal Experimentation.

Although many more invertebrates than vertebrates are used, these experiments are largely unregulated by law. The most used invertebrate species are *Drosophila melanogaster*, a fruit fly, and *Caenorhabditis elegans*, a nematode worm. In the case of *C. elegans*, the worm's body is completely transparent and the precise lineage of all the organism's cells is known, while studies in the fly *D. melanogaster* can use an amazing array of genetic tools.

These animals offer great advantages over vertebrates, including their short life cycle and the ease with which large numbers may be studied, with thousands of flies or nematodes fitting into a single room. However, the lack of an adaptive immune system and their simple organs prevent worms from being used in medical research such as vaccine development. Similarly, flies are not widely used in applied medical research, as their immune system differs greatly from that of humans, and diseases in insects can be very different from diseases in vertebrates.

Non-Primate Vertebrates

In the U.S., the numbers of rats and mice used is estimated at 20 million a year. Other rodents commonly used are guinea pigs, hamsters, and gerbils. Mice are the most commonly used vertebrate species because of their size, low cost, ease of handling, and fast reproduction rate.

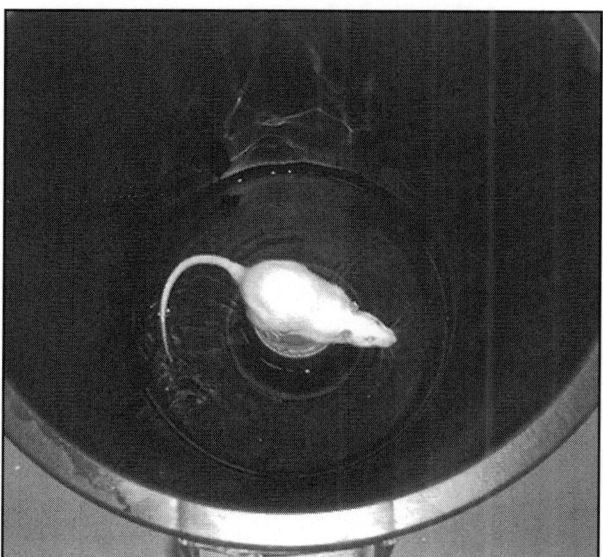

Fig. This Rat is Being Deprived of Restful REM Sleep by a Researcher Using a Single Platform ("flower pot") Technique.

The water is within 1 cm of the small flower pot bottom platform where the rat sits. At the onset of REM sleep, the rat would either fall into the water only to clamber back to its pot to avoid drowning, or its nose would become submerged into the water shocking it back to an awakened state.

Mice are widely considered to be the best model of inherited human disease and share 99 per cent of their genes with humans. With the advent of genetic engineering technology, genetically modified mice can be generated to order and can provide models for a range of human diseases.

Rats are also widely used for physiology, toxicology and cancer research, but genetic manipulation is much harder in rats than in mice, which limits the use of these rodents in basic science.Nearly 200,000 fish and 20,000 amphibians were used in the UK in 2004. The main species used is the zebrafish, *Danio rerio*, which are translucent during their embryonic stage, and the African clawed frog, *Xenopus laevis*. Over 20,000 rabbits were used for animal testing in the UK in 2004.

Albino rabbits are used in eye irritancy tests because rabbits have less tear flow than other animals, and the lack of eye pigment in albinos make the effects easier to visualize. Rabbits are also frequently used for the production of polyclonal antibodies.

Cats and Dogs

Cats are most commonly used in neurological research. Over 25,500 cats were used in the U.S. in 2000, around half of whom were used in experiments which, according to the American Antivivisection Society, had the potential to cause "pain and/or distress".

Dogs are widely used in biomedical research, testing, and education — particularly beagles, because they are gentle and easy to handle. They are commonly used as models for human diseases in cardiology, endocrinology, and bone and joint studies, research that tends to be highly invasive, according to the Humane Society of the United States. The U.S. Department of Agriculture's Animal Welfare Report for 2005 shows that 66,000 dogs were used in USDA-registered facilities in that year. In the U.S., some of the dogs are purpose-bred, while most are supplied by so-called Class B dealers licensed by the USDA to buy animals from auctions, shelters, newspaper ads, and who are sometimes accused of stealing pets.

Non-Human Primates

Non-human primates (NHPs) are used in toxicology tests, studies of AIDS and hepatitis, studies of neurology, Behaviour and cognition, reproduction, genetics, and xenotransplantation. They are caught in the wild or purpose-bred. In the U.S. and China, most primates are domestically purpose-bred, whereas in Europe the majority are imported purpose-bred. Rhesus monkeys, cynomolgus monkeys, squirrel monkeys, and owl monkeys are imported; around 12,000 to 15,000 monkeys are imported into the U.S. annually. In total, around 70,000 NHPs are used each year in the United States and European Union.

Most of the NHPs used are macaques; but marmosets, spider monkeys, and squirrel monkeys are also used, and baboons and chimpanzees are used in the U.S; in 2006 there were 1133 chimpanzees in U.S. primate Centres. The first transgenic primate was produced in 2001, with the development of a method that could introduce new genes into a rhesus macaque. This transgenic technology is now being applied in the search for a treatment for the genetic disorder Huntington's disease. Notable studies on non-human primates have been part of the polio vaccine development, and development of Deep Brain Stimulation, and their current heaviest non-toxicological use occurs in the monkey AIDS model, SIV.

In 2008 a proposal to ban all primates experiments in the EU has sparked a vigorous debate.

SOURCES

Animals used by Labouratories are largely supplied by specialist dealers. Sources differ for vertebrate and invertebrate animals. Most Labouratories breed and raise flies and worms themselves, using strains and mutants supplied from a few main stock Centres.

For vertebrates, sources include breeders who supply purpose-bred animals; businesses that trade in wild animals; and dealers who supply animals sourced from pounds, auctions, and newspaper ads. Animal shelters also supply the Labouratories directly. Large Centres also exist to distribute strains of genetically-modified animals; the National Institutes of Health *Knockout Mouse Project*, for example, aims to provide knockout mice for every gene in the mouse genome.

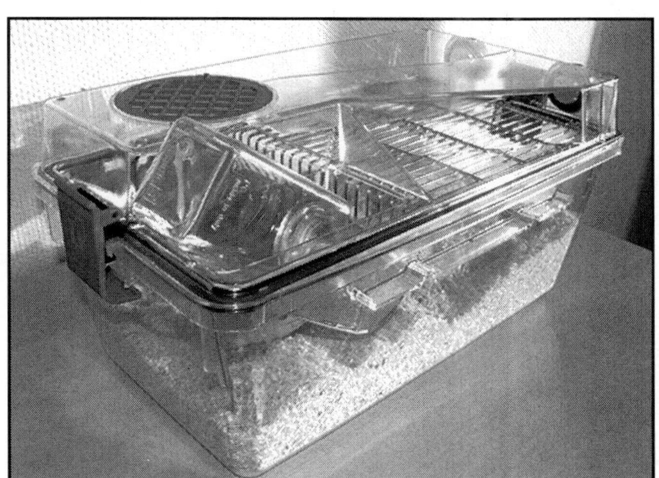

Fig. A Labouratory Mouse Cage. Mice are Either Bred Commercially, or Raised in the Labouratory.

In the U.S., Class A breeders are licensed by the U.S. Department of Agriculture (USDA) to sell animals for research purposes, while Class B dealers are licensed to buy animals from "random sources" such as auctions, pound seizure, and newspaper ads. Some Class B dealers have been accused of kidnapping pets and illegally trapping strays, a practice known as *bunching*. It was in part out of public concern over the sale of pets to research facilities that the 1966 Labouratory Animal Welfare Act was ushered in — the Senate Committee on Commerce reported in 1966 that stolen pets had been retrieved from Veterans Administration facilities, the Mayo Institute, the University of Pennsylvania, Stanford University, and Harvard and Yale Medical Schools.

The USDA recovered at least a dozen stolen pets during a raid on a Class B dealer in Arkansas in 2003.Four states in the U.S. — Minnesota, Utah, Oklahoma, and Iowa — require their shelters to provide animals to research facilities. Fourteen states explicitly prohibit the practice, while the remainder either allow it or have no relevant legislation.

In the European Union, animal sources are governed by *Council Directive 86/609/EEC*, which requires lab animals to be specially bred, unless the animal has been lawfully imported and is not a wild animal or a stray. The latter requirement may also be exempted by special arrangement. In the UK, most animals used in experiments are bred for the purpose under the 1988 Animal Protection Act, but wild-caught primates may be used if exceptional and specific justification can be established. The United States also allows the use of wild-caught primates; between 1995 and 1999, 1,580 wild baboons were imported into the U.S. Over half the primates imported between 1995 and 2000 were handled by Charles River Labouratories, Inc., or by Covance, which is the single largest importer of primates into the U.S

Pain and Suffering

The extent to which animal testing causes pain and suffering, and the capacity of animals to experience and comprehend them, is the subject of much debate.

According to the U.S. Department of Agriculture, in 2006 about 670,000 animals (57 per cent) (not including rats, mice, birds, or invertebrates) were used in procedures that did not include more than momentary pain or distress. About 420,000 (36 per cent) were used in procedures in which pain or distress was relieved by anesthesia, while 84,000 (7 per cent) were used in studies that would cause pain or distress that would not be relieved.

In the UK, research projects are classified as mild, moderate, and substantial in terms of the suffering the researchers conducting the study say they may cause; a fourth category of "unclassified" means the animal was anesthetized and killed without recovering consciousness, according to the researchers.

In December 2001, 39 per cent (1,296) of project licenses in force were classified as mild, 55 per cent (1,811) as moderate, two per cent (63) as substantial, and 4 per cent (139) as unclassified. There have, however, been suggestions of systemic underestimation of procedure severity.

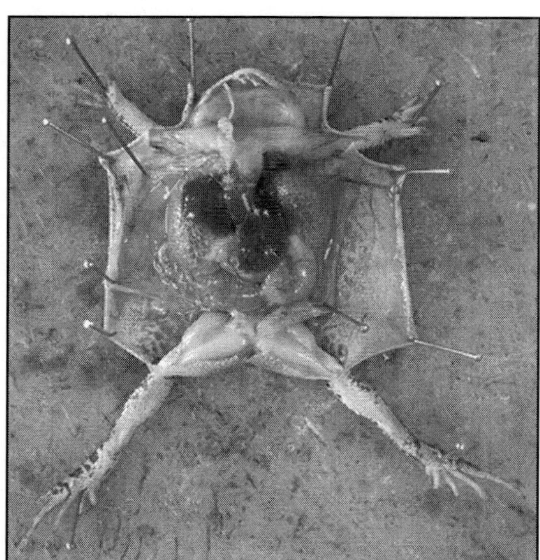

Fig. Prior to Vivisection for Educational Purposes, Chloroform was Administered to this Common Sand Frog to Induce Terminal Anesthesia.

The idea that animals might not feel pain as human beings feel it traces back to the 17th-century French philosopher, René Descartes, who argued that animals do not experience pain and suffering because they lack consciousness. Bernard Rollin of Colourado State University, the principal author of two U.S. federal laws regulating pain relief for animals, writes that researchers remained unsure into the 1980s as to whether animals experience pain, and that veterinarians trained in the U.S. before 1989 were simply taught to ignore animal pain. In his interactions with scientists and other veterinarians, he was regularly asked to "prove" that animals are conscious, and to provide "scientifically acceptable" grounds for claiming that they feel pain.

Carbone writes that the view that animals feel pain differently is now a minority view. Academic reviews of the topic are more equivocal, noting that although the argument that animals have at least simple conscious thoughts and feelings has strong support, some critics continue to question how reliably animal mental states can be determined. The ability of invertebrate species of animals, such as insects, to feel pain and suffering is also unclear.

The defining text on animal welfare regulation, "Guide for the Care and Use of Labouratory Animals" defines the parameters that govern animal testing in the USA. It states "The ability to experience and respond to pain is widespread in the animal kingdom.Pain is a stressor and, if not relieved, can lead to unacceptable levels of stress and distress in animals." The Guide states that the ability to recognize the symptoms of pain in different species is vital in efficiently applying pain relief and that it is essential for the people caring for and using animals to be entirely familiar with these symptoms.

On the subject of analgesics used to relieve pain, the Guide states "The selection of the most appropriate analgesic or anesthetic should reflect professional judgment as to which best meets clinical and humane requirements without compromising the scientific aspects of the research protocol". Accordingly, all issues of animal pain and distress, and their potential treatment with analgesia and anesthesia, are required regulatory issues in receiving animal protocol approval.

EUTHANASIA

There is general agreement that animal life should not be taken wantonly, and regulations require that scientists use as few animals as possible. However, while policy makers consider suffering to be the central issue and see animal euthanasia as a way to reduce suffering, others, such as the RSPCA, argue that the lives of Labouratory animals have intrinsic value. Regulations focus on whether particular methods cause pain and suffering, not whether their death is undesirable in itself. The animals are euthanized at the end of studies for sample collection or post-mortem examination; during studies if their pain or suffering falls into certain categories regarded as unacceptable, such as depression, infection that is unresponsive to treatment, or the failure of large animals to eat for five days; or when they are unsuitable for breeding or unwanted for some other reason.

Methods of euthanizing Labouratory animals are chosen to induce rapid unconsciousness and death without pain or distress. The methods that are preferred are those published by councils of veterinarians. The animal can be made to inhale a gas, such as carbon monoxide and carbon dioxide, by being placed in a chamber, or by use of a face mask, with or without prior sedation or anesthesia. Sedatives or anesthetics such as barbiturates can be given intravenously, or inhalant anesthetics may be used. Amphibians and fish may be immersed in water containing an anesthetic such as tricaine. Physical methods are also used, with or without sedation or anesthesia depending on the method.

Recommended methods include decapitation (beheading) for small rodents or rabbits. Cervical dislocation (breaking the neck or spine) may be used for birds, mice, and immature rats and rabbits. Maceration (grinding into small pieces) is used on 1 day old chicks. High-intensity microwave irradiation of the brain can preserve brain tissue and induce death in less than 1 second, but this is currently only used on rodents. Captive bolts may be used, typically on dogs, ruminants, horses, pigs and rabbits. It causes death by a concussion to the brain.

Gunshot may be used, but only in cases where a penetrating captive bolt may not be used. Some physical methods are only acceptable after the animal is unconscious. Electrocution may be used for cattle, sheep, swine, foxes, and mink after the animals are unconscious, often by a prior electrical stun. Pithing (inserting a tool into the base of the brain) is usable on animals already unconscious. Slow or rapid freezing, or inducing air embolism are acceptable only with prior anesthesia to induce unconsciousness.

RESEARCH CLASSIFICATION OF ANIMALS

PURE RESEARCH

Basic or pure research investigates how organisms behave, develop, and function. Those opposed to animal testing object that pure research may have little or no practical purpose, but researchers argue that it may produce unforeseen benefits, rendering the distinction between pure and applied research — research that has a specific practical aim — unclear.

Pure research uses larger numbers and a greater variety of animals than applied research. Fruit flies, nematode worms, mice and rats together account for the vast majority, though small numbers of other species are used, ranging from sea slugs through to armadillos.

Examples of the types of animals and experiments used in basic research include:

- Studies on *embryogenesis* and *developmental biology*. Mutants are created by adding transposons into their genomes, or specific genes are deleted by gene targeting. By studying the changes in development these changes produce, scientists aim to understand both how organisms normally develop, and what can go wrong in this process. These studies are particularly powerful since the basic controls of development, such as the homeobox genes, have similar functions in organisms as diverse as fruit flies and man.
- Experiments into *Behaviour*, to understand how organisms detect and interact with each other and their environment, in which fruit flies, worms, mice, and rats are all widely used. Studies of brain function, such as memory and social Behaviour, often use rats and birds. For some species, Behavioural research is combined with enrichment strategies for animals in captivity because it allows them to engage in a wider range of activities.
- Breeding experiments to study *evolution* and *genetics*. Labouratory mice, flies, fish, and worms are inbred through many generations to create strains with defined characteristics. These provide animals of a known genetic background, an important tool for genetic analyses. Larger mammals are rarely bred specifically for such studies due to their slow rate of reproduction, though some scientists take advantage of inbred domesticated animals, such as dog or cattle breeds, for comparative purposes. Scientists studying how animals evolve use many animal species to see how variations in where and how an

organism lives (their niche) produce adaptations in their physiology and morphology. As an example, sticklebacks are now being used to study how many and which types of mutations are selected to produce adaptations in animals' morphology during the evolution of new species.

Applied Research

Applied research aims to solve specific and practical problems. Compared to pure research, which is largely academic in origin, applied research is usually carried out in the pharmaceutical industry, or by universities in commercial partnerships. These may involve the use of animal models of diseases or conditions, which are often discovered or generated by pure research Programmemes. In turn, such applied studies may be an early stage in the drug discovery process. Examples include:

- Genetic modification of animals to study disease. Transgenic animals have specific genes inserted, modified or removed, to mimic specific conditions such as single gene disorders, such as Huntington's disease. Other models mimic complex, multifactorial diseases with genetic components, such as diabetes, or even transgenic mice that carry the same mutations that occur during the development of cancer. These models allow investigations on how and why the disease develops, as well as providing ways to develop and test new treatments. The vast majority of these transgenic models of human disease are lines of mice, the mammalian species in which genetic modification is most efficient. Smaller numbers of other animals are also used, including rats, pigs, sheep, fish, birds, and amphibians.
- Studies on models of naturally occurring disease and condition. Certain domestic and wild animals have a natural propensity or predisposition for certain conditions that are also found in humans. Cats are used as a model to develop immunodeficiency virus vaccines and to study leukemia because their natural predisposition to FIV and Feline leukemia virus. Certain breeds of dog suffer from narcolepsy making them the major model used to study the human condition. Armadillos and humans are among only a few animal species that naturally suffer from leprosy; as the bacteria responsible for this disease cannot yet be grown in culture, armadillos are the primary source of bacilli used in leprosy vaccines.
- Studies on induced animal models of human diseases. Here, an animal is treated so that it develops pathology and symptoms that resemble a human disease. Examples include restricting blood flow to the brain to induce stroke, or giving neurotoxins that cause damage similar to that seen in Parkinson's disease. Such studies can be difficult to interpret, and it is argued that they are not always comparable to

human diseases. For example, although such models are now widely used to study Parkinson's disease, the British anti-vivisection interest group BUAV argues that these models only superficially resemble the disease symptoms, without the same time course or cellular pathology. In contrast, scientists assessing the usefulness of animal models of Parkinson's disease, as well as the medical research charity *The Parkinson's Appeal*, state that these models were invaluable and that they led to improved surgical treatments such as pallidotomy, new drug treatments such as levodopa, and later deep brain stimulation.

XENOTRANSPLANTATION

Xenotransplantation research involves transplanting tissues, or organs from one species to another, as a way to overcome the shortage of human organs for use in organ transplants.

Current research involves using primates as the recipients of organs from pigs that have been genetically-modified to reduce the primates' immune response against the pig tissue. Although transplant rejection remains a problem, recent clinical trials that involved implanting pig insulin-secreting cells into diabetics did reduce these people's need for insulin.

The British Home Office released figures in 1999 showing that 270 monkeys had been used in xenotransplantation research in Britain during the previous four years.

Documents leaked from Huntingdon Life Sciences to *The Observer* in 2003 showed, between 1994 and 2000, wild baboons were imported to the UK from Africa to be used in experiments that involved grafting pigs' hearts and kidneys onto the primates' necks, abdomens, and chests. *The Observer* reports that some baboons died after suffering strokes, vomiting, diarrhea, and paralysis, while others died *en route* to the UK. The experiments were conducted by Imutran Ltd, a subsidiary of Novartis Pharma AG in conjunction with Cambridge University and Huntingdon Life Sciences. Novartis told the newspaper that developing new cures for humans invariably means experimenting on live animals.

The newspaper also wrote that researchers were deliberately underestimating the suffering in order to obtain licences. A report from Imutran said: "The Home Office will attempt to get the kidney transplants classified as 'moderate,' ensuring that it is easier for Imutran to receive a licence and ignoring the 'severe' nature of these Programmemes."

TOXICOLOGY TESTING

Toxicology testing, also known as safety testing, is conducted by pharmaceutical companies testing drugs, or by contract animal testing facilities, such as Huntingdon Life Sciences, on behalf of a wide variety of customers.

According to 2005 EU figures, around one million animals are used every year in Europe in toxicology tests; which are about 10 per cent of all procedures. According to *Nature*, 5,000 animals are used for each chemical being tested, with 12,000 needed to test pesticides. The tests are conducted without anesthesia, because interactions between drugs can affect how animals detoxify chemicals, and may interfere with the results.

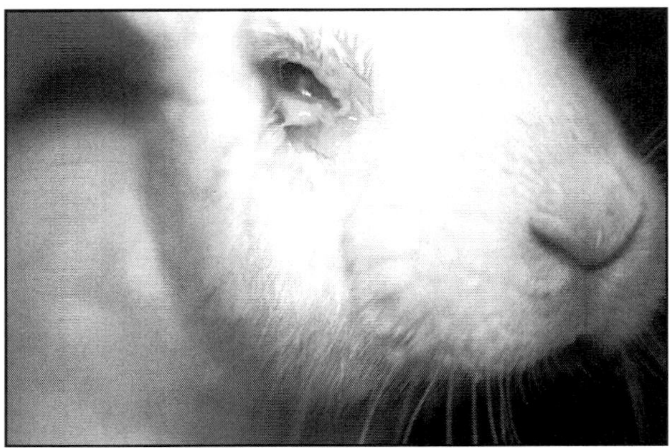

Fig. A Rabbit During a Draize Test.

Toxicology tests are used to examine finished products such as pesticides, medications, food additives, packing materials, and air freshener, or their chemical ingredients.

Most tests involve testing ingredients rather than finished products, but according to BUAV, manufacturers believe these tests overestimate the toxic effects of substances; they therefore repeat the tests using their finished products to obtain a less toxic label.

The substances are applied to the skin or dripped into the eyes; injected intravenously, intramuscularly, or subcutaneously; inhaled either by placing a mask over the animals and restraining them, or by placing them in an inhalation chamber; or administered orally, through a tube into the stomach, or simply in the animal's food. Doses may be given once, repeated regularly for many months, or for the lifespan of the animal.

There are several different types of acute toxicity tests. The LD50 ("Lethal Dose 50 per cent") test is used to evaluate the toxicity of a substance by determining the dose required to kill 50 per cent of the test animal population. This test was removed from OECD international guidelines in 2002, replaced by methods such as the fixed dose procedure, which use fewer animals and cause less suffering.

Nature writes that, as of 2005, "the LD50 acute toxicity test. still accounts for one-third of all animal [toxicity] tests worldwide." Irritancy is usually measured using the Draize test, where a test substance is applied to an animal's eyes or skin, usually an albino rabbit. For Draize eye testing, the recommended protocol involves observing the effects of the substance at intervals and grading any damage or irritation, but that the test should be halted and the animal killed if it shows "continuing signs of severe pain or distress". The Humane Society of the United States writes that the procedure can cause redness, ulceration, hemorrhaging, cloudiness, or even blindness. This test has also been criticized by scientists for being cruel and inaccurate, subjective, over-sensitive, and failing to reflect human exposures in the real world. Although no accepted *in vitro* alternatives exist, a modified form of the Draize test called the *low volume eye test* may reduce suffering and provide more realistic results, but it has not yet replaced the original test.

The most stringent tests are reserved for drugs and foodstuffs. For these, a number of tests are performed, lasting less than a month (acute), one to three months (subchronic), and more than three months (chronic) to test general toxicity (damage to organs), eye and skin irritancy, mutagenicity, carcinogenicity, teratogenicity, and reproductive problems. The cost of the full complement of tests is several million dollars per substance and it may take three or four years to complete.

These toxicity tests provide, in the words of a 2006 United States National Academy of Sciences report, "critical information for assessing hazard and risk potential".

However, as *Nature* reported, most animal tests either over- or underestimate risk, or do not reflect toxicity in humans particularly well, with false positive results being a particular problem. This variability stems from using the effects of high doses of chemicals in small numbers of Labouratory animals to try to predict the effects of low doses in large numbers of humans. Although relationships do exist, opinion is divided on how to use data on one species to predict the exact level of risk in another.

COSMETICS AND DRUG TESTING OF ANIMALS

Cosmetics testing on animals is particularly controversial. Such tests, which are still conducted in the U.S., involve general toxicity, eye and skin irritancy, phototoxicity (toxicity triggered by ultraviolet light) and mutagenicity.

Cosmetics testing is banned in the Netherlands, Belgium, and the UK, and in 2002, after 13 years of discussion, the European Union (EU) agreed to phase in a near-total ban on the sale of animal-tested cosmetics throughout the EU from 2009, and to ban all cosmetics-related animal testing. France, which is home to the world's largest cosmetics company, L'Oreal, has protested the proposed ban by lodging a case at the European Court of Justice in Luxembourg, asking that the ban be quashed.

The ban is also opposed by the European Federation for Cosmetics Ingredients, which represents 70 companies in Switzerland, Belgium, France, Germany and Italy.

DRUG TESTING

Before the early 20th century, laws regulating drugs were lax. Nowadays all new pharmaceuticals undergo rigorous animal testing before being licensed for human use. Tests on pharmaceutical products involve:

- *Metabolic tests*, investigating pharmacokinetics - how drugs are absorbed, metabolized and excreted by the body when introduced orally, intravenously, intraperitoneally, intramuscularly, or transdermally.
- *Toxicology tests*, which gauge acute, sub-acute, and chronic toxicity. Acute toxicity is studied by using a rising dose until signs of toxicity become apparent. Current European legislation demands that "acute toxicity tests must be carried out in two or more mammalian species" covering "at least two different routes of administration". Sub-acute toxicity is where the drug is given to the animals for four to six weeks in doses below the level at which it causes rapid poisoning, in order to discover if any toxic drug metabolites build up over time. Testing for chronic toxicity can last up to two years and, in the European Union, is required to involve two species of mammals, one of which must be non-rodent.
- *Efficacy studies*, which test whether experimental drugs work by inducing the appropriate illness in animals. The drug is then administered in a double-blind controlled trial, which allows researchers to determine the effect of the drug and the dose-response curve.
- Specific tests on *reproductive function*, *embryonic toxicity*, or *carcinogenic potential* can all be required by law, depending on the result of other studies and the type of drug being tested.

Education, Breeding, and Defence

Animals are also used for education and training; are bred for use in Labouratories; and are used by the military to develop weapons, vaccines, battlefield surgical techniques, and defensive clothing. For example, in 2008 the United States Defence Advanced Research Projects Agency used live pigs to study the effects of improvised explosive device explosions on internal organs, especially the brain.

There are efforts in many countries to find alternatives to using animals in education. Horst Spielmann, German director of the Central Office for Collecting and Assessing Alternatives to Animal Experimentation, while describing Germany's progress in this area, told German broadcaster ARD in 2005: "Using animals in teaching curricula is already superfluous. In many countries, one can become a doctor, vet or biologist without ever having performed an experiment on an animal."

ETHICS

The ethical questions raised by performing experiments on animals are subject to much debate, and viewpoints have shifted significantly over the 20th century. There remain strong disagreements about which animal testing procedures are useful for which purposes, as well as disagreements over which ethical principles apply, and to which species of animals. The dominant ethical position, worldwide, is that achievement of scientific and medical goals using animal testing is desirable, provided that animal suffering and use is minimized. The British government has additionally required that the cost to animals in an experiment be weighed against the gain in knowledge.

A wide range of minority viewpoints exist as well. The view that animals have moral rights (animal rights) is a philosophical position proposed by Tom Regan, who argues that animals are beings with beliefs, desires and self-consciousness. Such beings are seen as having inherent value and thus possessing rights. Regan still sees clear ethical differences between killing animals and killing humans, and argues that to save human lives it is permissible to kill animals.

However, some such as Bernard Rollin have taken his position further and argue that any benefits to human beings cannot outweigh animal suffering, and that human beings have no moral right to use an individual animal in ways that do not benefit that individual. Another prominent position is articulated by Peter Singer, who sees no convincing reason to include a being's species in considerations of whether their suffering is important in utilitarian moral considerations. Although these arguments have not been widely accepted, in response to these concerns some governments such as the Netherlands and New Zealand have outlawed invasive experiments on certain classes of non-human primates, particularly the great apes.

Some medical schools and agencies in China, Japan, and South Korea have built cenotaphs for killed animals. In Japan there are also annual memorial services (*Ireisai* pa—my) for animals sacrificed at medical school.

PROMINENT CASES

In 1997, People for the Ethical Treatment of Animals (PETA) filmed staff inside Huntingdon Life Sciences (HLS) in the UK, Europe's largest animal-testing facility, hitting puppies, shouting at them, and simulating sex acts while taking blood samples. The employees were dismissed and prosecuted, and HLS's licence to perform animal experiments was revoked for six months. The broadcast of the undercover footage on British television in 1997 triggered the formation of Stop Huntingdon Animal Cruelty, an international campaign to close HLS, which has been criticized for its sometimes violent tactics.

In February 1997 a team at the Roslin Institute in Scotland announced the birth of Dolly the sheep, a ewe that had been cloned from tissue taken from another adult sheep. Dolly was produced through nuclear transfer to an unfertilised oocyte, and was the only lamb that survived from 277 attempts at this technique. Dolly appeared to be a normal sheep, living for six years and giving birth to several lambs, but was euthanized in 2003 after contracting a progressive lung disease. Although the production of Dolly was a scientific breakthrough, it was controversial, since it showed that not only could cloned animals be produced for use in farming, but also that it would now be, in principle, possible to clone a human being.

Covance

In 2004, German journalist Friedrich Mülln shot undercover footage of staff in Covance, Münster, Europe's largest primate-testing Centre, making monkeys dance in time to blaring pop music, handling them roughly, and screaming at them. The monkeys were kept isolated in small wire cages with little or no natural light, no environmental enrichment, and high noise levels from staff shouting and playing the radio (video). Primatologist Dr. Jane Goodall described the living conditions of the monkeys as "horrendous." Primatologist Stephen Brend told BUAV that using monkeys in such a stressed state is "bad science," and trying to extrapolate useful data in such circumstances an "untenable proposition." Covance obtained a restraining order preventing Mülln from performing any further undercover research against the company for three years, and required him and PETA to turn over the material they obtained from Covance. PETA is further prevented from attempting to infiltrate Covance for five years.

The British Union for the Abolition of Vivisection (BUAV) raised concerns about primate experiments at the University of Cambridge in 2002. In a series of court cases, the BUAV alleged that monkeys had undergone surgery to induce a stroke, and were left alone after the procedure for 15 hours overnight. Researchers had trained the monkeys to perform certain tasks before inflicting brain damage and re-testing them.

The monkeys were only given food and water for two hours a day, to encourage them to perform the tasks. The judge hearing BUAV's application for a judicial review rejected the allegation that the Home Secretary had been negligent in granting the university a license. The British government's chief inspector of animals conducted a review of the facilities and experiments. It concluded the veterinary input at Cambridge was "exemplary"; the facility "seems adequately staffed"; and the animals afforded "appropriate standards of accommodation and care."

One of the cases of alleged abuse involved Britches, a macaque monkey born in 1985 at the University of California, Riverside, removed from its mother at birth, and left alone with its eyelids sewn shut, and a sonar sensor on its head, as part of an experiment to test sensory substitution devices for blind people. 260 animals, including Britches, were stolen from the Labouratories at the University of California, Riverside in a raid by the Animal Liberation Front. The university alleged that damage to the monkey's eyelids, caused by the sutures according to the ALF, had in fact been caused by an ALF veterinarian, and that the sonar device had been removed and re-attached by the activists. The ALF reported that Britches was later transferred to a sanctuary in Mexico. University officials reported that hundreds of thousands of dollars of damage was done by the theft, and by smashing Labouratory equipment, and years of medical research were lost.

COLUMBIA UNIVERSITY

CNN reported in October 2003 that a post-doctoral "whistleblowing" veterinarian at Columbia University approached the university's Institutional Animal Care and Use Committee about experiments being carried out by an assistant professor of neurosurgery, E. Sander Connolly. Connolly was allegedly causing strokes in baboons by removing their left eyeballs and using the eye sockets to reach a critical blood vessel to their brains. A clamp was placed on the blood vessel until the stroke was induced, after which Connolly would try to treat the condition with an experimental drug.

In a letter to the National Institute of Health, PETA cited the case of a baboon they said was unable to sit up or eat, and remained slouched over in its cage, before dying two days later. An investigation by the United States Department of Agriculture found the experiments did not violate federal guidelines. Connolly abandoned the research saying he felt under attack after receiving a threatening e-mail, but continued to believe his experiments were humane and potentially valuable.

THREATS TO RESEARCHERS

In 2006, a primate researcher at the University of California, Los Angeles (UCLA) shut down the experiments in his lab after threats from animal rights activists.

The researcher had received a grant to use 30 macaque monkeys for vision experiments; each monkey was anesthetized for a single physiological experiment lasting up to 120 hours, and then euthanized. The researcher's name, phone number, and address were posted on the website of the Primate Freedom Project. Demonstrations were held in front of his home. A Molotov cocktail was placed on the porch of what was believed to be the home of another UCLA primate researcher; instead, it was accidentally left on the porch of an elderly woman unrelated to the university.

The Animal Liberation Front claimed responsibility for the attack. As a result of the campaign, the researcher sent an email to the Primate Freedom Project stating "you win," and "please don't bother my family anymore." In another incident at UCLA in June 2007, the Animal Liberation Brigade placed a bomb under the car of a UCLA children's ophthalmologist who experiments on cats and rhesus monkeys; the bomb had a faulty fuse and did not detonate. UCLA is now refusing Freedom of Information Act requests for animal medical records.

These attacks, as well as similar incidents that caused the Southern Poverty Law Centre to declare in 2002 that the animal rights movement had "clearly taken a turn toward the more extreme," this prompted the US government to pass the Animal Enterprise Terrorism Act and the UK government to add the offense of "Intimidation of persons connected with animal research organisation" to the Serious Organised Crime and Police Act 2005. Such legislation, and the arrest and imprisonment of extremists may have decreased the incidence of attacks.

3

Digestive System

The digestive system is one of the body's major organ systems. All animals - with the exception of some endoparasites such as tapeworms - have a digestive system. In this section we're going to look at digestion in ruminants, and compare their guts with those of other, non-ruminant, mammals.

WHAT IS THE RUMEN?

The rumen underpins much of our agricultural industry. Without this stomach chamber, cows and other ruminants would be much less efficient at turning grass into milk, meat and wool. A cow's rumen has a capacity of up to 95 litres and contains billions of bacteria and other microbes. These microbes produce the enzymes that digest cellulose into sugars and fatty acids for their hosts to use. A less desirable by-product is the potent greenhouse gas, methane: a single cow can produce up to 280 litres of methane a day.

The rumen is one of four stomach compartments found in ruminants. Ruminants are animals such as cattle, sheep, goats and deer. (In comparison, animals such as pigs, dogs and horses have only a single stomach compartment and are called nonruminants, or monogastric animals.) The rumen allows grazing animals to digest cellulose, a very common carbohydrate in plants.

Three of the four ruminant stomach compartments make up the forestomach. These three compartments – the rumen, reticulum, and omasum – are an extension of the lower oesophagus. The rumen, the first of the forestomach chambers, stores and processes plant material. It can be a very large structure indeed: in large ruminants, the rumen may store up to 95 litres of undigested food (Brooker et al. 2008). The rumen holds plant material until it has been broken down, releasing volatile fatty acids, and fermentation of protein and carbohydrates has begun.

Why is the rumen so big? Because most plants, especially grasses, have a high cellulose content. A cellulose molecule is a polymer, made up of a long chain of subunits called simple sugars, or monosaccharides. Vertebrate animals lack the enzyme, called cellulase, needed to break down cellulose and release these sugars. Instead, they use symbiotic anaerobic bacteria that do possess the enzyme cellulase. Huge numbers of these bacteria are present in the rumen and the reticulum: with each gram of rumen fluid contains 10 - 50 billion bacteria.

The ruminant digestive system is a very efficient adaptation for extracting as much energy as possible from a high cellulose diet. Because food is held in a ruminant's gut for a relatively long time, symbiotic bacteria are able to grow and release nutrient sources that are not otherwise available to vertebrates.

THE RUMINANT DIGESTIVE SYSTEM

The Oesophagus

The oesophagus is a muscular tube that connects the mouth with the forestomach. Food passes down the oesophagus by contraction of the muscles in the walls that push the food along in a series of waves called peristalsis. The ruminant oesophagus is also capable of reversed peristalsis or antiperistalsis. This allows food to be easily regurgitated from the rumen and chewed.

The reticulorumen

The reticulorumen is composed of the rumen and the reticulum. The reticulorumen is partially separated from the rumen by the reticular fold, which allows mixing between the two compartments. The contents of the reticulorumen are mixed by contractions of the reticulorumen wall. The mixing recirculates undigested material preventing the rumen becoming clogged and distributing symbiotic bacteria throughout the ingested material. The reticulorumen becomes colonized by symbiotic bacteria in the first week after birth. The bacteria help to break down the food and release nutrients by a fermentation process.

The omasum

When food has been broken down enough, it passes from the reticulorumen through the reticulo-omasal orifice to the omasum. The omasum wall is highly folded, giving a large surface area which allows for the efficient absorption of water and salts released from the partially digested food. The omasum also acts as a type of pump, moving the food from the reticulorumen to the true stomach, the abomasum, where acid digestion takes place.

The abomasum

Unlike a ruminant's three forestomachs, the abomasum is a 'secretory stomach'. This means that cells in the abomasum wall produce enzymes and hydrochloric acid which hydrolyse proteins in the food and also in the microbes mixed in with the food. Hydrolysis breaks the proteins into smaller sub-units (e.g. dipeptides and amino acids), ready for further digestion and absorption in the small intestine.

Because ruminants eat such large amounts of plant material, there is an almost continuous flow of food through the abomasum. In comparison, activity in the stomach of monogastric animals generally has a circadian rhythm associated with food intake (Djikstra, 2005).

The small intestine

The small intestine is an elongated tube running from the abomasum to the large intestine. In ruminants, the small intestine is about 20 times longer than the length of the animal - so a cow two metres in length would have a small intestine 40 metres long!

A large proportion of the digestion and absorption of nutrients and water occurs in the small intestine. Enzymes in the small intestine break nutrient molecules down into their building blocks. Carbohydrates are broken down to simple sugars (monosaccharides), fats into fatty acids and monoglycerides, nucleic acids into nucleotides and proteins into amino acids. Some of these enzymes are on the surfaces of intestinal cells, while others are secreted into the small intestine, primarily from the liver and pancreas.

The small intestine has three regions: the duodenum, the jejunum and the ileum. Partially digested food passes from the duodenum along the small intestine by way of peristaltic muscle contractions that start at the part where the abomasum is joined to the duodenum.

Duodenum

The liver and pancreas both secrete materials through ducts into the duodenum. The common bile duct carries bile salts, a greenish fluid that is manufactured in the liver, stored in the gall bladder (the ruminant gall bladder does very little to concentrate the bile), and released into the duodenum to digest fats. The main pancreatic duct carries digestive secretions, which are rich in enzymes and bicarbonate. The bicarbonate neutralises acid from the stomach, which would otherwise inactivate many of the duodenum's digestive enzymes.

Jejunum

The lining of the jejunum is specialised for the absorption of carbohydrates and proteins. Its inner surface is covered in finger-like projections called villi, which increase the surface area available to absorb nutrients from the gut contents. The villi in the jejunum are much longer than in the duodenum or ileum. The epithelial cells which line these villi possess even larger numbers of microvilli, known collectively as the brush border. The combination of villi and microvilli increases the surface area of the small intestine, increasing the chance of a food particle encountering a digestive enzyme and being absorbed across the epithelium and into the blood stream.

Nutrients can cross the intestine wall by either passive or active transport. In passive transport molecules diffuse into the intestinal cells down a concentration gradient (i.e. they move from a region where they are in high concentration to an area of low concentration.) The sugar xylose enters the blood by passive transport. Active transport requires energy. Amino acides, small peptides, vitamins, and most glucose are moved across the intestine lining by active transport. Once nutrients have moved through the epithelial cells, they are taken up by either capillaries or lacteals and then transported around the body.

Ileum

The ileum's main function is absorption of vitamin B12, bile salts and whatever nutrients that were not absorbed by the jejunum. At the point where the ileum joins the large intestine there is a valve, called the ileocaecal valve, which prevents materials flowing back into the small intestine.

The caecum

The caecum is a pouch connected to the large intestine and the ileum. It is separated from the ileum by the ileocaecal valve, and is considered to be the beginning of the large intestine. In herbivores the caecum is greatly enlarged and serves as a storage organ that permits bacteria and other microbes time to further digest cellulose. Partially digested food enters the caecum through the ileoacecal valve, which is normally closed. The valve occasionally opens to allow food material in. As there is only one opening to the caecum, digesta must move in and out to the caecum through the same opening.

The large intestine

In addition to the caecum the large intestine is made up of the ascending colon, transverse colon, sigmoid colon, rectum, and anus. Much of the large intestine comprises the colon, which is shorter in length but larger in diameter than the small intestine. The colon is involved in the active transport of sodium, and absorption of water by osmosis, from the digested material that it contains. It also provides an environment for bacteria to grow and reproduce. These symbiotic bacteria produce important vitamins such as vitamin K, thiamine, and riboflavin, required by the animal for proper growth and health. Finally, the large intestine eliminates wastes. Undigested and unabsorbed food, as well as other body wastes, leave the intestine in the form of faeces, via the rectum & anus.

CONSISTS OF DIGESTIVE SYSTEM

The digestive system consists of the teeth, mouth, gullet (oesophagus), stomach, liver, intestine, pancreas, and rectum. Digestion begins in the mouth where feed is broken down into small pieces by the teeth and mixed with saliva before being swallowed. In the stomach feed is mixed with the juices to form a soft paste. This then passes into the intestine where bile from the liver and juices from the pancreas are added. The action of these juices is to break down the feed and allow the nourishment it contains to be absorbed by the blood in the walls of the intestine.

Waste matter collects in the rectum and passes out of the body through the anus (or cloaca in birds). Many herbivores do not have upper incisors (the teeth on the top jaw in the very front that cut food), cutting the plants with their lips instead. However, all herbivores need their molars (the big flat teeth at the back of the mouth) for grinding the mouthfuls of food.

A herbivore's molars are big and ridged for better grinding. Herbivore skulls have spaces for big muscles to be attached to move their jaws for so much chewing. Plants, particularly grasses, are very hard to digest. Animals that eat plants need to have a particular bacteria inside their bodies to help break down the tough plants so that they release nutrients. This process is called fermentation.

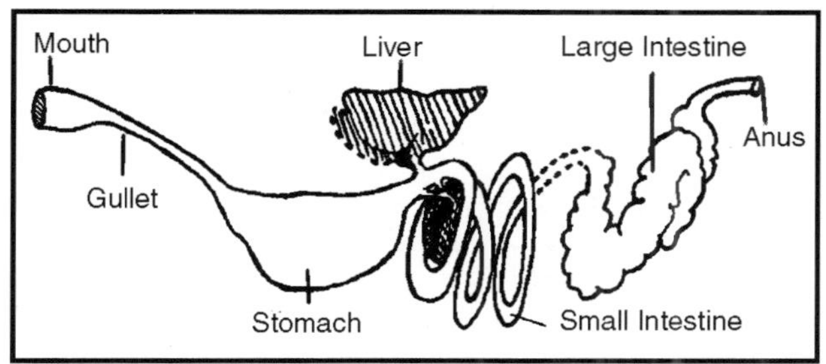

A dog's digestive system is a highly specialized anatomical structure. To gain an understanding of how it operates and what it requires it helps if you understand how it compares to the other types of digestive systems in the animal kingdom.

Herbivores (plant eaters) have the longest digestive tract in the mammalian kingdom. Some of them like, cows have multiple stomachs that are used to break down and ferment various plant materials. True herbivores have the ability to digest plant and vegetable cellulose and can rely on plants for complete nutrition. They have flat blunt teeth, which they use to grind cellulose and grain. Their jaws have the ability to move sideways and grind their food. Of course dogs don't fall in this category and their digestive organs were never designed to assimilate or catabolise plant based materials.

Omnivores: (plant and meat eaters) have one stomach and their intestines are shorter than the cow but longer than the dog. They have the ability to digest vegetation but they have enough enzymes and acid in their gut to digest animal protein as well. Their ability to break down cellulose is limited and they need both vegetation and animal protein for complete nutrition. Omnivores have a combination of sharp teeth used for tearing and ripping flesh and flat molars used for grinding grains and plants. *Carnivores*: (meat eaters) like the dog has the shortest digestive system in the kingdom of mammals. Their jaws are hinged and contain sharp jagged blade like molars, which allows them to swallow large chunks of meat and gorge themselves. This ability enables dogs to consume a great deal of food and then rest until the next kill. Dogs are direct decedents of the wolf and they require meat protein to stay healthy and vibrant. Dogs do not have the ability to digest or assimilate cellulose and have no real need or craving for grain or vegetable based food. The dog is a carnivore with a digestive system and process designed to break down and assimilate protein, bones, and fat. Their stomachs have a much higher level of hydrochloric acid to digest and assimilate meat protein. Many commercial grade dog foods are produced on the premise that a dog's digestion is similar to humans. Because it's cheaper to make dog food with grains and plant materials many times the main ingredient in the dog food is corn, wheat, or some other type of plant-based carbohydrate. Many veterinarians believe commercial grade dog food is garbage or even poison. Some of them have stated carbohydrates are not required at all for the nutritional need of dogs. It's not hard to understand if you consider a wolf will starve before it will eat corn or any other vegetable. Dogs require a vast array of amino acids that are only found in meat. To feed them vegetable products will only shorten their life and ruin their health.

DIGESTIVE SYSTEMS IN DIFFERENT ANIMALS

Different species of animals have different digestive systems which are adapted to their unique requirements. The type of food, method of food gathering and energy needs are some factors that influence the type of digestive system an animal needs in order to survive.

Herbivores have a more specialised digestive system than that of a carnivore because it is more difficult to digest vegetation than meat. The teeth are flat so that grass and plant material can be ground down, rather than the sharp teeth of carnivores designed to tear flesh.

Animals which eat both plants and meat, such as humans, have both types of teeth so that they can perform both functions. In simple animals the digestive system is not complex, usually containing a single tube. As the animal becomes more complex organs with specialised functions develop. Higher order animals require a storage organ, such as the stomach, which allows them to take in large amounts of food in one feeding and then use its energy over a long period of times. This makes it possible for them to devote time to activities other than feeding.

BIRD

Birds need a high body temperature which requires a large amount of energy to maintain. This means that birds need to eat larger amounts of food to gain the energy they need every day to survive.

In order to do this they have a specialised digestive system where there is an efficient absorption of energy. Food passes through very quickly and is all absorbed, leaving little waste. Birds have no teeth so digestion does not begin in the mouth, all of the food breakdown must occur within the digestive system. Food enters through the mouth where it passes down the esophagus into the crop. This organ is where the food is stored and begins to soften. From here it moves into the stomach, which is called the proventriculus.

This acts as a true stomach where digestive juices continue to chemically break down food. The partially digested food moves into the muscular gizzard, which has a rough lining to break down the food further. It sometimes contains sand or pebbles which have been swallowed by the bird, which add to the grinding process.

The food moves into the intestine, first into the small intestine and then onto the large intestine. At the point where the small and large intestine meet are two pouches or caeca, which absorb the water from the food. In herbivores this is the site of cellulose deposition. The food becomes harder and enters into a chamber called the cloaca. It then passes out of the body through the cloacal lining.

HORSE

An adult horse, over five years old, has 40-42 teeth which include incisors, canines and cheek teeth. The incisors work together with the lips to grasp and move food around the mouth. The molars are used to grind down food, making it easier to digest. The digestive system has developed to effectively break down and digest fodder, with the stomach being smaller than that of other cud chewing animals.

The average adult horse is able to hold 7.5-9.5 litres (2-2.5 gallons) of chyme in their stomach. The small intestine is 18-21 metres (60-70 feet) long, while the large intestine is enormous, adapted to digesting grass and hey. The caecum is a pocket between the large and small intestine and is able to hold 15-65 litres (4-17 gallons) while the large colon can hold 60-150 litres (16-34 gallons). In the large intestine food is broken down through fermentation by both bacteria and protozoa. Food may remain in the intestine for up to 55 hours.

INSECT

The digestive system in insects is basically a tube that begins at the mouth and ends at the rectum. It can be divided into a pharynx, esophagus, stomach, intestine, colon and rectum. The stomach or midgut has glands called the gastric ceca which secrete the digestive juices.

The malpighian tubes removes the nitrogen rich waste from the blood. Each tube empties at the connection between the stomach and large intestine, producing an end product of uric acid, which is passed with faeces. Insects such as the praying mantis are carnivorous and begin to digest their food by chewing.

Other insects such as wasps paralyse their pray and lay their eggs in the bodies. This provides a living food supply for the young, providing their immediate source of food. Termites gain their energy from wood and begin to digest the cellulose before it enters the digestive system. Protozoans are released onto the wood and begin its breakdown, continuing to act on the wood once it is passed onto the stomach. Flatworms have a simple digestive system, with a single tube serving as both mouth and anus.

CRUSTACEAN

The digestive system of a crustacean varies depending on the species. In simple species it is a single tube, while others have a specialised system with chambers and organs, each with a specialised function. This often reflects their feeding habits, some animals are scavengers and their food is often beginning to decay. Others require more complex systems as they fully digest the food.

SNAKE

Snakes eat all parts of their pray and need a specialised digestive system to gain the most nutrients from their food. Their teeth are very thin and usually curve backwards. Their function is not to grind down food as it is in most animals, rather it is to capture prey. The food is swallowed whole, thus the teeth perform a specialised function. They have powerful digestive enzymes to break down the hair, feathers, bones, organs and other parts of their food.

The salivary glands also produce strong enzymes which are also used to kill the organism. If saliva enters the wounds of the animal it will begin the digestive process and cause severe tissue damage, which can often lead to the death of the animal. These toxic substances are found in the saliva of many non poisonous snakes. In poisonous snakes it is the salivary glands which have developed into venom sacks, with the venom being a highly toxic form of saliva.

MOLLUSK

The mollusk digestive system has millions of microscopic hair like fibres along the main digestive tract and has several divisions for the different organs.

The first section contains the mouth and esophagus and is the site of the initial breakdown of food. There is a specialised filelike radual found in the mouth, which acts like teeth or a tongue in the food breakdown.

Oysters, clams and muscles do not feature the radula, as they are filter feeders, the food is already filtered when it enters the mouth and continues down the digestive tract. It reaches the liver and stomach, which continues the digestion. In many mollusks the stomach has a flexible rod, which is made up of mucus and proteins in a crystalline structure. This secretes the digestive juices and enzymes and acts as a kind of stirring stick, mixing up the stomach contents to aid digestion. The final section of the digestive tract contains the intestine and anus, from which the waste is removed.

DIGESTIVE SYSTEM OF HORSE

The horse is a non-ruminant herbivore. Non-ruminant means that horses do not have multi-compartmented stomachs as cattle do. Instead, the horse has a simple stomach that works much like a human's. Herbivore means that horses live on a diet of plant material. The equine digestive tract is unique in that it digests portions of its feeds enzymatically first in the foregut and ferments in the hindgut.

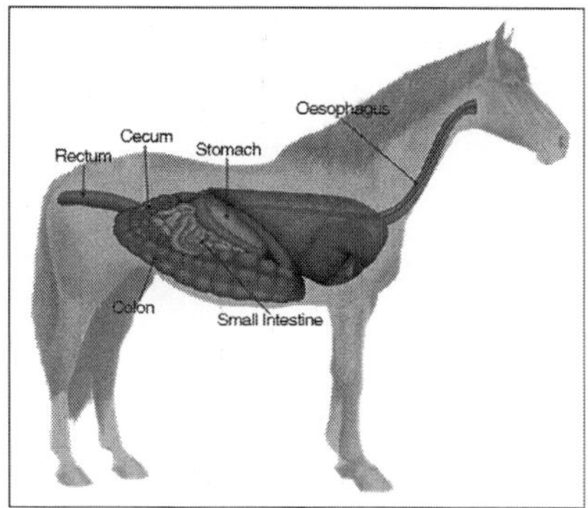

The horse's digestive system really should be thought of as being in two sections. The first section has similarities to the pre-caecal digestive system of a monogastric animal such as the dog, man or pig. The second section is more like the rumen of a cow. This has profound effects on the way we need to think about feeding the horses in our care. However, the horse is neither a dog nor a ruminant or even a direct combination of both. It is unique and needs to be considered as such. The cow benefits by having the microbial breakdown of fibrous food at the start of the GIT (gastrointestinal tract) and nutrient absorption can then take place along the entire intestine. Dietary protein is not utilised efficiently because the microbial fermentation breaks down protein plus some carbohydrate. In the horse unlike in the ruminant the microbial fermentation occurs after the 'monogastric' like section rather than before. This has a great impact on how we should feed a horse and explains in part why the horse and cow differ so much in their nutritional efficiencies and requirements.

MOUTH

Horses grasp food using a combination of the lips, tongue and the teeth. Horses' lips are extremely tactile when it comes to consuming feed. They can be quite selective as many of us would have seen powdered supplements or pellets in a nice little pile at the bottle of the feed bin.

Feeds are mixed with saliva in the mouth to make a moist bolus that can be easily swallowed. Three pairs of glands produce saliva - the parotid, the submaxillary, and the sublingual. Horses will produce between 20-80 litres of saliva per day. Salvia contains bicarbonate which buffers and protects amino acids in the highly acidic stomach. Saliva also contains small amounts of amylase which assist with carbohydrate digestion. The mouth contains 36 teeth (females) and 40 teeth (males). Wolf teeth are not included as not all horses have them. The horses upper jaw is wider than the bottom jaw to allow for a chewing motion that is quite complex. The chewing action of the horse is a sweeping action which incorporates both lateral forward and backwards motions and vertical motions. This allows the feed to be effectively ground and mixed with saliva to initiate the digestive process.

The texture of the feeds fed to horses will dramatically influence the chewing rate (jaw sweeps) and rate of ingestion. An average horse with general take 60,000 jaw sweeps per day when grazing. This amount will be dramatically reduced when confined to a stable and large amounts of grain are fed.

The size of the horse also effects the time and amount of jaw sweeps it takes to sufficiently masticate the feed. The average 500kg horse generally takes 40 minutes and 3400 jaw sweeps to consume one kilogram of hay. Ponies will generally take twice as long to consume this amount of hay. Oats on the other hand only take 10 minutes and 850 jaw sweeps for the mature horse and up to five times longer for ponies. When horses chew fibrous feeds such as hay or pasture it is a long jaw sweep action. This is why horses continually out on pasture rarely develop sharp edges on their teeth. Grains are consumed in a shorter sweep which does not extend past the outer edge of the teeth. When large amount of grain are fed, horses chewing action will be changed and the teeth will not be worn evenly. Hooks or sharp edges will start to form on the outside edge of the teeth. If teeth are not properly 'floated' or rasped the rate of intake, chewing efficiency, appetite and temperament can be seriously affected. If feed are not masticated correctly the bolus (feed and salvia) may lodge in the oesophagus and cause choke.

ESOPHAGUS

This is a simple muscular tube that takes food from the mouth to the stomach. The esophagus is around 1.5m in length in a mature horse. As the esophagus is quite long and the horse has very little reflux capacity, incorrectly chewed are large pieces of feed such as carrots etc can lodge inside the horse's esophagus and can cause choke. This is why it is important to maintain horses' teeth correctly to ensure horses chew their feed sufficiently as well as stopping horses 'bolting' their feed down without chewing their feed. By adding chaff to a horses' feed or putting a brick or large stone in to a horses feed bin will slow horses rate of intake and reduce the risk of choke from a horse 'bolting' its' feed.

STOMACH

The stomach of the horse is small in relation to the size of the animal and makes up only 10 per cent of the capacity of the digestive system or 9-15 litres in volume. The natural feeding habit of the horse is to eat small amounts of roughages often. Domestication has brought a change to all this. Horses are now expected to eat large amounts of grain feed once or twice a day to suit our lifestyle. This greatly undermines the horse's digestive capabilities and health. It has been established that we can improve the digestive efficiency of a horse by feeding small meals often (assimilate natural grazing), but this has been weighed against the labour costs of doing so. In the stomach, feed is mixed with pepsin (an enzyme to digest proteins) and hydrochloric acid to help break down solid particles. The rate of passage of feed through the stomach is highly variable, depending on how the horse is fed. Passage time may be as short as 15 minutes when the horse is consuming a large meal. If the horse is fasted, it will take 24 hours for the stomach to clear.

It has long been a question as to what you should feed a horse first, grain or hay. Because of their density, grains tend to stay in the stomach longer, but it has not been proved to be advantageous to feed either first. For fast eaters chaff can be added to the feed to bulk the feed out which slows the rate of consumption. Another question is whether a horse should get water before or after a meal. If you leave it up to the horse, it will usually drink a little as it eats, if consuming dry feeds. The best recommendation is to offer fresh clean water at all times.

The stomach has 3 main areas; the saccus caecus, fundic and pyloric regions. Each is quite unique in structure and function. The saccus caecus region is located at the entrance of the stomach and the oesophagus. When food enters the stomach it begins to come under the influence of hydrochloric acid and pepsin - a protein digesting enzyme. However, this feed, (especially if it is predominantly grass), is already releasing soluble sugars for absorption and undergoing bacterial fermentation to produce lactic acid. Under normal circumstances, as the hydrochloric acid mixes in with the stomach ingesta, the pH drops, fermentation slows down and eventually stops. This is an important process - because if it does not occur and fermentation continues, the relatively non-distensible, fixed-volume stomach will very quickly fill with gas and, with little ability to release pressure through the oesophagus gastric colic may result or in extreme cases a ruptured stomach lining.

As the feed moves through the stomach the next section of the stomach is the fundic region. The pH level decreases to around 5.4 and fermentation begins to halt. Pepsin and stomach acid initiates the digestion and degradation of lipids (fats) and proteins (amino acids). The final section of the stomach is the pyloric region where the stomach joins the small intestine. The pH drops further to 2.6 which virtually eliminates all fermentable lacto-bacteria. The proteolytic activity (protein digestion) in this area is 15-20 times that of the fundic region.

Changed feeding practices have led to long periods of the day where horses' stomachs are virtually empty. The mixture of feed and saliva mixes with the acid produced by stomach. When the horses' stomach is empty the acid destroys the non- protected squamous cells of the saccus caecus region of the stomach. This causes the stomach lining to ulcerate. Studies have shown that over 80 per cent of thoroughbreds have some degree of stomach ulceration. Stomach ulcers can affect horse's appetite, behaviour and performance. Feeding horses a higher proportion of roughage in their diet, small frequent meals and allow them ability to graze will dramatically reduce the frequency and severity of stomach ulcers.

SMALL INTESTINE

Digesta passes from the stomach into the small intestine. The small intestine is approximately 28 per cent of the horses' digestive tract, is 15-22m long and has a volume of 55-70 litres. This is the major site of digestion in the modern performance horse. The small intestine is broken into 3 sections; the duodenum, jejunum and the ileum.

The saliva of a horse contains only small amounts of amylase and there is little actual digestion that occurs in the stomach of most horses. Most digestion therefore occurs in the small and large intestines. Although the intestine itself secretes some enzymes, the pancreas releases by far the greatest amount. In the small intestine the digestive processes (enzymatic breakdown of proteins, fats, starches and sugars) are similar to those of other monogastric animals but the activity of several of the enzymes in the chyme (food mix), in particular amylase, are lower than in other monogastric animals.

There are many components to this digestive process. Pancreatic enzymes will help digest the food; carbohydrates digest sugars and starches; proteases break proteins down into amino acids; lipases and bile from the liver is added to emulsify (break into smaller units) fats and to suspend the fat in water. Bile constantly flows into the small intestine from the liver because the horse does not have a gall bladder in which to store it. The pancreatic juice also contains some alkali and bicarbonates, which buffer the acid ingesta (feed bolus) leaving the stomach, and help maintain an optimal environment for the functioning of the digestive enzymes.

After the feed has been digested, it is absorbed through the walls of the small intestine and carried off by the blood stream to whatever cells need the nutrients. Nearly 30-60 per cent of carbohydrate digestion and absorption and almost all amino acid absorption occur in the small intestine. Fat soluble vitamins A, D E and K are absorbed in the small intestine as well as some minerals such as calcium and some phosphorous. Changing the structure of carbohydrates of the feed by processes such as micronization greatly increases the grains digestibility in the small intestine to around 90 per cent. This reduces the burden on the large intestine and can reduce the risk of over loading the digestive tract and incidences of colic, laminitis and acidosis.

It can take as little as 30 to 60 minutes for food to pass through the small intestine, as most digesta moves at a rate of approximately 30cm per minute.

However, feed generally take 3-4 hours to pass through the small intestine. The quicker the digesta moves through the small intestine the less time the enzymes have to act.

The addition of oil to a horses' diet has shown to reduce the flow of feed through the small intestine thus allowing the digestive enzymes more time to process starches, proteins and fats thereby increasing the total tract digestibility of these nutrients and maximizing the small intestines digestive efficiency.

Horses are very susceptible to colic or death from toxic materials in the feed. Unlike the cow that has bacteria in the rumen that can detoxify materials before they reach the small intestine, toxic material a horse may consume enters the intestine and is absorbed into the blood stream before it can be detoxified. Therefore, it is very important not to feed horses mouldy or spoiled feeds. Urea is a feed supplement fed to cattle that can be utilized in their rumen to make protein. Horses cannot use this feed supplement because it is absorbed in the small intestine before it can get to the cecum where it could be used. Urea can be toxic to the horse, but the horse can tolerate the level at which it is added to most cattle feeds.

Microbial protein, which is synthesised in the large intestine, cannot be utilised to any great extent by the horse. This means that animals with a high demand for protein (foals, lactating mares and probably intensively exercising horses) must be fed high quality protein which can be broken down and absorbed primarily in the small intestine. In a practical sense this does not mean we need to necessarily increase the crude protein content of our horses feed but to increase the quality of it. This may mean ensuring that the correct levels of essential amino acids such as lysine, methionine and threonine are in sufficient levels to meet the demands of the horse.

THE HIND GUT

The hindgut or large intestine, to which it is commonly referred to, consists of the caecum, large (or ascending colon, small colon, rectum and anus. Here is where a bulk of the digestive more is done. The hindgut comprises of 62 per cent of the entire gut is approximately 7 meters in length and has a volume of 140-150L. Digestion in the hindgut is largely microbial rather than enzymatic. Digestion in the hindgut is performed by billions of symbiotic bacteria which efficiently break down plant fibres and undigested starches into simpler compounds call volatile fatty acids (VFA's) which can be absorbed through the gut wall.

Compared with the digestive tract of ruminants the horse is not as well suited to digesting products of grass with high crude fibre content, low-grade protein and low levels of carbohydrates, starch and fat. They are however much better at it than man or pigs! And equids have reduced these disadvantages by selectively grazing large amounts of feed each day.

CAECUM

The caecum is a blind sack approximately 1.2m long that can hold around 28-36 litres of feed and fluid. The caecum is a microbial inoculation vat, similar to the rumen in a cow. The microbes break down feed that was not digested in the small intestine, particularly fibrous feeds like hay or pasture.

The caecum is odd in design because its entrance and exit are both at the top of the organ. This means that the feed enters at the top, mixes throughout, and is then expelled up at the top. This design is the cause of problems if an animal eats a lot of dry feeds without adequate water or if a rapid change of diet occurs. Both may cause a compaction in the lower end of the caecum, this in turn produces pain (colic). The microbial population in a caecum is somewhat specific as to what feedstuffs it can digest. It can take up to 2-3 weeks for the microbial population of the caecum to adjust to a new diet and return to normal function.

This is why you will read on bag labels to slowly introduce new feeds to a horse over 7-14 days. Feed will remain in the caecum for about seven hours, allowing bacteria time to start breaking it down using the fermentation process. The microbes will produce vitamin K, B-complex vitamins, proteins, and fatty acids. The vitamins and fatty acids will be absorbed, but little if any protein will be absorbed.

LARGE COLON

The large colon consists of the right and left ventral colons and dorsal colon is about 3-3.5m long and will hold 86 litres. Microbial digestion (fermentation) continues, and most of the nutrients made through microbial digestion are absorbed here as well as B group vitamins produced by the bacteria and some trace minerals and phosphorous.

The ventral colons have a "sacculated" construction that resembles a series of pouches. This design facilitates the digestion of large quantities of fibrous materials but due to its design can become a large risk factor for colic. The pouches can easily become twisted and fill with gas due to fermentation of the feed. Feed may reach here in as little as seven hours and will stay here for 48-65 hours.

SMALL COLON, RECTUM AND ANUS

The small colon is approximately the same length as the large colons but only has diameter of roughly 10cm. By now the vast majority of the nutrients have been digested, and what is left can not be digested or used by the horse. The main function of the small colon is to reclaim excess moisture and return it to the body. This results in fecal balls being formed. These fecal balls, which are the undigested and mostly indigestible portion of what was fed some 36-72 hours ago are then passed to the rectum and expelled as manure through the anus.

DIGESTIVE TIGHTROPE

The equine gastrointestinal tract functions well under normal constant conditions. However as all horse people know the equine GUT is extremely sensitive and easy to upset and colic is the number one cause for equine death.

Any sudden change in diet can compromise and change the bacteria population in the horse's hindgut, potentially resulting in colic and at least a reduced digestive efficiency of the diet. Keeping the microflora happy can be difficult if a horse is under stress, travelling large distances, suffered illness or injury, received antibiotics, weaned foal or a high performance horse being fed large amounts of grain. It is imperative that we treat the horse hindgut with respect and monitor the diet of ours horses and there general health. Trying to feed your horses as close to their natural grazing habit as possible, (small meals frequently) will greatly reduce the risk of gastrointestinal tract disorders. This will allow you to enjoy your horse to its fullest potential.

DIGESTIVE SYSTEM OF BOVINE

The bovine digestive system, also known as the gastrointestinal tract, is amazing. Along with camels, deer, giraffes, goats and sheep, cattle belong to a small suborder of grazing, two-toed, hoofed animals called ruminants that have four stomach compartments.

Like other mammals, cows have nutritional requirements for water, vitamins, minerals, carbohydrates and proteins. Such requirements depend on their age, available pastures, pregnancy status, stage of lactation and the season of the year.

Ruminants process grass, hay or grain by unique mechanisms. In cows, food works its way through stomach sections called the reticulum, the rumen and the omasum. The reticulum is closest to the esophagus and is a skull-cap shaped collector of feed and wire scraps that can cause hardware disease. The rumen occupies the left rear abdominal cavity and is the largest of the four stomach compartments. Initial digestive processes occur in the rumen with the help of bacteria, parasites and muscle contractions that cause tossing, turning and breakdown of feed.

While in the rumen, food is repeatedly regurgitated into the mouth and re-chewed in a process called "chewing the cud," a chore cows spend hours on daily. The re-chewed food is digestible when it reaches the abomasum, (the only true stomach) and the intestines, where it is absorbed into the blood stream. Food then moves through the intestines via muscle-contractions and arrives in the rectum as soft dung.

Diseases of bovine GI tract include bloat, food overload, diarrhea, twisted bowels, ruptures, tears and hardware disease that infect the lining of the abdominal cavity due to a wire puncturing the reticulum. Cows can also develop metabolic diseases called acetonemia and milk fever due to dietary excesses designed to increase milk production. Antibiotics and hormonal growth promotants are controversial components of bovine management. Both are sometimes administered to salves or cattle to hasten their maturity, weight gain or milk production.

It has been suggested that antibiotics may increase the presence of antibiotic-resistant microbes in milk and meat. Other concerts indicate that hormones in meat can increase hormone levels in children. Suggested regulations to increase these components in milk and meat are gradually emerging.

DIGESTIVE SYSTEM OF DOG

A dog digestive system is different than a human's and therefore dogs process and eat differently than us. This is important to know and understand so that you can feed your dog the correct diet and be aware when something goes wrong.

THE MOUTH

In humans, the role of the mouth, teeth and saliva play an important part in the digestion of food. In canines, this is not true. Dogs' mouths are designed to bite off and chew large pieces and to eat quickly. Dogs have hinged jaws and large teeth, meant to ingest large chunks of meat, bones and fat products that are usually a part of the dog diet.

ESOPHAGUS TO STOMACH

Since the mouth is not really a part of the digestive process, per se, the stomach is really more vital to the digestion of a dog's food. The food passes through the esophagus on its way to the stomach.

Once food reaches the dog stomach it is processed with a high level of hydrochloric acid. This is important because this allows the breakdown of the large pieces of protein and bones that dogs ingest. Dogs also have a natural regurgitation instinct which allows them to spit out food that has not been processed correctly, then to re-swallow it.

STOMACH TO SMALL INTESTINE

After food has been processed in the stomach with the aid of the hydrochloric acid, it then passes through to the small intestine in the form of liquid. This is where the main part of the digestion occurs and where the food is assimilated into nutrients for the dog body.

SMALL INTESTINE TO LARGE INTESTINE

From the small intestine, the unassimilated food passes through to the large intestine. The large intestine is the last stop before the waste is passed through rectum in the form of feces.

OTHER CONSIDERATIONS

The dog actually has the shortest digestive system of mammals and it takes roughly 8-9 hours for the whole digestive process. Of course, that number is smaller for puppies, which do not have the mature system of adolescent and adult dogs. The digestive system of canines is important and can be a good indicator when something is not working correctly or when illness is present. You should be familiar with your dog's eating habits and pooping habits as well. If your dog is acting out of sorts, has dog bloat, or is not eating or pooping as usual, there is probably something going on inside. Although most dogs experience some gas, just as humans do, particularly unpleasant gas is usually an indication of a poor diet. This can cause other problems so be consistent with your dog's diet and feeding habits.

LIVER DISEASE IN DOGS

The liver is an important organ for your dog. It helps with digestion and blood clotting, and it removes toxins from his system. If it's not working right, it can make your companion sick. But liver disease can often be treated and managed.

Symptoms

It's easy to miss the symptoms of liver disease. They're similar to those for other problems.

Your dog's symptoms may include:

- Loss of appetite
- Weight loss
- Vomiting or diarrhea
- Increased thirst
- An unstable walk
- Increased need to pee
- Confusion
- Yellowish eyes, tongue, or gums (jaundice)
- Signs of weakness
- Blood in his pee or poop
- Seizures
- Ascites (a build-up of fluid in the belly)

If your dog's liver disease isn't caught early, it can lead to a serious brain condition called hepatic encephalopathy.

What Causes Liver Problems?

Sometimes liver disease can happen as a result of aging. Sometimes it's genetic. But it can also be brought on by infection or trauma to the area. Some diseases and medications can hurt your dog's liver.

Other causes of liver disease may include:

- Some plants and herbs such as ragwort, certain mushrooms, and blue-green algae
- Molds that grow on corn
- Untreated heartworms
- Diabetes
- Issues with the pancreas
- Long-term use of painkillers
- Fatty foods

If your dog has some symptoms of liver problems, your vet may ask you about his diet and medications. The vet may want to do blood tests and X-rays or an ultrasound to get a picture of what is going on with your dog's liver. He may also want to take a biopsy -- remove a small tissue sample for testing.

Treatment

Your dog's treatment will depend on how soon you catch the problem and what caused it.

A vet will need to see how much damage there is to the liver:

- Diet changes often help. Your dog may need a special diet to make sure he's getting the nutrients and calories needed to help his liver.
- Supplements such as SAM-E or milk thistle may help the liver recover.
- Medications may help control his liver problems. You may also need to change your dog's other medications or reduce how much he takes.
- Surgery may be an option for dogs with tumors or cysts.

Work closely with your vet to manage the disease and avoid liver failure.

Prevention

You can help your dog avoid getting liver disease. Take him to the vet for his yearly exams and vaccinations. Make sure your vet is aware of any drugs or supplements he may take. Be mindful of what you feed your dog. Fatty foods can hurt his liver. And don't let your dog roam free in areas where there may be poisonous plants or insects.

CAVITY ADJACENT OF THE LIVER

The liver is situated in the abdominal cavity adjacent to the diaphragm. It is the largest single organ of the body and has over 100 known functions.

Its most important digestive functions are:

- The production of bile to help the digestion of fats (described above) and
- The control of blood sugar levels

Glucose is absorbed into the capillaries of the villi of the intestine. The blood stream takes it directly to the liver via a blood vessel known as the hepatic portal vessel or vein. The liver converts this glucose into glycogen which it stores. When glucose levels are low the liver can convert the glycogen back into glucose. It releases this back into the blood to keep the level of glucose constant. The hormone insulin, produced by special cells in the pancreas, controls this process.

Other functions of the liver include:

- Making vitamin A,
- Making the proteins that are found in the blood plasma (albumin, globulin and fibrinogen),
- Storing iron,
- Removing toxic substances like alcohol and poisons from the blood and converting them to safer substances,
- Producing heat to help maintain the temperature of the body.

In spite of the fact that distinctions between various sciences and their subdivisions may be more or less arbitrary, each branch of knowledge has to a greater or less extent a reason for existence. Perhaps one can think of each scientific subject as representing an attempt to answer a question. Thus, in biological science, anatomy covers the question of form. It tells us what organisms or their parts look like. Physiology, on the other hand, is concerned with the problem of function. It attempts to describe the actions of various organs or tissues and, more than this, it attempts to explain this action in terms of known chemical and physical forces. In such explanation, moreover, there is an effort to relate the phenomena in terms of cause and effect. Obviously there are various branches of physiological science. Because of its intimate relation to the science and art of medicine, human physiology has been studied since the very beginning of human learning. Our knowledge of the physiology of other forms of life has been focused on certain types rather than others. Insect physiology is now rather widely studied; plant physiology is an old and well-developed subject.

Some groups of organisms have been neglected, and there is comparatively little information about the physiology of certain invertebrate phyla. Sometimes it is convenient to lump together the physiological knowledge of all sorts of organisms into a subject known as "comparative physiology." The point of view of this subject is to emphasize the differences rather than the resemblances between various types of living material. Opinions may differ as to the proper definition of general physiology. To some it may be little more than a diluted vertebrate or human physiology. It attempts to answer the question, "What is life?" The general physiologist believes that all life has something in common; his search is often for the least common denominator of living processes.

That such a search may not be entirely futile is indicated by the recent history of biological thought. Modern progress in biological science has resulted largely from the fortunate realization that living things, no matter how diverse they appear in externals, are fundamentally much alike. There is an underlying unity which has proved of tremendous importance. Cytologists learned to know cell division and chromosomes from a study of cells best suited for their purposes. Fertilization was studied first in the egg cells of marine invertebrates, and only later was the same process shown to occur in widely different types of organisms. The fundamental facts of genetics were discovered first for plants, and modern study in this field for the most part contents itself with work on these forms which are easy to raise and which breed rapidly. And yet no one doubts that genetic science is capable of universal application. In physiology, on the other hand, the tendency has been to stress the study of vertebrate or mammalian tissues. Physiology is so close to medicine and its facts are so certain of practical application that there is a strong desire to study animals close to man.

The field of mammalian or human physiology has had a marvelous development, and it would be absurd to belittle its striking achievements. And yet, in spite of the fact that students of the physiology of mammals have accumulated a vast store of precise and valuable information, the ultimate mechanisms underlying the activity of mammalian cells and tissues are but little understood. The physiologist has been loath to accept the method of attack so fruitful in other branches of biology. If students of genetics or cytology had insisted on studying mammals or vertebrates and no other organisms, these sciences would scarcely have developed far. Great advances in theoretical biology are made by study of that type of living material particularly adapted to the problem at hand. Cells of mammals or vertebrates are often more difficult to study than those of simpler forms. The general physiologist, in his search for fundamental information, uses whatever material he can find best suited for his purpose.

It is the aim of the general physiologist to discover, in so far as possible, the nature and mechanism of living matter. This is the *raison d'être* of the science. Its students are more or less convinced that, if one could discover the essential principles which govern the activities and life of any one living cell or living material, the same principles could be used, with minor adjustments and modifications, to explain the life of practically every type of cell. This may seem almost too much to ask, but the progress of biology has repeatedly shown the deep underlying similarity of what seem at first the most diverse manifestations of the living process. The extreme difficulty of biological research is thus to some extent compensated by the underlying unity of living materials. Although there may be a million different species of animals, there are not a million different biologies, but rather one fundamental science with variations. In general the cell is the unit of living matter, and the life of an organism is to all intents and purposes the sum total of the life of its constituent cells. It seems clear therefore that vital machinery must be interpreted in terms of cells, and general physiology thus becomes cellular physiology. This point of view was strongly emphasized by Verworn, who states over and over again that, if physiology is to attempt fundamental explanation of vital activity, it must be a cell physiology. There are, however, possible exceptions to this point of view. It may be argued that not all living matter is truly cellular. Thus only by a stretch of the imagination can some of the smaller bacteria be regarded as cells; and filtrable viruses which are beyond the limits of microscopic vision, and which may or may not be alive, are certainly not cells in any ordinary sense.

This argument seems to have very little force. Biologists generally realise that the cell doctrine is not absolutely true, and that there are forms of living matter which are not truly cellular. Nevertheless, the cell doctrine is true for all practical purposes, and it forms the basis for such sciences as histology, pathology, embryology, etc. Because ultramicroscopic forms of life may exist, neither the histologist nor the embryologist has seen fit to throw over the cell theory. In the same way physicists and physical chemists cling to the second law of thermodynamics, although it is well known that there are special conditions under which the law does not hold. There is also another reason sometimes given for not identifying general physiology with cell physiology. In investigating the activity of a mass of living matter, it is often much simpler to study great numbers of cells rather than individual units. This is especially true of chemical study, for chemical properties of cells are usually additive.

Thus if one is attempting to discover the change in the glycogen content of cells during activity, one can do this best by analyzing great numbers of cells. The analysis is, therefore, conducted on tissues rather than on cells, and in this sense, from the standpoint of method or technic, the study is no longer truly cellular. But the primary interest of the investigation is the glycogen change in the individual cell, so that this argument seems rather a superficial one. At the present time, in many branches of physiology, there is an increasing tendency to study the individual cells in so far as this is possible. Muscle physiologists are giving more and more attention to the isolated single muscle fibre, and students of nerve are attempting as best they can to isolate single nerve fibres. As a matter of fact, these recent studies of muscle and nerve physiologists have been inspired more by a desire to avoid the complexities which arise from the existence of many fibres not always in perfect time accord, rather than from any desire to study the single fibre from the viewpoint of the student of cell protoplasm.

Nevertheless, they indicate a growing realization that the ultimate mechanism responsible for any form of vital activity lies inherent in the individual cells. Whether or not we regard general physiology as synonymous with cell physiology is of no great consequence. A science is whatever its devotees choose to make it. No one could be excluded from the field of general physiology because he did not think in terms of cells. There is, however, a growing realization that an understanding of cells and cell protoplasm is essential for the interpretation of the various vital processes as they occur in animal and plant organisms. Much of the hope for the future of general physiology lies in the possibility of using simpler types of protoplasm in order to discover the general characteristics of living substance. The field of the general physiologist is as broad as all life itself.

How broad this is, at the present time it is impossible to state, for there is no agreement as to the lower limits of life. Numerous submicroscopic filtrable viruses exist, many of them causing diseases in animals and plants. But whether these viruses are alive or not is a question still being argued. True, they reproduce and some of the larger ones resemble bacteria. On the other hand, unlike bacteria they are incapable of growth on simple synthetic media and they can only exist within bacterial, plant or animal cells. Moreover, Stanley found that the virus which causes tobacco mosaic disease is a protein molecule, and since then all the plant viruses that have been studied have been found to be protein molecules. However, although some animal viruses seem to consist wholly of protein, others like vaccinia virus contain fat and carbohydrate as well as protein. Viruses vary widely in size and shape. Some are so small that their molecular diameter is only about 25 mm (0.000,025 mm.). The largest virus has a volume approximately 10,000 times that of the smallest. Such large viruses can be as large or larger than small bacteria. Some viruses are spherical, some are rod-shaped; one has been found to be tadpole-shaped, with a spherical head and a slender elongate tail. In a study of these diverse, extremely tiny, living or partly living organisms or substances, much can doubtless be learned concerning the nature of life processes.

A considerable body of information has already been accumulated. General physiology is a theoretical science just as physical chemistry is. But whereas practical chemists and chemical engineers have long since learned to depend on physicochemical principles, medical scientists and students of applied human physiology and pharmacology have sometimes been slow to realise the relation of their subjects to general physiology.

It is interesting to note that a leading student of pharmacology, which is one of the most practical of biological sciences, has stated that "The manner in which drugs exert their action on cells has become one of the most important fundamental problems of physiology. Fortunately, at the present time, especially among the younger medical men, there is an ever-growing realization of the importance of basic general physiology. The primary object of the general physiologist is to interpret and explain vital phenomena. Obviously the explanations he seeks must be in terms of known scientific concepts. As best he can, the general physiologist attempts to give a complete description of living substance in terms of its physical and chemical properties; and more than that, he attempts to show exactly what physical and chemical changes occur during vital activity.

But mere description is not enough. He must aim to find causal relations between the physical and chemical phenomena observable in the living material and the life itself; in other words he is interested in discovering mechanism. This is his most difficult task. To measure mechanical, thermal, electrical or chemical change in plant and animal tissues is not too hard, but to find out exactly which changes are primarily responsible for definite phases of vital activity is always exceedingly difficult and often, at our present stage of progress, impossible.

Even in the simplest types of vital activity so many changes occur that it is hard to know which ones are intimately responsible for what is happening. Similar difficulties exist even for non-living machinery. We know how an automobile works because it has been constructed by human hands, but if we were obliged to explain the action of an automobile by what we could see, we might be inclined to believe that its movement was due to the noise it made, the heat it produced or the breeze it generated. As scientists, general physiologists are concerned only with explanations in terms of what is known or what can be known.

Whether or not life can be explained in terms of known or knowable chemical and physical forces is a philosophical rather than a scientific question and it should perhaps be left to the philosophers. For them, and for thoughtful people generally, it is a question of tremendous interest. "Since a man must needs live before he can be a philosopher, no problem of philosophy is more fundamental than the nature of life." For many years, those who believe that eventually explanations of the nature of life processes can be obtained in terms of chemistry and physics have been called mechanists.

On the other hand, those who deny that physical and chemical forces can ever provide a complete explanation have been called vitalists. Between mechanists and vitalists, the arguments have often been bitter—among working biologists generally, the term vitalist is often used as a term of reproach—and hence in recent years there has been a semantic attempt to alter the terminology or to abandon it altogether. But the terms are still properly understood in their original meaning, and it is doubtful if other words or other definitions of the old words will make the arguments any less bitter. To some modern vitalists, the chief characteristic of living material, the one most difficult to explain chemically or physically, is the extremely complex organization of living systems. The distinguished general physiologist Lillie believes that living material has a "directiveness" quite different from the "randomness" of inanimate material. The mechanist is impressed with the fact that because of our newer knowledge of viruses there is no longer any sharp and clear-cut distinction between living and non-living, and he also likes to argue that vital phenomena once thought highly mysterious have now been explained, to some extent at least, in physical and chemical terms.

To the hard-working physiologist, intent on obtaining at least a partway explanation of some physiological process in physiochemical terms, the validity of the mechanist point of view scarcely seems worth discussing. He is not concerned with the ultimate truth sought by the philosopher. But, unfortunately, when some elderly biologist loses faith in physiochemical interpretation as an answer to all the ultimate problems of biology and leaves his laboratory to publish defeatist or vitalistic views in philosophical journals, these views are promptly read by the philosophers, who by and large have very little acquaintance with biological journals and biological thought and who commonly are convinced that the vast majority of biologists are vitalists. Nothing could be farther from the truth.

4

Respiratory System

The respiratory system performs several functions. Most importantly, it delivers oxygen to the cardiovascular system for distribution to the body and it removes carbon dioxide. Gas transfer occurs in the alveoli of the lungs, where the air-blood barrier is a thin, permeable membrane. Failure or major dysfunction of gas transfer due to disease processes that compromise this membrane or its air or blood supply have serious effects.

In addition to gas exchange, the respiratory system performs numerous other functions, including maintaining acid-base balance, acting as a blood reservoir, filtering and probably destroying emboli, metabolizing some bioactive substances (eg, serotonin, prostaglandins, corticosteroids, and leukotrienes), and activating some substances (eg, angiotensin). The respiratory system also protects its own delicate airways by warming and humidifying inhaled air and by filtering out particulate material. The upper airways also provide for the sense of smell (olfaction) and play a role in temperature regulation in panting animals.

Large, airborne particles are usually deposited on the mucous lining of the nasal passages, larynx, trachea, and bronchi, after which they are carried by the mucociliary "blanket" to the pharynx to be swallowed or expectorated. Small particles may be deposited as deep as the alveoli, where they are phagocytized by macrophages.

Defence against invasion by microorganisms and other foreign particles is provided by anatomic structures and by both non-specific and immunologic mechanisms (both cellular and humoral). These are the factors that determine species and individual susceptibility to disease and that may be manipulated by using various management techniques, vaccines, antimicrobials, and other agents such as interferons and lymphokines. Other mechanical factors include the tortuosity of nasal passages; presence of hairs, cilia, and mucus; the cough reflex; and bronchoconstriction. Cellular defences include macrophages, which phagocytize invaders and present them (or at least their important antigens) to lymphocytes for stimulation of an immune response, and neutrophils, which often die in their fight against invaders and must be removed along with their potentially damaging enzymes. Secretory defences include interferon for antiviral defence, complement for lysis of invaders, surfactant lining the alveoli to prevent their collapse and to facilitate macrophage function, fibronectin to modulate bacterial attachment, antibodies, and mucus.

The respiratory system must perform many functions, preferably while expending minimal energy. The required effort is increased by processes that oppose expansion of the lung (eg, fibrosis or hydro-, chylo-, pneumo-, or hemothorax), impede the flow of air (eg, obstructive nasal disease, bronchiolitis, bronchoconstriction, laryngeal paralysis, or pulmonary edema), or thicken the air-blood interface (eg, interstitial pneumonia due to viruses or toxins, pulmonary edema).

The anatomy of the respiratory tract differs markedly among species in the following features: 1) shape of both the upper and lower respiratory tract; 2) extent, shape, and pattern of the turbinate bones; 3) branching patterns of bronchi; 4) anatomy of terminal bronchioles, including collateral ventilation; 5) lobation and lobulation; 6) thickness of pleura; 7) completeness of the mediastinum; 8) relationship of pulmonary arteries to bronchial arteries and bronchioles; 9) presence of vascular shunts; 10) distribution of mast cells; and 11) blood supply to the pleura. Each variation in anatomic structure implies variation in function, which can influence the pathogenesis of respiratory disease in a particular species. The three main groups of species that have similar subgross anatomy of the lung are 1) cattle, sheep, and pigs; 2) dogs, cats, monkeys, rats, rabbits, and guinea pigs; and 3) horses and people.

Marked physiologic variations also exist between different species. For example, cattle are prone to retrograde drainage from the pharynx, are predisposed to pulmonary hypertension and reduced ventilation in a cold environment, have relatively small lungs with low tidal volume and functional residual capacity, and are more sensitive to changes in environmental temperatures than are most other species.

These anatomic and physiologic differences largely determine why some pathogens affect only some species (eg, Mannheimia haemolytica affects cattle but not pigs) and why pneumonia is very important in some species (cattle, pigs) but less so in others (dogs, cats).

Hypoxia (lowered oxygenation, often termed anoxia) causes clinical signs of respiratory disease. It can result from the following: 1) reduced oxygen-carrying capacity of the blood (anemic anoxia, as in carbon monoxide or nitrite poisoning, or true anemia due to various causes); 2) reduced blood flow (stagnant anoxia, as in congestive heart failure or shock); 3) insufficient alveolar ventilation, mismatching between ventilation and perfusion, shunt or diffusion impairment (hypoxic anoxia, as in pneumonia, pulmonary edema, chronic congestion, pneumothorax, or paralysis of respiratory muscles); or 4) inability of tissues to use available oxygen (eg, histotoxic anoxia, as in cyanide poisoning).

Compensatory mechanisms for hypoxia include increased depth and rate of breathing, which is mediated by chemoreceptors located in the carotid and aortic bodies; contraction of the spleen, which forces more RBC into the circulation; and increased cardiac stroke volume and heart rate. If cerebral hypoxia develops, respiratory function may be reduced even further due to depression of neuronal activity. Erythropoiesis is also stimulated with chronic hypoxia, although the degree of polycythemia is species dependent. In addition, myocardial, renal, and hepatic functions may be reduced, as may motility and secretions of the intestine. If compensatory mechanisms are inadequate, a vicious cycle may begin in which all body tissues function less efficiently.

SURFACES OF RESPIRATORY

All animals need to take in O_2 and eliminate CO_2. *Lungs* are membranous structures designed for gas exchange in a terrestrial environment. *Gills* are designed for gas exchange in an aquatic environment. Oxygen must be dissolved in water before animals can take it up. Therefore, the respiratory surfaces of animals must always be moist. This is true of all animals. Very small organisms donot need respiratory surfaces because they have a high surface:volume ratio.

SKIN

The skin can be used as a respiratory surface but it does not have much surface area compared to lungs or gills. Animals that rely on their skin as a respiratory organ are small and either have low metabolic rates or they also have lungs or gills. Like all respiratory surfaces, the skin must remain moist to function in gas exchange. Amphibians, most annelids, some mollusks, and some arthropods use their skin as a respiratory organ.

Gills

Gills provide a large surface area for gas exchange in aquatic organisms. It is difficult to circulate water past gills because water is dense and the O_2 concentration in water is low. There is 5% as much oxygen in water as there is in air. To circulate water past the gills, amphibian larvae physically move their gills, mollusks pump water into mantle cavity which contains the gills, and some crustacean gills are attached to branches of the walking legs. The flow of blood in the gills of fish is in the opposite direction that water passes over the gills. This arrangement enables fish to extract more oxygen from the water than if blood moved in the same direction as the passing water. Gills cannot be used in air because they lack structural support; they would collapse. Their use in air would also result in too much water loss by evapouration. Gills greatly increase the surface area for gas exchange. They occur in a variety of animal groups including arthropods, annelids, fish, and amphibians. Gills typically are convoluted outgrowths containing blood vessels covered by a thin epithelial layer. Typically gills are organized into a series of plates and may be internal or external to the body. Gills are very efficient at removing oxygen from water: there is only 1/20 the amount of oxygen present in water as in the same volume of air. Water flows over gills in one direction while blood flows in the opposite direction through gill capillaries. This countercurrent flow maximizes oxygen transfer.

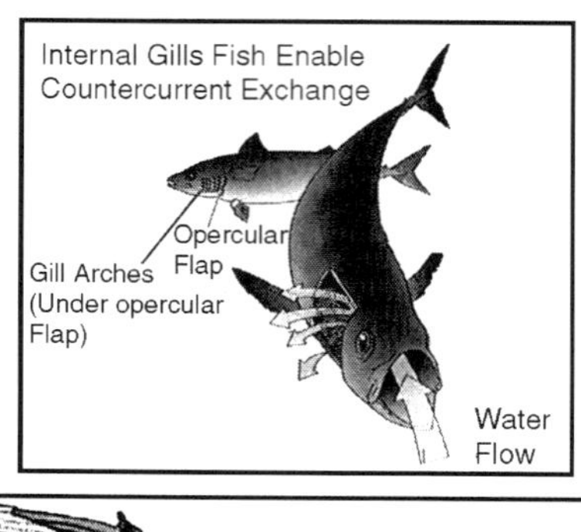

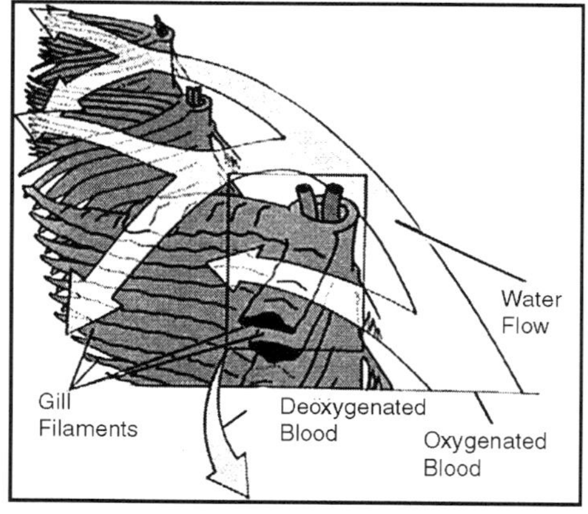

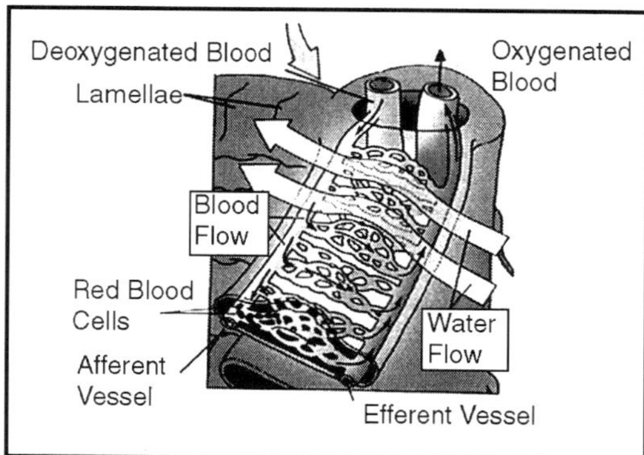

Fig. Countercurrent Flow in a Fish.

Tracheal System

Insects, centipedes, and some mites and spiders have a tracheal respiratory system. Tracheae are a network of tubules that bring oxygen directly to the tissues and allow carbon dioxide to escape. The openings to the outside, called spiracles, are located on the side of the abdomen. Trachea and lungs are internal to reduce water loss. Many terrestrial animals have their respiratory surfaces inside the body and connected to the outside by a series of tubes.Tracheae are these tubes that carry air directly to cells for gas exchange.

Spiracles are openings at the body surface that lead to tracheae that branch into smaller tubes known as tracheoles. Body movements or contractions speed up the rate of diffusion of gases from tracheae into body cells. However, tracheae will not function well in animals whose body is longer than 5 cm.

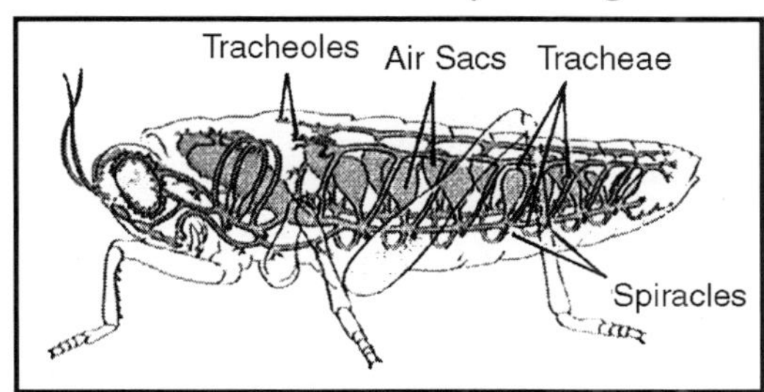

Fig. Respiratory System in an Insect.

Vertebrate Lungs

- Simple lungs evolved 450 million years ago in fish.
- Some evolved into swim bladders.
- Others evolved into more complex lungs.
- Paired lungs are the respiratory surfaces in all reptiles, birds, and mammals.

Amphibians

lung is a simple convoluted sac have small lungs but obtain much O_2 by diffusion across moist skin ventilate lungs by positive pressure; (reptiles, birds and mammals use negative pressure)

Reptiles

- The skin is watertight; it is not used as a respiratory surface.
- The lungs possess alveoli.
- All diffusion occurs across the alveolar surface.

Birds and Mammals

The lungs of birds and mammals are more branched with smaller, more numerous alveoli.

Birds

Birds have one-way flow of air in their lungs. As a result, the lungs receive fresh air during inhalation and again during exhalation. *Advantages of one-way flow*: no residual volume; all old (stale) air leaves with each breath crosscurrent flow (crosscurrent = 90° ; countercurrent = 180°; crosscurrent is not as efficient but is still more efficient than mammalian lung) One-way flow is accomplished by the use of air sacs as illustrated below. During inspiration, the air sacs fill. During expiration, they empty.

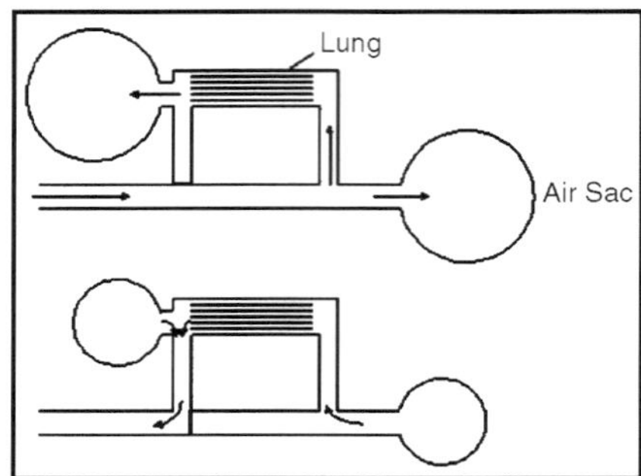

PROCESS OF RESPIRATORYSYSTEM

Respiration (breathing) consists of inspiration (breathing in) and expiration (breathing out). There are two lungs which are found in the chest protected by the bony cage of the ribs. The windpipe carries air from the nostrils to the lungs which are spongy because of air spaces in them. As the animal breathes, air moves in and out of the lungs. Inside the lungs oxygen needed by the body passes into the blood in the walls of the lungs and water and carbon dioxide pass out of the blood into the air which is then breathed out.

THE RESPIRATORY SYSTEM

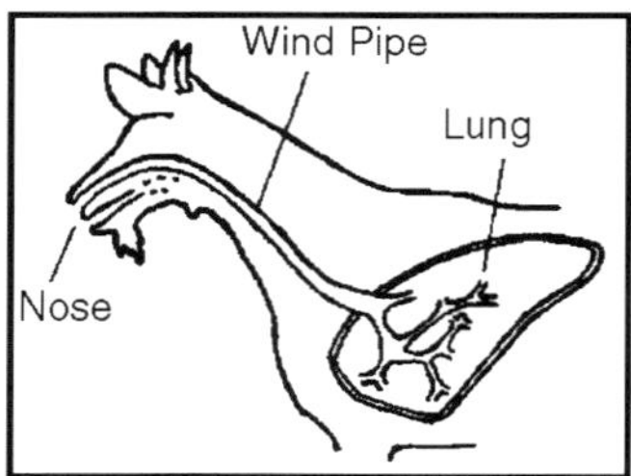

Flatworms and annelids use their outer surfaces as gas exchange surfaces. Earthworms have a series of thin-walled blood vessels known as capillaries. Gas exchange occurs at capillaries located throughout the body as well as those in the respiratory surface.

Amphibians use their skin as a respiratory surface. Frogs eliminate carbon dioxide 2.5 times as fast through their skin as they do through their lungs.

Eels (a fish) obtain 60% of their oxygen through their skin. Humans exchange only 1% of their carbon dioxide through their skin. Constraints of water loss dictate that terrestrial animals must develop more efficient lungs.

Lungs

Lungs are ingrowths of the body wall and connect to the outside by as series of tubes and small openings. Lung breathing probably evolved about 400 million years ago. Lungs are not entirely the sole property of vertebrates, some terrestrial snails have a gas exchange structures similar to those in frogs.

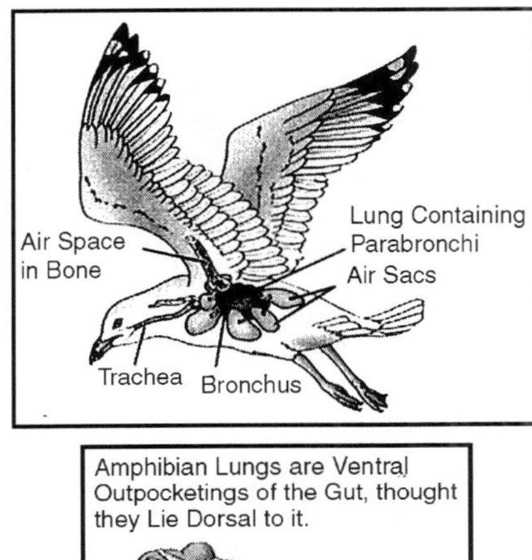

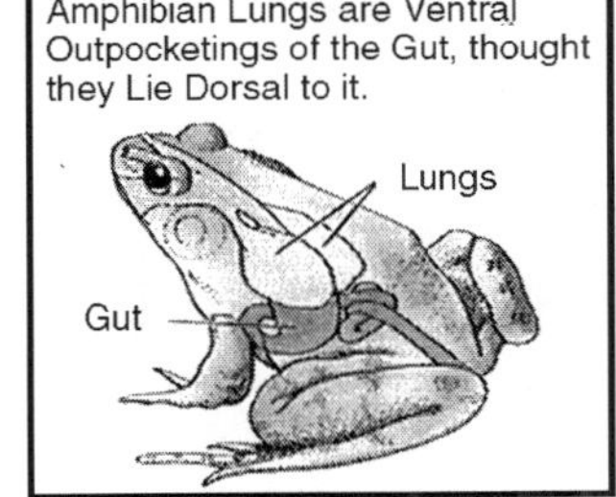

Fig. Lungs in a Bird (top) and Amphibian (Bottom).

Lungs and Pleura

Palpation - The only evidence of disease manifested on palpation is that of pain. Percussion - Sound on percussion is best noted over thin chest walls. The sound is resonant normally and is clearer about the middle of the chest in large animals. The sound is clear through-out in small animals. In some diseases, the resonance is more extensive and very clear such as Pulmonary Emphysema or Pneumothorax. The sound is dull and flat over area of consolidation in Pneumonia, in tumors or cysts, in Hydrothorax or in Pleurisy with effusion. In the latter two conditions, the dull sound is made outing the lower portion of the chest up to the upper level of the fluid. The outline of the dull areas is irregular in Pneumonia.

Auscultation

The sounds of lungs are intensified by exercise. The normal sounds are:

1. Vesicular murmur
2. Bronchial sounds

The vesicular murmur is a short sound noted specially on inspiration and is due to stretching of the walls of the vesicles. The vesicular murmur is intensified in dyspnoea and in bronchitis in' the early stage. It is diminished in thickening of thoracic walls and in pulmonary congestion. It is absent over areas of consolidation in pneumonia, tumours or cysts and over pleural exudates ortransudates. In the latter case; the absence of sound is due partly to displacement of the lungs and partly to collapse. In pneumonia, the solid area is surrounded by a zone in which feeble crepitating sound may be heard. The bronchial sounds are formed by the larynx. They are blowing sounds and most marked at the middle portion of the lungs. The bronchial sounds like the other lung sounds are synchrony-nous with respiration and most marked during inspiration. Various abnormal bronchial sounds are heard and are called 'Bales' and distinguished as dry and moist.

Dry Rales

Are due to passage of air over tough bronchial secretion or over swollen bronchial mucous membrane. They are humming, hiss-in, wheezing or whistling and are noted in the early stages of Acute Bronchitis, Chronic Bronchities and, to a slight extent, in Emphysema or in Compression of the bronchi with nodules or cysts.

Moist Rales

These rile are gurgling or bubbling. They appear in the stage of exudation in bronchitis and are due to the passage of air through or over the fluid present. They are most marked towards the end of inspiration.

The Crepitate Rales

Fine crackling noises due to separating of adhesive walls of the small bronchial tubes. They are noted in bronchiolitis, in pulmonary edema and in the early stage and the stage of resolution in pneumonia. In the latter case, they are often called secondary crepitationsounds. In Acute Pleurisy, during the early stages, that is, in the dry stages, friction sounds may behead comparable with the rustling of silk due to rubbing of dry pulmonary pleura on the costal pleura. These sounds are synchronous with the respiration. When the fluid accumulates in the pleural sac, trickling or splashing sounds synchronous with the respiration at the upper level of the fluid may be noted. In examination of the lungs, Borborygmous and the sounds produced by regurgitation of food or gas through the esophagus must be distinguished.

RESPIRATORY SYSTEM OF THE DOG

The respiratory system includes the:

- Mouth and nose
- Trachea
- lungs and smaller airways (bronchi and bronchioles)

The respiratory system is responsible for taking in oxygen and eliminating waste gases like carbon dioxide. Because dogs and cats do not sweat through the skin, the respiratory system also plays an important role in regulation of temperature.

MOUTH

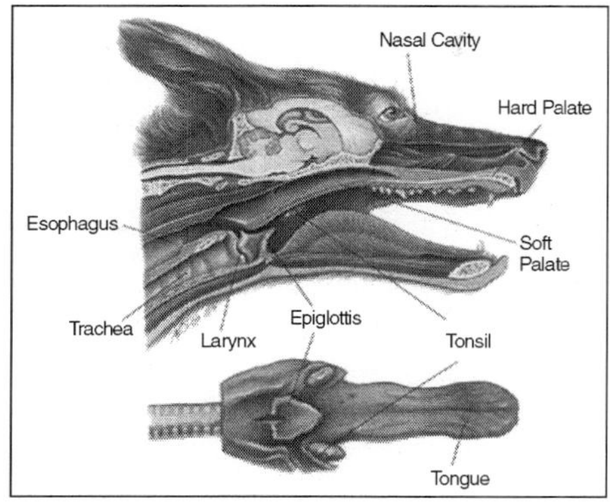

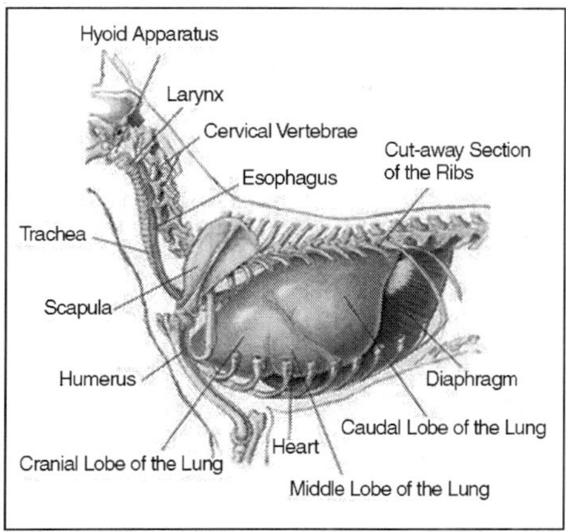

LUNGS

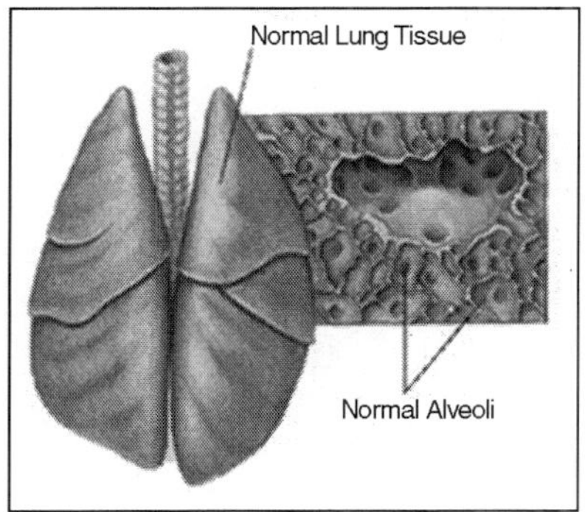

TECHNIQUES OF DIAGNOSTIC

Clinical history and physical examination should help to determine the possible cause and site of respiratory disease. Lateral cervical and thoracic radiographs may be helpful when obstructive upper airway disease or fixed airway obstruction is suspected (eg, tracheal foreign body, masses, foreign bodies, or stenosis). Thoracic radiographs are essential in any animal exhibiting lower respiratory signs (eg, cough, rapid shallow breathing, dyspnea) but diagnostic value may be limited in animals that have a large thorax (eg, adult horse or cattle). Arterial blood gas analysis or pulse oximetry may help assess the need for oxygen therapy in an animal with severe dyspnea.

When obstructive upper airway disease is suspected, the diagnostic procedure of choice is endoscopy of the respiratory tract, preferably without sedation. Laryngeal function should be assessed, and the presence of obstructive lesions within the nasopharynx, oropharynx, larynx, trachea, or principal bronchi should be identified.

With diffuse or lobar lung disease, diagnostic procedures include transtracheal wash, bronchoscopy with bronchoalveolar lavage or endobronchial biopsy, and transthoracic fine needle aspirates of lung or lung biopsy. When bacterial pneumonia is suspected, bacterial culture of transtracheal wash is recommended. Cytologic evaluation of transtracheal or bronchoalveolar lavage fluid may aid in the diagnosis of fungal, parasitic, or allergic lung diseases.

Transthoracic fine needle aspirates of lung often are useful in the diagnosis of fungal pneumonia but have lower yields in the definitive diagnosis of solitary pulmonary lesions. Solitary pulmonary masses often require transthoracic lung biopsy or surgical excision for definitive diagnosis. Transthoracic ultrasonography is a sensitive diagnostic tool for pleural disease (eg, pleural effusion, pneumothorax) and for parenchymal lung disease when lesions are adjacent to the pleural surface.

In dogs or cats with pleural effusions, thoracocentesis should be performed for cytologic and potentially microbiologic evaluation of fluid. In cats, pleural effusions often occur with cardiac disease, so an echocardiography should be performed. In animals suspected to have a chylous effusion, serum and fluid triglyceride levels should be determined. Chylous effusions are associated with fluid triglyceride levels greater than that in serum.

Acute nasal discharge, sneezing, or both, may suggest the presence of infection (viral or bacterial) or a nasal foreign body. Chronic nasal discharge warrants further investigation via radiography (nose, guttural pouches in horses), nasal CT, rhinoscopy, nasopharyngoscopy, or nasal biopsy. Rhinoscopy may be of limited value if copious thick discharge or hemorrhage is present. Bacterial cultures of nasal tissue may be of value if bacterial rhinitis is suspected; however, in some species (eg, dogs and cats) primary bacterial rhinitis is rare and typically occurs secondary to other nasal conditions.

Cytologic evaluation of nasal tissue may help diagnose nasal fungal infections. Serologic testing for fungal respiratory infections may be considered, but these findings should correlate with the animal's clinical signs and documentation of the presence of fungal organisms because false-positive and false-negative tests can occur.

RESPIRATORY MALFUNCTION

Congenital anomalies of the respiratory tract are rare but do occur. Examples include cysts in the sinuses and turbinates, tracheal hypoplasia, nasopharyngeal turbinates, and accessory lungs. A common cause of upper respiratory tract malfunction is rhinitis (which results in exudation of neutrophils, macrophages, and fluids), or erosion and ulceration (or both) of the nasal mucosa.

It may be caused by viral, bacterial, fungal, or parasitic agents, as well as by hypersensitivity reactions, such as localized allergies and anaphylaxis. Atrophy of the turbinates (eg, in atrophic rhinitis of pigs) removes a major filtration function and exposes the lungs to much heavier loads of dust and microorganisms. The nasal cavity may be obstructed by tumors, granulomas, abscesses, or foreign bodies. Sinusitis can be a complication of upper respiratory infections, tooth root infection, or dehorning.

Laryngitis, tracheitis, and bronchitis result in coughing and possibly inspiratory or expiratory dyspnea. Coughing may be non-productive if the irritation is caused by mucosal erosion, or productive if caused by copious exudate in the major airways. Severe pulmonary edema and emphysema cause extreme respiratory insufficiency.

The most common respiratory disease is pneumonia, which is defined as inflammation of the lungs. There are many systems to classify the various types of pneumonia. One useful method is to classify according to the distribution of lesions in the lungs. Focal pneumonia has one or more discrete foci in a random pattern, eg, abscessation due to emboli from other sites, tuberculosis, or actinomycosis.Lobular pneumonia accentuates the anatomic pattern of lobules, as in bronchopneumonia caused byPasteurella multocida. Lobar pneumonia covers large areas of lobes and is often severe (eg, fibrinous pneumonic pasteurellosis of cattle). Diffuse or interstitial pneumonia often involves the entire lung, as in maedi of sheep or in hypersensitivity reactions. The appearance or cause of a particular pneumonia can be described further, eg, gangrenous, parasitic (verminous), aspiration, etc.

Infection may develop as a result of one or a combination of factors: 1) defence mechanisms are overwhelmed, 2) the infectious agent is highly virulent, 3) the size of the inoculum is large, and/or 4) the animal's defence mechanisms are compromised. The initial problem in many pneumonias is thought to be a sudden change in the normal nasal bacterial flora, which results in a sudden dramatic increase in one or more species of bacteria. Bacterial proliferation is usually caused by a breakdown of the host defences as a result of stress (eg, transportation, concurrent illness) or cellular insult (eg, viral infection, toxicity). These bacteria are breathed into the lung in large numbers and may overwhelm the normal defence mechanisms, localize, multiply, and initiate inflammation. In addition, stress is often a precursor of viral respiratory infections, particularly in groups of animals that have recently been congregated and stressed by travel, handling, and mixing. Some respiratory viral infections can cause temporary dysfunction of phagocytic mechanisms of the alveolar macrophages. This usually occurs several days after viral exposure. Inhaled bacteria proliferate and pneumonia ensues, often with an overwhelming infection and massive exudation into the alveoli.

Pneumonia also can be caused by direct infection with viruses, bacteria, and fungi, as well as by toxins arriving hematogenously, by inhalation, or by aspiration of food or gastric contents.

Through natural processes, possibly aided by appropriate therapy, the exudate may be removed from the lungs, and the mucosal lesions of the air passages may heal. However, serious sequelae can persist.Bronchiectasis is a chronic lesion of the bronchi and parenchyma characterized by irreversible cylindrical or saccular dilatation, secondary infection, and atelectasis. Ulceration of bronchioles caused by viral agents may lead to organized plugs of connective tissue in small bronchioles, a lesion calledbronchiolitis obliterans, which may cause permanent obstruction, atelectasis, and severe respiratory insufficiency. Constriction of bronchi and bronchioles in chronic allergic bronchitis and bronchiolitis results in similar clinical signs. However, administration of bronchodilators results in rapid relief of airway obstruction in cases of allergic bronchitis (eg, heaves in horses). Some chronic pneumonias (eg, maedi in sheep) are characterized by firm diffuse lesions due to hyperplasia of lymphoid follicles, hyperplasia of smooth muscle around bronchioles, diffuse fibrosis, and diffuse lymphocytic infiltration. Aspiration pneumonia often leads to gangrene, with severe toxemia accompanying the acute inflammatory reaction.

Most infectious pneumonias develop in the anteroventral portions of the lungs. However, infectious agents, as well as neo-plasms, can invade the lungs via the blood, which may extensively impair pulmonary function, as can pulmonary edema from chronic heart failure. Pleuritis, empyema, hydrothorax, chylothorax, atelectasis, diaphragmatic hernia, or pneumothorax can also seriously impair respiratory function. Pulmonary thrombosis leads to acute, often fulminant, respiratory failure as a result of a lack of pulmonary arterial blood flow to ventilated regions of the lung. Infarction of the lung can reduce respiratory function but is rare because of the dual blood supply of the organ. Toxic injury, such as in 3-methylindole toxicity in cattle, causes edema, emphysema, and necrosis of alveolar epithelium, followed by compensatory hyperplasia of these cells; the effects on gas exchange result in severe hypoxia and dyspnea. Although pneumonia is most important, several other thoracic conditions can cause respiratory dysfunction. Pulmonary edema, the abnormal accumulation of fluid in the interstitial tissue, airways, or alveoli of the lungs, may occur in conjunction with circulatory disorders, particularly left ventricular failure or increased capillary permeability, occasionally in anaphylactic and allergic reactions, and in some infectious diseases. Head trauma can cause pulmonary edema in dogs. Dyspnea and open-mouth breathing may occur. Animals stand in preference to lying down, lie only in sternal recumbency, or may assume a sitting position. Auscultation of the chest may reveal wheezing and fluid sounds.

Pleuritis (pleurisy) may be caused by any pathogen that gains entrance to the pleural cavity, but it is often an extension of pneumonia. Rapid shallow breathing, fever, and thoracic pain are suggestive of pleuritis. Auscultation of the chest may reveal friction sounds.

Empyema (purulent exudate in the pleural cavity) is caused by pyogenic bacteria or fungi reaching the thoracic cavity via the blood or by extension of a pneumonia, traumatic reticulitis, or penetrating wound of the chest. Cough, fever, pain, and dyspnea may be present.

Hemothorax (the accumulation of blood in the pleural cavity) is usually caused by trauma to the thorax, systemic coagulopathy, or thoracic neo-plasia. Hydrothorax (the accumulation of transudate in the pleural cavity) is usually due to interference with venous blood flow or lymph drainage. Chylothorax (the accumulation of chyle in the pleural cavity) is relatively rare and is seen most often in cats. It may be caused by rupture of the thoracic duct but often is idiopathic. The signs of all three conditions include respiratory embarrassment (eg, rapid shallow breathing with inspiratory dyspnea) and weakness.

Pneumothorax (air in the pleural cavity, see Treatment) may be of traumatic or spontaneous origin. Air can enter the pleural cavity through penetrating wounds of the thoracic wall or by extension from pulmonary emphysema or ruptured bullae. The lung collapses if a large volume of air enters the pleural cavity. Bilateral pneumothorax may develop if the mediastinum is weak or incomplete. Inspiratory dyspnea or rapid, shallow breathing is evident.

RESPIRATORY DISEASE AND PRINCIPLES OF THERAPY

Respiratory disease is often characterized by abnormal production of secretions and exudates and by a reduced ability to remove them. The primary goal of therapy is to reduce the volume and viscosity of the secretions and to facilitate their removal.

This can be accomplished by controlling infection and inflammation, modifying the secretions, and when possible, improving postural drainage and mechanically removing the material. Therapeutic methods include altering the inspired air and administering expectorants, antitussives, bronchodilators, antimicrobials, diuretics, and other drugs. However, expectorants have shown little or no beneficial effects in clinical trials. Hydration should be maintained.

Inhalation of humidified air may facilitate removal of airway secretions. Expectorants are sometimes used with the intention of liquefying these secretions. However, they should be used in conjunction with ancillary respiratory therapy such as improved postural drainage, mild exercise, and thoracic percussion, which (in addition to coughing) encourages expectoration and removal of secretions. Mechanical removal of tenacious and viscid secretions by aspiration may be necessary in severe airway obstruction.

Antitussive agents are indicated to relieve the discomfort associated with non-productive coughing but are contraindicated when secretion of airway mucus is excessive. Products that contain atropine also are contraindicated, at least in theory, because atropine increases the viscosity of airway secretions.

Increased airway resistance caused by bronchial smooth muscle contraction can be alleviated with bronchodilators, which may be indicated in animals with asthma-like conditions and chronic respiratory disease. Methylxanthines, such as theophylline and aminophylline, are effective bronchodilators in species other than cattle (and possibly dogs); however, the therapeutic index is relatively narrow and they are less efficacious than β_2-agonists.

Isoproterenol, clenbuterol, and epinephrine are also generally effective, and sodium cromoglycate may be used in horses with inflammatory airway disease. Corticosteroids are highly effective in allergic conditions, but systemic use may result in adverse effects. Aerosolized corticosteroids are efficacious and associated with few to no adverse effects; however, they require an aerosol delivery device (eg, face mask) for proper administration. Antihistamines can be used to alleviate the bronchoconstriction caused by histamine release; however, they are of limited value in large animals. Bronchospasm also can be reduced significantly by removing irritating factors, using mild sedatives, or reducing periods of excitement.

In bacterial infection, antimicrobial therapy should be instituted. The goal is to select either the most effective agent against a specific organism or the least toxic agent of several alternatives. Culture and sensitivity testing of airway secretions provide a worthwhile, although not infallible, guide to determining the appropriate antibiotic. Knowledge of tissue penetration and pharmacokinetic characteristics of the antimicrobial agents is important as well.

The following agents have proved effective in the listed species: cattle-oxytetracycline, cephalosporins, fluoroquinolones, macrolides, florfenicol, penicillins, and sulfonamides; sheep and goats-oxytetracycline, cephalosporins, macrolides, penicillins, and sulfonamides; pigs-lincomycin, spectinomycin, penicillins, and sulfonamides; dogs and cats-cephalosporins, chloramphenicol, amoxicillin-clavulanate, aminoglycosides, trimethoprim-sulfamethoxazole, fluoroquinolones, macrolides, and tetracyclines; horses-penicillins, aminoglycosides, cephalosporins, fluoroquinolones, sulfonamides, and tetracyclines (the latter with caution due to an occasional adverse effect of severe diarrhea). Aminoglycosides are useful but can be nephrotoxic. Trimethoprim, usually in combination with a sulfonamide, is useful for respiratory therapy in most species but is not licensed for food-producing animals in the USA. Drugs such as enrofloxacin (approved for small animals and cattle but not for horses in the USA) and ceftiofur are effective for pneumonia.

Broad-spectrum antibiotics should be used if specific bacteria cannot be identified, and once begun, a full course of therapy should be completed. Multiple antimicrobial agents should be used only with full knowledge of the potential drug interactions. Because of residues in food-producing animals, veterinarians must use these products according to label instructions and provide sound advice to producers. Extra-label use of antimicrobials is permitted in some situations and is regulated by the Animal Medicinal Drug Use Clarification Act of 1994.

The hypoxemia caused by most lung disorders usually can be corrected by administering oxygen. However, continuous administration of high concentrations increases the tendency for regional resorption atelectasis, thus worsening the hypoxemia, and can cause pneumonitis on its own. Hypoxemia is often accompanied by variable degrees of hypercapnia and acidemia. Endotracheal intubation and mechanical ventilation may be necessary in animals with acute respiratory failure or in animals that are comatose or apneic. Arterial blood gas and pH determinations, when practicable, are extremely valuable to monitor treatment. Diuretics are indicated in pulmonary edema. The osmotic diuretics have a minimal action on diuresis, carbonic anhydrase inhibitors (eg, acetazolamide) have a moderate effect, and loop diuretics (eg, furosemide) have a profound effect.

RESPIRATORY DISEASE AND ITS CONTROL

Sudden dietary changes, weaning, cold, drafts, dampness, dust, high levels of ammonia, poor ventilation in general, and the mixing of widely divergent age groups all play a role in respiratory disease in groups of animals. Stress and mixing of animals from several sources should be avoided or minimized. Establishing individual animal identification, making accurate clinical and postmortem diagnoses, and maintaining a record system of diagnosis and treatment are important to minimize or control outbreaks of pneumonia. Transportation over long distances is another stress factor that plays a major role in the pathogenesis of respiratory infections in large animals.

Immunization can help control respiratory infection. However, control may be compromised by improper timing, use of ineffective or inappropriate vaccines, or overwhelmingly negative management practices. In most cases, severe insults to the natural defences cannot be reversed later by therapeutic agents and biologicals.

The mucosal surfaces of the respiratory tract contain lymphoid follicles that exchange cells with other parts of the body. However, most of the lymphocytes in the respiratory lining produce only IgA, whereas the cells in the lymph nodes of the respiratory tract produce IgM and IgG. Depending on the agent involved, various cell- and antibody-mediated immune responses occur in the respiratory tract and include opsonization, agglutination, immobilization, neutralization of toxins and viruses, blockage of adherence to cells, lysis, and chemotaxis. The type of immune response varies because of age, species, and the means to respond to specific virulence mechanisms of the pathogens involved.

Species vary in the type of immune response available at different sites in the respiratory tract. Large antigen droplets may immunize the upper tract with IgA, but small replicating particles may be necessary to immunize the lower tract. To develop adequate antibody levels to protect the lungs, repeated doses of antigen plus adjuvant, or a replicating antigen, are often necessary. These results are seldom achieved under field conditions (eg, many field trials using respiratory vaccines in cattle have not demonstrated statistically significant efficacy).

Environmental management is an essential part of therapy in allergic respiratory diseases. For example, clinical signs in horses with heaves or cattle with hypersensitivity pneumonitis may be effectively controlled by preventing exposure to molds present in hay.

5

Urinary System

Primary functions of the urinary system include: 1) excretion of waste products of metabolism; 2) maintenance of a constant extracellular environment through conservation and excretion of water and electrolytes; 3) production of the hormone erythropoietin, which regulates hematopoiesis, 4) production of the enzyme renin, which regulates blood pressure and sodium reabsorption; and 5) metabolism of vitamin D to its active form (1,25-dihydroxycholecalciferol).

Many abnormalities of the urinary system can be diagnosed from the signalment, history and physical examination findings, serum chemistry profile, urinalysis, and aerobic bacterial urine culture. The history should include information regarding changes in water consumption, frequency of urination, volume of urine produced, appearance of urine, and behaviour of the animal. It is also important to obtain information about historical and current drug administration, appetite, diet, changes in body weight, and previous illnesses or injuries.

The physical examination should include palpation of the bladder and examination of external genitalia. In dogs, rectal examination should be performed to evaluate the urethra in both sexes and the prostate in male dogs. Rectal examination in cats may not be feasible because of their small size; however, the kidneys are generally easier to palpate in cats than in dogs. A full neurologic examination should be performed on all animals with micturition disorders. Additional diagnostic tests, such as CBC, blood gas analysis for acid-base status, blood pressure, urine protein:creatinine ratio, iohexol clearance test, survey abdominal radiography, abdominal ultrasonography, contrast studies of the upper and lower urinary tract, cystoscopic examination of the urinary bladder, and renal biopsy may also provide valuable information.

URINALYSIS

One of the most important diagnostic tests for evaluation of urinary tract disorders is a urinalysis. Urine may be collected by one of four methods: spontaneous micturition, manual compression of the urinary bladder, catheterization, and cystocentesis. Each method has advantages and disadvantages. A urinalysis should include method of collection, urine specific gravity, colour, turbidity, pH, glucose, ketones, bilirubin ictotest, occult blood, protein, and leukocytes (urine dipstick leukocyte tests are unreliable in cats). Urine specific gravity should be obtained using a refractometer. Microscopic examination of urine sediment should include RBCs, WBCs, epithelial cells, renal casts, bacteria, yeast, parasitic ova, fat, sperm, and crystals. Delay in analyzing urine samples can result in artifacts (eg, changes in urine pH, formation of crystals, etc), so it is important to note the time when the sample was collected and the time when it was analyzed. If a sample will not be analyzed immediately, it should be refrigerated.

Protein in urine should be evaluated in light of the specific gravity. Protein in a concentrated urine sample may not be significant, whereas the same amount in a dilute sample may be significant.

In dogs, the following International Renal Interest Society (IRIS) guidelines should be used for interpretation of urine protein:creatinine ratios. In dogs, <0.2 = non-proteinuric, 0.2-0.5 = borderline proteinuric, and >0.5 = proteinuric; in cats, <0.2 = non-proteinuric, 0.2-0.4 = borderline proteinuric, and >0.4 = proteinuric.

MAIN ORGANS OF URINARY SYSTEM

The main organs are the two kidneys, which lie against the backbone, and the bladder. Waste materials and water are taken out of the blood in the kidneys. This forms urine. Urine collects in the bladder then passes out of the body.

Primary functions of the urinary system include:

- Excretion of waste products of metabolism;
- Maintenance of a constant extracellular environment through conservation and excretion of water and electrolytes;
- Production of the hormones erythropoietin and renin, which regulate hematopoiesis, blood pressure, and sodium reabsorption;
- Metabolism of vitamin D to its active form (1,25-dihydroxycholecalciferol).

Many abnormalities of the urinary system can be diagnosed from the signalment of the patient, history and physical examination findings, serum chemistry profile, urinalysis, and aerobic bacterial urine culture. The history should include information regarding changes in water consumption, frequency of urination, volume of urine produced, appearance of urine, and behaviour of the patient. It is also important to obtain information about historical and current drug administration, appetite, diet, changes in body weight, and previous illnesses or injuries. The physical examination should include palpation of the bladder and examination of external genitalia.

In dogs, rectal examination should be performed to evaluate the urethra in both sexes and for evaluation of the prostate in male dogs. Rectal examination in cats may not be feasible due to their small size; however, the kidneys are generally easier to palpate in cats than in dogs. A full neurologic examination should be performed on all animals with micturition disorders. Additional diagnostic tests, such as CBC, blood gas analysis for acid-base status, blood pressure, urine protein:creatinine ratio, iohexol clearance test, survey abdominal radiography, abdominal ultrasonography, contrast studies of the upper and lower urinary tract, cystoscopic examination of the urinary bladder, and renal biopsy may also provide valuable information.

Protein in urine should be evaluated in light of the urine specific gravity. Protein in a concentrated urine sample may not be significant, whereas the same amount in a dilute sample may be significant. Urine dipsticks provide a semiquantitative assessment of protein and can be influenced by urine pH. Therefore, they should be used only as a screening test for protein, not as a definitive diagnosis of proteinuria. A urine protein:creatinine ratio from a single urine sample or from a 24-hr urine sample is required to quantitate the amount of protein in urine. In dogs, the following guidelines should be used for interpretation of urine protein:creatinine ratios: 0.0-0.3 = normal; 0.3-1.0 =questionable; and >1.0 = abnormal. In cats, a urine protein:creatinine ratio <0.7 is considered normal. Urine protein:creatinine ratios must be interpreted in the context of other information from the urinalysis. Inflammation and hematuria can falsely elevate urine protein:creatinine ratios. The urinary system is responsible for filtering wastes from the blood and both forming and secreting urine. These functions help to maintain the composition and volume of body fluids.

Although it has far-reaching effects, the urinary system is relatively simple anatomically and consists of:

- Kidneys
- Ureters
- Bladder
- Urethra

The main organs are the kidneys, which filter blood and produce urine. The other parts are simply accessory structures for the transport and storage of urine. During the normal breakdown of protein and nucleic acids, nitrogen is released into the bloodstream. Some of this nitrogen is recycled to make new cellular products, but most of it is disposed of. The body has to have a way to rid itself of this unused nitrogen, as high levels in the blood can be toxic.

Most of the nitrogen is bound with hydrogen as NH_3 (ammonia), which is readily dissolved in water. For this reason, fish are able to excrete much of their nitrogen by simple diffusion into the surrounding water. The build-up of nitrogen in the water is one of the reasons that tank water needs to be changed regularly. Terrestrial animals have a different way of ridding their bodies of excess nitrogen. It is either excreted as uric acid or urea. Animals that are concerned about water loss, such as birds and reptiles, excrete the more concentrated uric acid as a pasty white material. Mammals, on the other hand, can excrete urea, along with more water. The mixture of urea, water, and other wastes is called 'urine.' Urine is still very concentrated in comparison to the blood, and the system that facilitates this concentration is the 'urinary system'.

A urinalysis is unreliable for ruling out a urinary tract infection (UTI). Not all UTI are associated with an inflammatory response. In addition, >10,000 bacterial rods/mL and >100,000 bacterial cocci/mL of urine are required to consistently find bacteria in a urine sample using light microscopy. Urine samples for bacterial culture may be obtained by the same methods used for obtaining samples for urinalysis; however, the preferred method is cystocentesis.

Urine obtained by cystocentesis should be sterile. If urine samples are collected by methods other than cystocentesis, a quantitative urine culture should be requested. If the sample is collected by spontaneous micturition or manual compression, significant numbers of bacteria are present if e"100,000 colony forming units (CFU)/mL of urine in dogs or e"10,000 CFU/mL of urine in cats are detected. Samples with >10,000-90,000 CFU/mL in dogs and >1,000-10,000 CFU/mL in cats are suspicious for a UTI. If the sample is collected by catheterization, e"10,000 CFU/mL in dogs and e"1,000 CFU/mL in cats is significant, while samples containing 1,000-10,000 CFU/mL in dogs and 100-1,000 CFU/mL in cats are suspicious for a UTI.

More sensitive methods for detecting renal dysfunction include plasma clearance tests (*e.g*, insulin clearance), radionuclide techniques, endogenous creatinine clearance, and exogenous creatinine clearance. However, these tests are impractical to perform routinely in clinical practice. The iohexol clearance test is a recently developed alternative for detecting renal dysfunction. It entails recording an accurate body weight, administering a precise amount of iohexol IV, and accurately timing collection of blood samples as directed following administration. This test does not require timed collection of urine samples or special equipment.

NEPHRONS

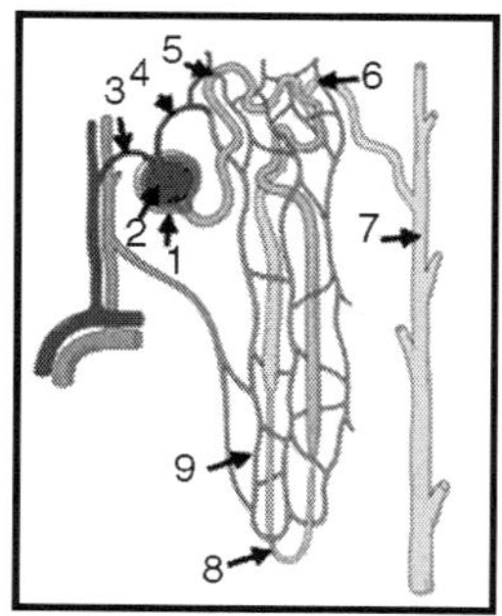

1. Bowman's capsule
2. Glomerulus

3. Afferent arteriole
4. Efferent arteriole
5. Proximal convoluted tubule
6. Distal convoluted tubule
7. Collecting duct
8. Loop of Henle
9. Peritubular capillary

KIDNEYS

The kidneys of mammals are round or bean-shaped organs. They are located outside of the peritoneum – the membrane that encloses the organs of the abdominal cavity. Because of this position, they are referred to as 'retroperitoneal'. They are surrounded by fat tissue known as 'perirenal fat'. A fibrous capsule covers the kidney. The indentation of the bean shape is called the 'hilum.' The hilum is the site where the renal artery enters the kidney and both the renal vein and ureter exit.

The kidney can be divided into two distinct regions – the outer cortex and the inner medulla. The cortex is where blood is actually filtered through small structures called 'glomeruli'. The medulla is where the urine is concentrated through a complex system of tubules. They accomplish this by absorbing the water and electrolytes while preventing waste products from being reabsorbed. One glomerulus and its corresponding set of tubules are called a 'nephron' – the microscopic functional unit of the kidney. The anatomy and function of the nephron will be discussed in detail below.

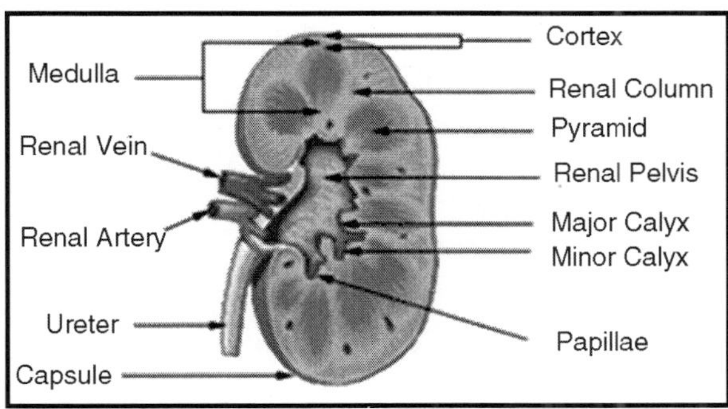

Fig. Anatomy of the Kidney

The tubules of multiple nephrons are grouped into larger visible portions of the kidney called 'pyramids'. The renal columns are spaces between the renal pyramids that provide a route for blood vessels traveling to the cortex. The tips of the pyramids are called 'papillae,' and they drain urine from nephron tubules into larger vessels called 'minor calyxes'. The minor calyxes converge into still larger vessels called the 'major calyxes'. These lead to the enlarged opening of the ureter. This collecting chamber is called the 'renal pelvis.'

URETERS

The ureters are muscular tubes that transport urine from the kidneys to the urinary bladder.

Ureters have three layers of tissue:

1. Fibrous outer coat
2. Muscular layer
3. Inner mucosal layer

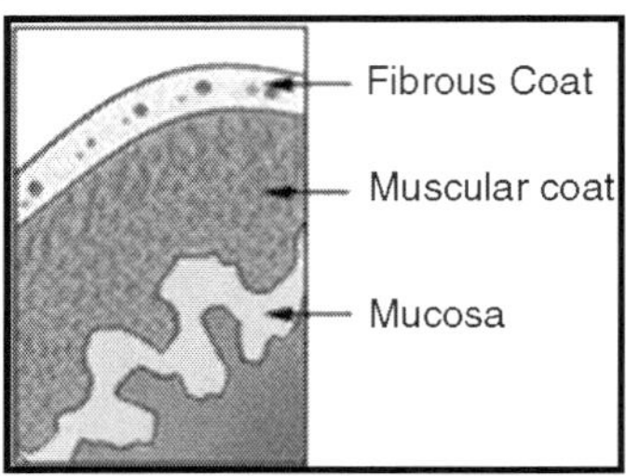

URINARY BLADDER

The urinary bladder is a sac for the temporary storage of urine. It is located in the pelvic cavity. The outer surface is covered with fibrous connective tissue. Inside the connective tissue is a muscular layer called the 'detrusor muscle.' This smooth muscle contracts to expel urine from the bladder.

The next tissue layer is the 'submucosa' an elastic fibrous membrane that supports the mucosa, which lines the inside of the bladder. The mucosa is composed of specialized cells called 'transitional epithelium.' When the bladder is empty, the mucosa has many folds termed 'rugae.' The rugae and transitional epithelium allow the bladder to stretch when filled with urine.

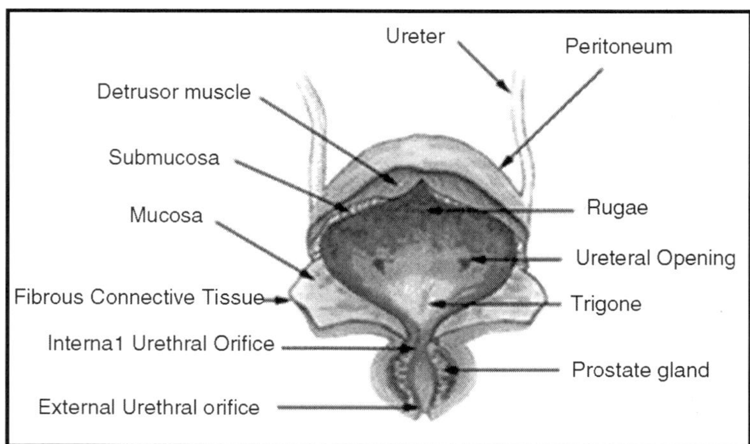

At the base of the bladder, a triangular structure called the 'trigone' is formed from the openings of the two ureters and the urethra. The opening of the urethra is surrounded by a band of detrusor muscle, forming an internal urethral sphincter. This sphincter is relaxed by involuntary muscle control, and is innervated such that when the bladder is approximately half full, the animal perceives the urge to urinate.

URETHRA

The final passageway for urine out of the bladder is through the thin-walled urethra. This tube runs from the base of the urinary bladder to the outside of the body. In the female, it is relatively short, connecting the bladder to external urethral sphincter. In males, however, it is longer.

It passes through the prostate gland (in those animals that have one) and travels the length of the penis before reaching the external sphincter. The external urethral sphincter is voluntarily controlled, and is relaxed by the animal when a suitable site and time for urination has been determined.

BACTERIAL CULTURE OF URINE

A urinalysis is unreliable to exclude a urinary tract infection (UTI). Not all UTIs are associated with an inflammatory response. In addition, >10,000 bacterial rods/mL and >100,000 bacterial cocci/mL of urine are required to consistently find bacteria in a urine sample using light microscopy. Approximately 25 per cent-30 per cent of all dogs with UTI have urine bacterial counts below these figures at the time of specimen collection, so urine culture is important to exclude a UTI.

Urine samples for bacterial culture may be obtained by the same methods used to obtain samples for urinalysis; however, the preferred method is cystocentesis. Urine obtained by cystocentesis should be sterile. If urine samples are collected by methods other than cystocentesis, a quantitative urine culture should be requested.

If the sample is collected by spontaneous micturition or manual compression, significant numbers of bacteria are present if ≥100,000 colony forming units (CFU)/mL of urine in dogs or ≥10,000 CFU/mL of urine in cats are detected.

Samples with >10,000-90,000 CFU/mL in dogs and >1,000-10,000 CFU/mL in cats are suspicious for a UTI. If the sample is collected by catheterization, ≥10,000 CFU/mL in dogs and ≥1,000 CFU/mL in cats is significant, whereas samples containing 1,000-10,000 CFU/mL in dogs and 100-1,000 CFU/mL in cats are suspicious for a UTI.

SERUM CHEMISTRY PROFILE

Evaluation of serum chemistries, including BUN, creatinine, calcium, phosphorus, bicarbonate, and serum electrolytes, is useful in many urinary tract disorders and can provide a crude indication of glomerular filtration rate (GFR). Although increases in BUN and creatinine are supportive of renal dysfunction, these tests are influenced by non-renal factors as well. For example, dehydration can cause increases in BUN and serum creatinine not associated with renal failure. BUN can also be influenced by diet and GI bleeding and is considered inferior to creatinine to evaluate GFR. Serum creatinine levels can be falsely decreased in animals with severe muscle wasting and falsely increased in patients with severe muscle damage.

Although BUN and serum creatinine increase as GFR decreases, this relationship is not linear. Large changes in GFR early in renal disease cause only small increases in BUN and serum creatinine, whereas small changes in GFR in advanced renal disease may be associated with large changes in BUN and serum creatinine.

ADDITIONAL DIAGNOSTIC TESTS

More sensitive methods to detect renal dysfunction include plasma clearance tests (eg, inulin clearance), radionuclide techniques, endogenous creatinine clearance, and exogenous creatinine clearance. However, these tests are impractical to perform routinely in clinical practice. The iohexol clearance test is a recently developed alternative to detect renal dysfunction. It entails recording an accurate body weight, administering a precise amount of iohexol IV, and accurately timing the collection of blood samples as directed after administration.

This test does not require timed collection of urine samples or special equipment. Plasma clearance of exogenous creatinine has also recently been validated for use in dogs.

Depending on the cause of the urinary tract disorder, radiographic procedures, sonographic examination, and cystoscopic examination of the bladder may provide additional valuable information. The kidneys have a limited range of responses to disease; therefore, renal biopsies are rarely useful when evaluating renal dysfunction. An exception to this is in animals with significant proteinuria. Blood gas analysis or serum bicarbonate levels provide useful information on acid-base status, especially in animals with renal dysfunction. Metabolic acidosis is a common problem in chronic renal failure and can result in protein catabolism.

URINARY DISEASE AND PRINCIPLES OF THERAPY

Diseases of the urinary system can result from a variety of pathologic processes, and appropriate therapy depends on the location, severity, and cause of the problem. If the condition is not life threatening, appropriate diagnostic samples should be collected before initiating therapy.

It is important to remember that some diagnostic tests and treatments have the potential to cause significant harm. If the specific cause cannot be determined, non-specific and supportive therapy (eg, monitoring fluids, treating acidosis) should be instituted.

URINARY SYSTEM OVERVIEW - ANATOMY AND PHYSIOLOGY

The urinary system includes the kidneys, the ureters which join the kidneys to the bladder, the bladder itself and the urethras which permit urine collecting in the bladder to be excreted - a process termed micturition. Understanding the physiology of kidney function is key when looking at the diseases that occur in this organ, and the anatomy of all the structures within the urinary sytem is significant as a foundation to understanding the pathology which affects them.

The kidneys also play a vital role in the excretion of many different types of veterinary drug; newborn and aged animals have altered kidney functional capacity and this is an important factor in drug excretion rates. At a molecular level, an understanding of the principles of diffusion and osmosiswill help to understand how water and other molecules can be redistibuted between the intracellular and extracellular spaces via the phospholipid bilayer that contains transport proteins that actively transport molecules such as sodium chloride.

THE KIDNEY

The function of the kidneys is to maintain the volume and composition of plasma, regulate water, ion and pH levels, retain nutrients and excrete waste, toxins and excess electrolytes. The kidneys achieve these functions via glomerular filtration, solute reabsorption, tubular secretion, water balance and acid-base regulation. The kidneys are paired organs which reside in the left hand side and right hand side of the dorsal abdomen respectively, and they form during development from the intermediate mesoderm. Their role is to filter the blood through the renal corpuscle; this comprises a capillary tuft known as a glomerulus which is surrounded by the Bownam's capsule within the nephron; the movement of fluid and soluble material across these structures forms what is known as the filtrate.

The filtrate is then mostly reabsorbed along the nephron until what is left comprises compounds superfluous to the requirements of the animal. Some compounds, normally fully reabsorbed, are occasionally present in the body in excess - the kidney tubules are able to respond to this excess and excrete such compounds in greater amounts. In this way the kidneys play a major role in the homeostasis of an animal. The kidneys also play a vital role in total water balance, varying their excretion of water in relation to the hydration status of the animal. Medically, the physiology of the kidneys can be manipulated using diuretic drugs, which inhibit the reabsorption of water from the tubules resulting in an increase in volume and therefore water loss in the urine.

The kidneys receive 25 per cent of cardiac output. From this they filter 20 per cent of the plasma forming a filtrate of which all but 1 per cent is reabsorbed. This equates to the entire circulatory volume being filtered and reabsorbed every 30 minutes. The kidneys respond dynamically to changes in blood pressure and hydration status, using several mechanisms of regulation including the Renin-Angiotensin-Aldosterone system which can alter the movement of sodium chloride and water in the vascular system and extracellular spaces. The kidneys are responsible for the production and release of two hormones - Erythropoietin and Renin, which are produced in the Juxtaglomerular Cells. The kidneys also regulate the activation of vitamin D.

THE LOWER URINARY TRACT

The lower urinary tract (LUT) is the collection of organs which convey the urine formed within the kidneys to the exterior of the body. Urine is not altered in this part of the system in species other than the horse (where mucous is added) but instead the function of the LUT is to collect and store urine until enough of it is collected for release to become necessary. This gives the animal urinary continence. Three major structures make up this tract; the ureters, the bladder and the urethras which are formed from the horizontal division of the primitive hind gut in the cloacal region during development. Urine gives valuable information to the veterinary practitioner regarding kidney function and other urinary system abnormalities such as crystals, casts and infections.

NON-MAMMALIAN RENAL SYSTEMS

The renal anatomy and physiology of fish, amphibians, birds and reptiles is significantly different to that of mammals. Fish, for example have only a single kidney, and in physiological terms the products of excretion vary between these animal groups from that of mammals.

Urinary System Overview - Anatomy and Physiology Learning Resources
Flashcards Test your knowledge using flashcard type questions
Urinary System Flashcards OVAM
Anatomy Museum Resources Urinary System Quiz
PowerPoint presentation on the urinary system and comparative kidneys.
Histology of renal organs

ANATOMY AND FUNCTION OF URINARY SYSTEM IN MAMMALS

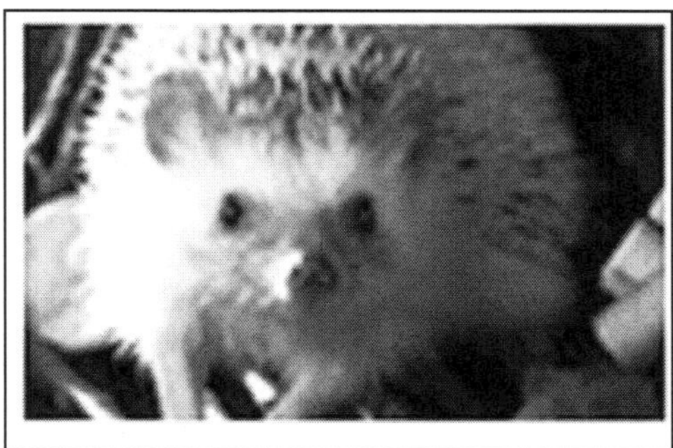

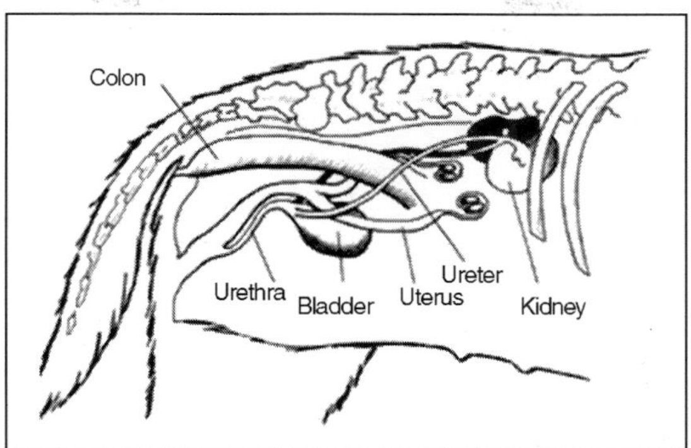

The urinary system is responsible for filtering wastes from the blood and both forming and secreting urine. These functions help to maintain the composition and volume of body fluids.

Although it has far-reaching effects, the urinary system is relatively simple anatomically and consists of:

- Kidneys
- Ureters
- Bladder
- Urethra

The main organs are the kidneys, which filter blood and produce urine. The other parts are simply accessory structures for the transport and storage of urine. During the normal breakdown of protein and nucleic acids, nitrogen is released into the bloodstream. Some of this nitrogen is recycled to make new cellular products, but most of it is disposed of. The body has to have a way to rid itself of this unused nitrogen, as high levels in the blood can be toxic. Most of the nitrogen is bound with hydrogen as NH3 (ammonia), which is readily dissolved in water. For this reason, fish are able to excrete much of their nitrogen by simple diffusion into the surrounding water. The build-up of nitrogen in the water is one of the reasons that tank water needs to be changed regularly. Terrestrial animals have a different way of ridding their bodies of excess nitrogen. It is either excreted as uric acid or urea. Animals that are concerned about water loss, such as birds and reptiles, excrete the more concentrated uric acid as a pasty white material. Mammals, on the other hand, can excrete urea, along with more water. The mixture of urea, water, and other wastes is called 'urine.' Urine is still very concentrated in comparison to the blood, and the system that facilitates this concentration is the 'urinary system.'

KIDNEYS

Anatomy of the Kidney

The kidneys of mammals are round or bean-shaped organs. They are located outside of the peritoneum - the membrane that encloses the organs of the abdominal cavity. Because of this position, they are referred to as 'retroperitoneal.' They are surrounded by fat tissue known as 'perirenal fat.' A fibrous capsule covers the kidney. The indentation of the bean shape is called the 'hilum.' The hilum is the site where the renal artery enters the kidney and both the renal vein and ureter exit.

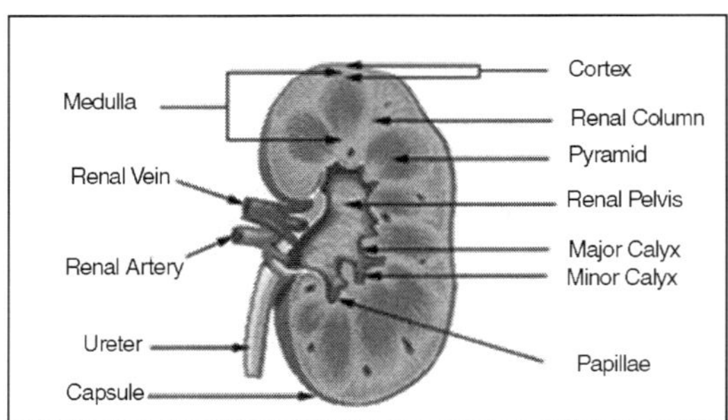

The kidney can be divided into two distinct regions - the outer cortex and the inner medulla. The cortex is where blood is actually filtered through small structures called 'glomeruli'. The medulla is where the urine is concentrated through a complex system of tubules. They accomplish this by absorbing the water and electrolyteswhile preventing waste products from being reabsorbed. One glomerulus and its corresponding set of tubules are called a 'nephron' - the microscopic functional unit of the kidney.

The tubules of multiple nephrons are grouped into larger visible portions of the kidney called 'pyramids'. The renal columns are spaces between the renal pyramids that provide a route for blood vessels traveling to the cortex. The tips of the pyramids are called 'papillae,' and they drain urine from nephron tubules into larger vessels called 'minor calyxes.' The minor calyxes converge into still larger vessels called the 'major calyxes'. These lead to the enlarged opening of the ureter. This collecting chamber is called the 'renal pelvis.'

Nephrons Microscopic Anatomy of a Nephron

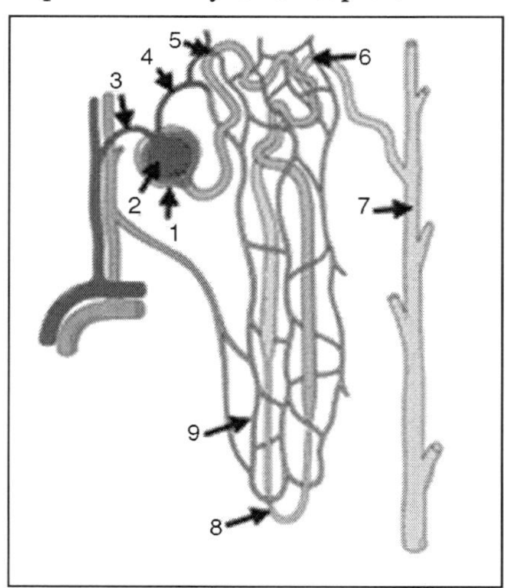

- Bowman's capsule
- Glomerulus
- Afferent arteriole
- Efferent arteriole
- Proximal convoluted tubule
- Distal convoluted tubule
- Collecting duct
- Loop of Henle
- Peritubular capillary

The nephrons are the actual filtration elements of the kidneys. Blood enters the kidneys through the renal artery and travels through branching arteries. These arteries coming into the nephron become smaller and smaller, and are finally called 'afferent arterioles.' The blood in these vessels is under high pressure. The afferent arteriole branches into the glomerulus - a cluster of capillaries within a shell called 'Bowman's capsule.' The pressure of the blood causes water, glucose, amino acids, and salts to leave the blood vessels and enter the Bowman's capsule. The blood cells and most proteins are too big to be filtered out, and remain inside the blood vessel to be carried out of the glomerulus via the efferent arteriole.

Bowman's capsule leads to the network of tubules that concentrate the filtrate into urine. The tubules are surrounded by small blood vessel called a 'capillary'. This capillary is where materials are reabsorbed back into the blood. The first part of the tubule is aptly named the 'proximal convoluted tubule' for its twisted shape. Here 99 per cent of the water is reabsorbed along with all of the glucose and amino acids. The presence of glucose or amino acids in the urine is a sign of disease. For example, diabetics that have too much glucose in their blood cannot reabsorb it all, so it is excreted in the urine.

The proximal convoluted tubule leads to the 'loop of henle,' a long looping structure that extends down into the medulla of the kidney. More water and electrolytes (salts) are absorbed here. Next, the filtrate is passed through the 'distal convoluted tubule,' where excess potassium ions, hydrogen ions, and some drugs or toxins are passed from the blood into the filtrate. The final product is then dumped into a large collecting duct, into which several nephrons empty. This collecting duct leads to the papillae of the pyramids, through the calyxes, and into the renal pelvis to be excreted through the ureter.

URETERS

Microscopic Anatomy of the Ureter The ureters are muscular tubes that transport urine from the kidneys to the urinary bladder.

Ureters have three layers of tissue:

1. Fibrous outer coat
2. Muscular layer
3. Inner mucosal layer

The muscle layer is the functional layer, using peristalsis to move the urine along. Peristalsis is a waving contraction of the muscles to propel the contents of a tube in one direction. In this case, the urine is propelled to an opening at the base of the bladder.

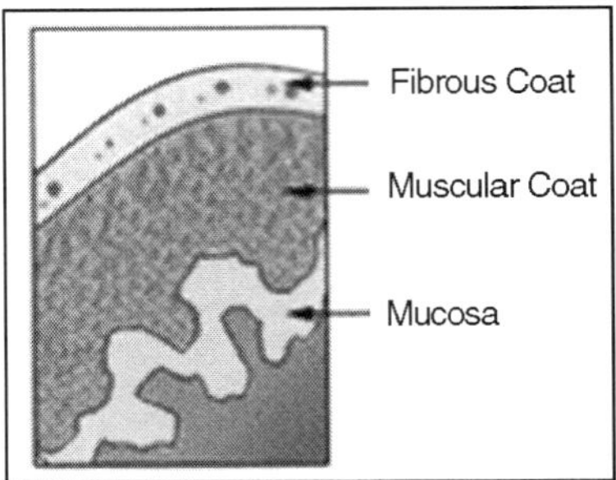

URINARY BLADDER

Anatomy of the Urinary Bladder

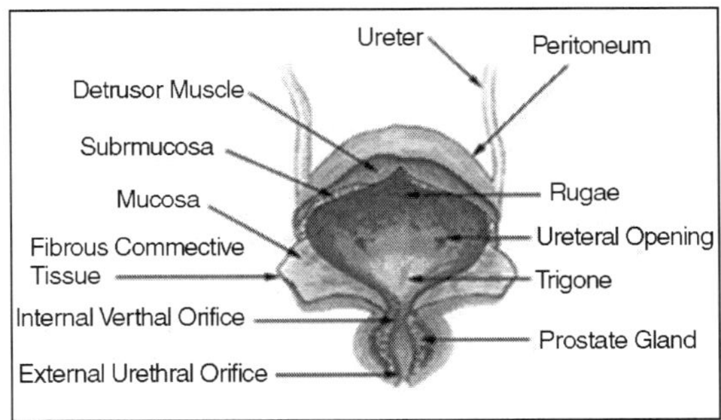

At the base of the bladder, a triangular structure called the 'trigone' is formed from the openings of the two ureters and the urethra. The opening of the urethra is surrounded by a band of detrusor muscle, forming an internal urethral sphincter. This sphincter is relaxed by involuntary muscle control, and is innervated such that when the bladder is approximately half full, the animal perceives the urge to urinate.

URETHRA

The final passageway for urine out of the bladder is through the thin-walled urethra. This tube runs from the base of the urinary bladder to the outside of the body. In the female, it is relatively short, connecting the bladder to external urethral sphincter.

In males, however, it is longer. It passes through the prostate gland (in those animals that have one) and travels the length of the penis before reaching the external sphincter. The external urethral sphincter is voluntarily controlled, and is relaxed by the animal when a suitable site and time for urination has been determined.

Interesting facts:

- Each kidney has over a million nephrons!
- The male urethra is also the pathway for products of the reproductive system.
- Even if 75% of the nephrons are lost, the kidney will still function. It is possible to live a healthy life with only one kidney.
- Urine was once used as a cleaning product!
- Normal urine is sterile (germ-free). It is composed of water, salts, and waste products.
- Reptiles have adapted a very long loop of henle to facilitate more water reabsorption and prevent dehydration.

6

Cardiovascular System: Anatomy and Physiology

The heart is the pump responsible for maintaining adequate circulation of oxygenated blood around the vascular network of the body. It is a four-chamber pump, with the right side receiving deoxygenated blood from the body at low presure and pumping it to the lungs (the pulmonary circulation) and the left side receiving oxygenated blood from the lungs and pumping it at high pressure around the body (the systemic circulation). The myocardium (cardiac muscle) is a specialised form of muscle, consisting of individual cells joined by electrical connections.

- These cells generate a rhythmical depolarisation, which then spreads out over the atria to the atrio-ventricular node.
- The atria then contract, pushing blood into the ventricles.
- The electrical conduction passes via the Atrio-ventricular node to the bundle of His, which divides into right and left branches and then spreads out from the base of the ventricles across the myocardium.
- This leads to a 'bottom-up' contraction of the ventricles, forcing blood up and out into the pulmonary artery (right) and aorta (left).

The atria then re-fill as the myocardium relaxes.

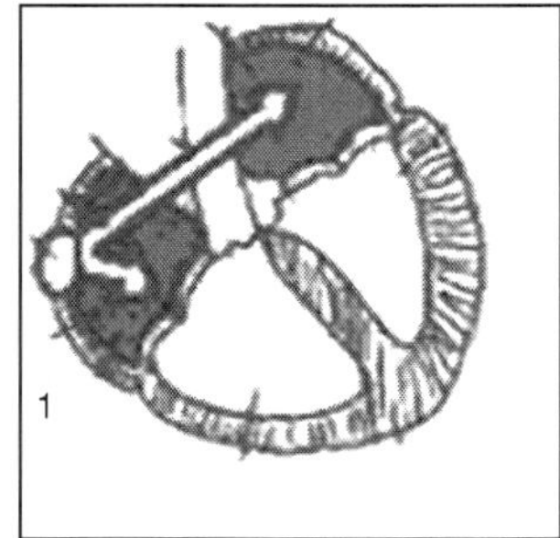

The contraction of each cell is produced by a rise in intracellular calcium concentration leading to spontaneous depolarisation, and as each cell is electrically connected to its neighbour, contraction of one cell leads to a wave of depolarisation and contraction across the myocardium. This depolarisation and contraction of the heart is controlled by a specialised group of cells localised in the sino-atrial node in the right atrium- the pacemaker cells.

The 'squeeze' is called systole and normally lasts for about 250ms. The relaxation period, when the atria and ventricles re-fill, is called diastole; the time given for diastole depends on the heart rate.

CARDIOVASCULAR SYSTEM OF HEART

The cardiovascular system comprises the heart, the veins, and the arteries. The atrioventricular (mitral and tricuspid) and semilunar (aortic and pulmonic) valves keep blood flowing in one direction through the heart, and valves in large veins keep blood flowing back towards the heart.

The rate and force of contraction of the heart and the degree of constriction or dilatation of blood vessels are determined by the autonomic nervous system and hormones produced either at the heart and blood vessels (ie, paracrine or autocrine) or at a distance from the heart and blood vessels (ie, endocrine).

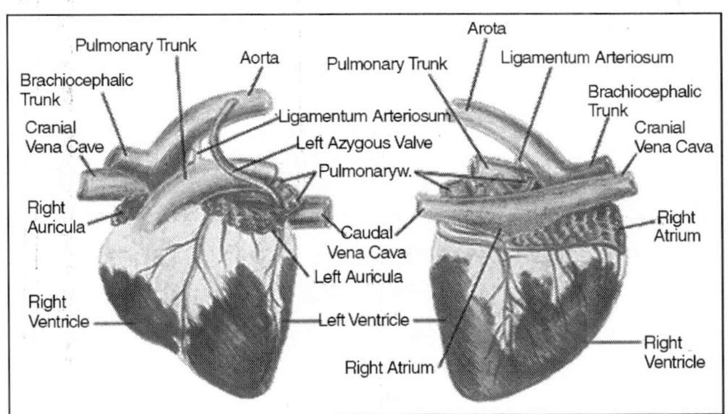

Fig. Normal bovine Heart. Illustration by Dr. Gheorghe Constantinescu.

Slightly >10 per cent of all domestic animals examined by a veterinarian have some form of cardiovascular disease. Similar to many chronic diseases of other organ systems, cardiovascular diseases generally do not resolve but progress and become more limiting, which may ultimately lead to death. Evaluation of the heart depends on heart sounds and murmurs, pressure pulses and the apex beat, the electrocardiogram, radiography, and echocardiography.

HEART RATE AND THE ELECTROCARDIOGRAM

The heart beats because of a wave of depolarization that originates in the sino-atrial (SA) node at the juncture of the cranial vena cava and the right atrium. At rest, the SA node discharges ≥15 times/min in the horse, >120 times/min in the cat, and 60-120 times/min in the dog. In general, the larger the species, the slower the rate of SA node discharge and the slower the heart rate.

The rate of SA node discharge increases when norepinephrine is released from the sympathetic nerves and binds to the ≥1-adrenoreceptors on the SA node. This cardioacceleration may be blocked by ≥-adrenergic blocking agents (eg, propranolol, atenolol, metoprolol, esmolol). The rate of SA node discharge decreases when acetylcholine released by the parasym-pathetic (vagus) nerves binds to the cholinergic receptors on the SA node. This vagally mediated cardiodeceleration may be blocked by a parasympatholytic (vagolytic) compound (eg, atropine, glycopyrrolate). When the SA node discharges and the wave of depolarization traverses the atria, the P wave of the ECG is produced. Subsequently the atria contract, ejecting a small volume of blood into the respective ventricles.

In quiet, healthy dogs, the variation of the heart rate with respiration is termed respiratory sinus arrhythmia (RSA); it results from decreased vagal activity during inspiration and increased vagal activity during expiration. Therefore, vagolytic compounds, as well as excitement, pain, fever, and congestive heart failure usually abolish or diminish RSA. Heart rate variability synchronized with respirations is a good indicator of cardiac health. It is rare to find an animal that has heart failure with an RSA.

Heart rate is also inversely related to systemic arterial blood pressure. When blood pressure increases, heart rate decreases; when blood pressure decreases, heart rate increases. This relationship is known as the Marey reflex and occurs by the following mechanism. When high-pressure arterial baroreceptors in the aortic and carotid sinuses detect increases in blood pressure, they send increased afferent volleys to the medulla oblongata, which increases vagal efferents to the SA node and causes the heart rate to decrease. In heart failure, the baroreceptors (laden with Na+/K+-ATPase) become fatigued, which reduces the afferent signals to the medulla oblongata. This results in less vagal efferent signaling.

Once the wave of depolarization reaches the atrioventricular (AV) node in the right atrium, it travels slowly through the AV node, giving the atria time to contract and to eject the blood into the ventricles. The depolarization then travels rapidly to the subendocardium of the ventricles and to the ventricular septum. From these points, it travels slowly through the ventricular myocardium, producing the QRS complex of the ECG with subsequent ventricular contraction. Under rare conditions, there may be depolarization without contraction; this is called electromechanical dissociation.

The interval on an ECG between the onset of the P wave and the onset of the QRS complex is termed the PQ or PR interval. It is a measure of the time it takes for the electrical wave of depolarization to begin at the SA node and reach the ventricles (lastly traversing the AV node).

Whatever speeds or slows the rate of discharge of the SA node (chronotropy) also speeds or slows conduction through the AV node (dromotropy). Thus, as the heart rate increases, the PR shortens; when heart rate slows, the PR lengthens. The T wave of the ECG represents repolarization of the ventricles. It is affected by electrolyte imbalance, myocardial injury, or ventricular enlargement. Repolarization of the atria (Ta wave) is rarely seen, because it occurs during the much larger QRS complex. Occasionally, it can be seen with AV nodal disease (AV block), appearing as a "hammock" after the P wave.

FORCE OF VENTRICULAR CONTRACTION

The force with which the ventricles contract is determined by many factors, including the end-diastolic volume (preload), which is the volume of blood within the ventricles just before they begin to contract, and myocardial contractility (inotropy), which is the rate of cycling of the microscopic contractile units of the myocardium.

The preload is determined by the difference in end-diastolic pressure between the ventricle and the pleural space, divided by the stiffness of the ventricular myocardium. The end-diastolic pressure of the ventricle is determined by the ratio of blood volume and the compliance of the myocardium.

Preload is regulated predominantly by low-pressure volume receptors in the heart and large veins. When these receptors are stimulated by an increase in blood volume or by distention of the structures the receptors occupy, the body responds by making more urine and by dilating the veins-an attempt to decrease blood volume and lower the pressures in the veins responsible for venous distention. Stretching of receptors in the atria and in the ventricles causes them to release natriuretic proteins, brain natriuretic peptide (BNP) from the ventricles and atrial natriuretic peptide (ANP) from the atria. These proteins, also called atriopeptin, are natriuretic, relax smooth muscle, and in general oppose vasopressin and angiotensin II.

Myocardial contractility is determined by the availability of ATP and calcium, which allows myosin-actin cross-bridging to occur. The rate of liberation of energy from ATP is determined, in part, by the amount of norepinephrine binding to ≥1-adrenergic receptors in the myocardium. One of the most important factors in heart failure is the down-regulation (decreased number) of ≥1-receptors.

OXYGEN AND THE MYOCARDIUM

Oxygen is essential for the production of energy that permits all body functions. The amount of oxygen available for production of this energy is termed the tissue oxygen content. The myocardial oxygen content is a balance between how much oxygen is delivered to the heart minus how much oxygen is consumed by the heart. The amount of oxygen delivered to the heart depends on how well the lungs function, how much hemoglobin (Hgb) is present to carry the oxygen, and how much blood carrying the Hgb flows through the heart muscle via the coronary arteries. If the lungs are functioning well and there is sufficient Hgb, coronary blood flow will determine how much oxygen is delivered to the myocardium. Coronary blood flow is determined by the difference in mean pressure between the aorta (normally 100 mm Hg), and the right atrium (normally 5 mm Hg), into which coronary blood empties. Because coronary flow is greatest during diastole, slower heart rates (which preferentially increase diastolic time) are associated with improved myocardial oxygen delivery.

The amount of oxygen consumed by the heart is termed myocardial oxygen consumption. It is determined, principally, by wall tension and heart rate. Wall tension is expressed by the law of LaPlace, in which tension increases with increases in pressure or diameter of the ventricle, and tension decreases with increases in wall thickness of the ventricle. Tension increases with conditions that increase afterload (pressure) such as pulmonic stenosis, subaortic stenosis, systemic or pulmonary hypertension, or preload (volume) including mitral valve insufficiency and dilated cardiomyopathy. In the absence of a stenotic lesion, afterload is determined by the relative stiffness of the arteries and by the degree of constriction of the arterioles.

The tone of vascular smooth muscle depends on many factors, some of which constrict the muscle (eg, adrenergic agonists, angiotensin II, vasopressin, endothelin) and some of which relax the muscle (eg, norepinephrine, atriopeptin, bradykinin, adenosine, nitric oxide). Afterload is often increased in heart failure, and therapy is often directed at decreasing it. Increases in heart rate result in increasing myocardial oxygen consumption while decreasing diastole when coronary blood flow is greatest. The combination can set the stage for an imbalance in myocardial oxygen demand and supply, leading to myocardial ischemia. Cardiac failure is characterized by an increase in sympathetic tone and relative increases in heart rate; the ultimate impact is an inefficient myocardium that can result in deleterious remodeling.

Oxygen is responsible for the production of the vast majority of ATP, which fuels both contraction and relaxation of the myocardium. Calcium must rapidly be released by intracellular stores (sarcoplasmic reticulum) to allow contraction, while equally rapid removal of calcium back into the sarcoplasmic reticulum is necessary for relaxation. Both processes of calcium cycling are energy dependent. In heart failure, inappropriate handling of calcium may be the most important factor that leads to both reduced force of contraction and reduced rate of relaxation (ie, reduced systolic as well as diastolic function).

HINDRANCE TO BLOOD FLOW

Blood flow from the heart, termed cardiac output, occurs from both the left and right ventricles. Blood flows through the systemic arterial (left ventricular) or pulmonary arterial (right ventricular) trees and is critical to satisfactory function of the heart and consequent perfusion of organs with adequate quantities of blood and the oxygen it contains. Most (>90 per cent) of the hindrance to blood flow is from the degree of constriction of the arterioles, termed the vascular resistance; however, some interference is from the stiffness of the portion of the great arteries closest to the ventricles, termed the impedance. The ventricles eject a stroke volume into the proximal portion of the great arteries, which expand to accommodate the stroke volume; when the ventricles are relaxed, the distended great arteries recoil and keep blood moving through the arterioles into the capillaries. The aortic and pulmonic valves close and prevent the stroke volume from returning to the ventricle that ejected it.

One of the most important features of heart failure that leads to morbidity is increased resistance of arterial, arteriolar, and venous smooth muscle because of increased angiotensin II, vasopressin, and endothelin. If the left ventricle is unable to eject a normal stroke volume or cardiac output, it is reasonable that the ventricular function might be improved by decreasing vascular resistance. Decreasing afterload (arterial vasodilation) is one therapeutic goal in heart failure therapy.

7

Musculoskeletal System: Anatomy and Physiology

The musculoskeletal system includes bones, joints, cartilage, muscles, ligaments and tendons. In order to describe anatomical landmarks for example for the purposes of surgery and to be able to describe different directional information, for example when recording the view of a recently taken x-ray, it is necessary to have a way of describing the planes and axes that can be applied to the musculoskeletal system to pinpoint a specific anatomical area.

THE TRUNK

The trunk consists of three segments: thorax, abdomen, and pelvis, each of which is bounded by body wall and contains a cavity. The thoracic cavity lies cranial to the diaphragm, whereas the abdominal cavity lies caudal. Dorsally, the roof of all three cavities is formed by the spinal column and associated muscles. The pelvic cavity is defined by the borders of the bony pelvis and communicates with the abdominal cavity. The bony thorax includes the ribs and sternum; the thoracic musculature is predominantly associated with respiration.

Knowledge of the abdominal musculature is important when performing surgery on abdominal organs, and these muscles are traditionally divided into ventrolateral and sublumbar groups.

THE HEAD AND NECK

The shape and size of the skull varies widely, not only between species but also with age, breed and sex of similar species. The skull is divided into three components- the neurocranium, the dermatocranium and the viscerocranium. The skull also includes the hyoid apparatus, mandible, ossicles of the middle ear and the cartilage of the larynx, nose and ear. The skull protects the brain and head against injury and supports the structures of the face. In some animals the skull is also used for defensive actions, for example in horned ungulates such as red deer stags.

MUSCULATORY SKELETAL SYSTEM

This system consists of the bones and the muscles (meat).The bones form the skeleton which is the framework within the body. It carries weight and supports the body. Bones are connected together so they can move. The places where this happens are called joints. The bones are held together at the joints by elastic strands called ligaments. Between the bones is a softer material called cartilage (gristle) which cushions the bones at the joints when the body moves. Bones are very hard and contain minerals. Each bone has a name such as the scapula (shoulder blade) and skull (head). There are about 200 bones in the body.

Muscles are joined at both ends to the bones. The muscles are the meat of the body and when they contract (shorten) or relax (lengthen) they make the bones move. Mammals are vertebrates by definition, this means that all mammals have an internal bony support structure to which muscles and ligaments are attached. This is what we call a skeleton.

The basic plan of the mammalian skeleton, as seen above, is fairly straight forward. It consists of a head at one end of a vertebral column from which extend ribs to support the working organs and four limbs for locomotion. The vertebral column ends in a tail. The huge range of lifestyles and habitats utilised by mammals means that a great deal of variety exists between different groups.

Some species lack a tail, others lack apparent hind limbs and the skull is very variable. Here we are giving a general outline of the mammalian skeleton with some notes to indicate particular variations. To understand the skeleton fully you should also have a look at the bones and joints.

THE SKULL

The vertebrate skull in general and the mammal skull in particular is a complex amalgam of bones, not just one or two but about 34 bones, if they all are present, make up the skull and lower jaw. Most of these bones are now fused together. Anyone who has looked carefully at a mammal skull wmust have noticed the crinkly lines where the once individual bones meet. Most of them come in pairs, one each side. The skull can be divided into 3 basic parts; the Braincase (enclosing the brain); the Rostrum (the snout and upper jaw); the Lower Jaw.

Some of the main bones of the skull are:

- Nasal bones - the roof of the nasal cavity
- Maxillary bones - the main bones of the upper jaw, including the Zygomatic arch; the bones to which the strong jaw muscles are attached and which form the boundaries of the eyes. The Zygomatic arches also contain the Jugal bones and the Squamosal bones.
- Frontal bones - the top of the skull in most mammals. These are the bones that horns and antlers grow from.

- Parietal bones - these form the roof and back of the Braincase.
- Occipital bones - the lower back of the braincase (actually 3 bones fused together; basioccipital, exoccipitals and the supraoccipital).
- Dentary bones - the lower jaw.

THE VERTEBRAE - SPINAL COLUMN

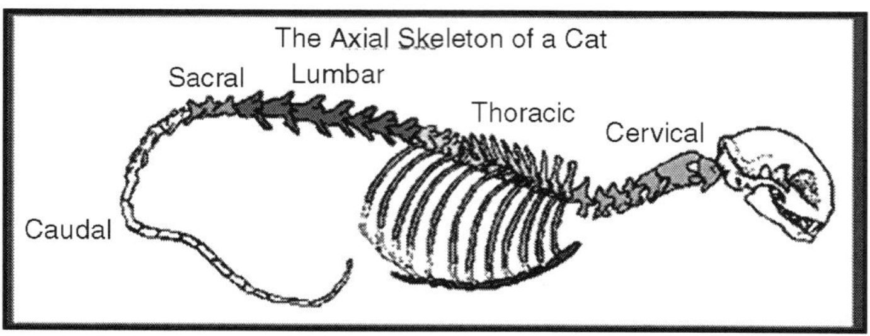

The spinal column in mammals, as in other vertebrates, is composed of a series of small bones with one or more holes through their centre. These holes are aligned to make a highly protected tube. This tube houses and protects the spinal chord a thick sheath of nerves and ganglia that is the unifying characteristics of the Phylum Chordata. The Phylum Chordata contains the Subphylum Vertebrata and hence the Class Mammalia.

In many mammals the vertebrae can be seen to be divided into five distinct regions, though in some groups such as the whales they are pretty indistinct. Where the adjacent vertebrae meet each other they have special smooth, flatish surfaces called zygopophyses.

These contact surfaces are also protected by cartilage. Cervical Vertebrae - the neck region of an animal is supported by the cervical vertebrae and normally in mammals there are 7 of them. The first vertebra, the one immediately behind the skull is called the 'Atlas'. It has two large depressions in its front face which accept (articulate with) the occipital condyles, two bumps unique to mammals found at the base of the skull. It also has a slot in the rear face to accept the odontoid process, a forward project of bone on the second vertebra. This second vertebra is called the 'Axis'.

The rest of the cervical vertebrae do not have special names. They are often cemented together for extra strength in digging and swimming mammals. Thoracic Vertebrae - these are the bones from which the rib bones extend. They often have large dorsal spines. These are usually 12-15 thoracic vertebrae.

The spines help support the muscles that lift and control the neck and head. Lumbar Vertebrae - the third part of vertebrae are the lumbar vertebrae. These are the rest of the spine down to where the back legs connect. Normally there are only 6 or 7 of them except in the toothed whales (Odontoceti) where there can be as many as 20. Lumbar vertebrae often have numerous spines and processes and can look quite complicated.

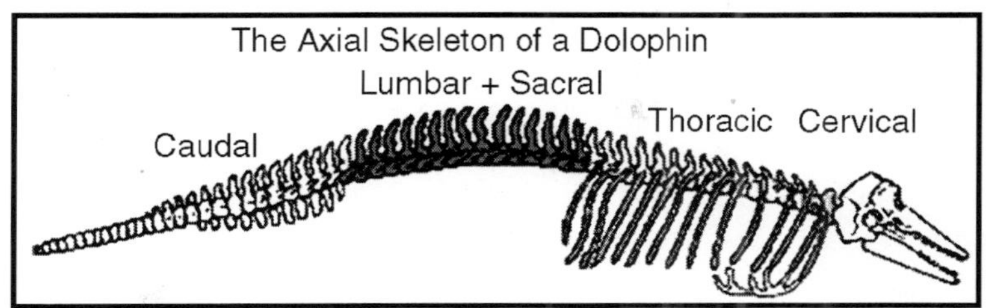

Sacral Vertebrae - these bones support the pelvic girdle and are often fused together. There are usually 3-5 in number but can be more, up to 10 in the Edentata for instance. Caudal Vertebrae - the last lot of vertebrae are the bones of the tail. They are generally smaller and less complicated than the rest of the vertebrae. They also do not contain the spinal column which ends at or before the Sacral vertebrae, though they do contain some nerves and blood vessels. In mankind and Chimpanzees, the Caudal vertebrae are reduced to 4 in number and are fused to form the Coccyx.

Rib bones - these support the vital organs, making a cage within which heart and lungs can be carried in protection. Ribs normally arise from the thoracic vertebrae but in a few groups (Edentata, Monotremata) some species have ribs arising from the cervical vertebrae.

Ribs end under or in front of the animal along each side of the sternum (breast bone). In many species the lower or posterior ribs do not meet the sternum, these are called floating ribs. In most groups articulated ribs (those which meet and join with the sternum) outnumber the floating ribs easily, but in Whales and Dolphins it is the other way around partly because of a reduced sternum (meeting in only 6 pairs of ribs as compared to 9 pairs in a cat) and partly because of a greater number of ribs; 15 pairs versus 12 pairs in a cat. The Sternum or breastbone is actually made up of a number of smaller bones called 'sternebrae'.

The front part of the sternum is keeled (to give a larger area for muscle attachment) in bats who need to flap their wings, and in many digging species who also need large muscles to work their forelimbs, *i.e.* moles. Most of the remaining bones are to do with limbs, either being part of them or supporting them. The two supporting areas are called girdles (Pelvic girdle and Pectoral girdle). The Pelvic girdle consists of two halves each of which is made up of three bones fused together.

These two halves are called the 'innominate bones'. The three pairs of bones which make up each innominate bone are the Ilium, the Ischium and the Pubic bones. In marsupials and monotremes another pair of bones are present called the Epipubic bones. The exact role that these play in the life of the Marsupials and Monotremes which possess them is unknown.

The pectoral girdle consists of two pairs of bones, the large flat Scapula (shoulder bone) and the much smaller and more slender Clavicle (collar bone).

The clavicle runs from the far end of the scapular to the sternum in most mammals, though in the Monotremata it meets the interclavicle instead.

Monotremes also have a pair of bones called the Epicoracoid or Precoracoid bones. In some mammals such as the Anisodactyla, Perissodactyla, Mysticeti and Odontoceti (Horses, Pigs, Deer, Buffaloes, etc. and Whales) the clavicle is absent. The scapula is the bone that the legs or arms start from, *i.e.* the humerus joins the far end of the scapula at the glenoid fossa.

LIMBS

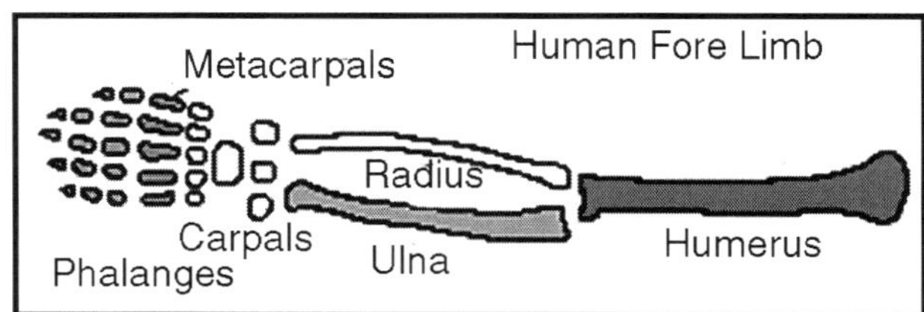

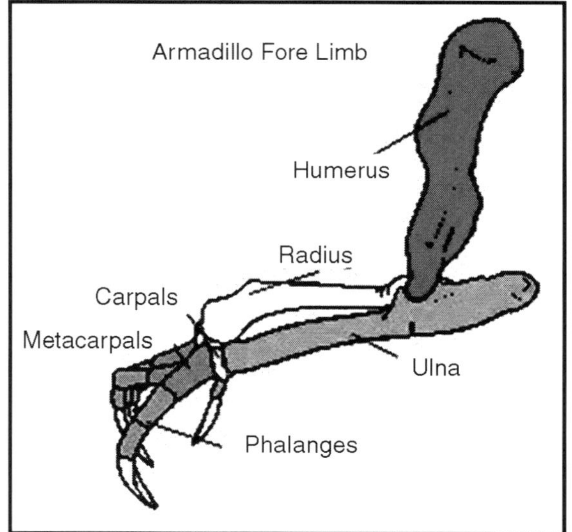

The basic vertebrate limb evolved as the first amphibian like fish left the warm seas for the new dry land. It is called the pentadactyl limb, from the Greek penta for five because it ends in five digits or phalanges.

This business of having five separate endings to a single limb was quite an important new development when it first occurred. It was obviously a good thing because it has been very successful. The pentadactyl limb supported the dinosaurs for millions of years and has played a major role in mankind's technological development.

It remains the same all across the vertebrate classes. In mammals it perhaps reaches its peak and greatest diversity. Though the fore and hind limbs are basically the same they have different names for the various bones.

Thus starting at the body and moving outwards the forelimbs consist of:

Humerus	Ulna + Radius	Carpel bones	Metacarpel bones or Digits	Phalanges
Upper arm	Fore arm	Wrist	Palm of hand	Fingers

Hind limbs consist of:

Femur	Patella	Fibula + Tibia	Tarsal bones bones	Metatarsal Digits	Phalanges or
Thigh	Knee	Shin	Ankle bones	Foot bones	Toes

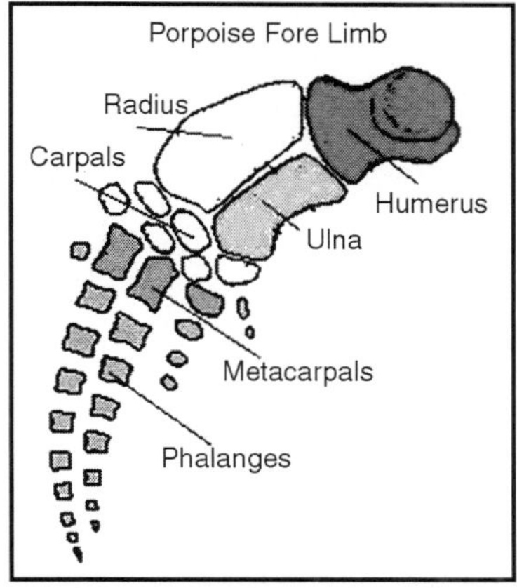

The lower part of both limbs consists of a pair of bones running parallel to each other. The Forearm consisting of the Ulna and Radius and the Shin consisting of the Fibula and Tibia. This arrangement allows for greater flexibility and stronger turning/twisting movements than a single bone would. Though this is not terrible important in some mammals which only use their limbs for walking on, for those who use their limbs, prticularly the fore limbs, for grasping, climbing and or digging it is of great value and has contributed greatly to the diversity of mammals. The Carpels and or Tarsals come in 3 rows see the Human fore limb above and make up the wrist. However as can be seen from the other fore limb images their number is often reduced and their role less important than it is in the classic design.

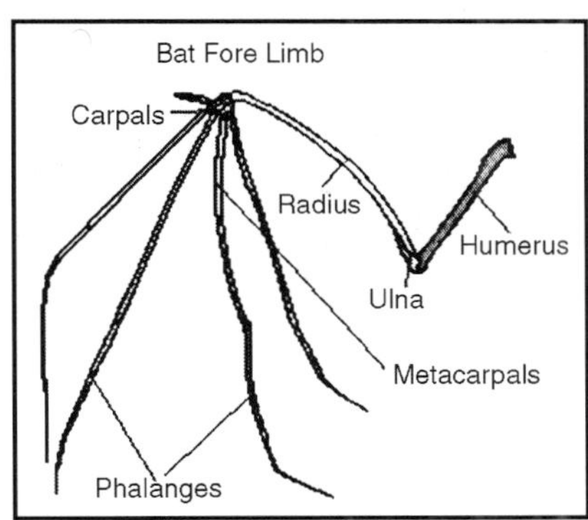

These various other limb bones also have varying degrees of importance in different families of mammals. They have all been modified by the forces of evolution to fulfil different roles relevant to the different way various animals use their limbs. In Whales and Dolphins, for instance the number of finger bones 'phalanges' in the forelimb has greatly increased. This is known as hyperphalangy. In some families not all the bones mentioned above still exist, some have been lost in the course of evolution. Like all bones, limb bones contain various 'processes' (special extensions of bones to aid muscle attachment) and fossae (smooth surfaces where two bones meet and articulate [move in relationship to each other]).

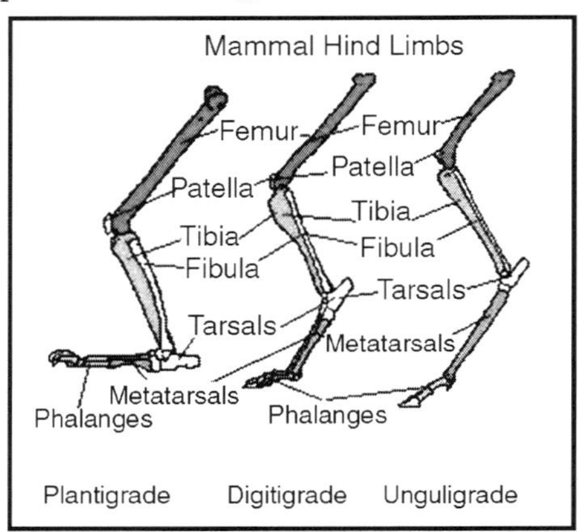

MUSCULOSKELETAL SYSTEM: BONES, CARTILAGE, MUSCLES, LIGAMENTS, AND TENDONS

The musculoskeletal system consists of bones, cartilage, muscles, ligaments, and tendons. Primary functions of the musculoskeletal system include support of the body, provision of motion, and protection of vital organs. The skeletal system serves as the main storage system for calcium and phosphorus and contains critical components of the hematopoietic system. Many other body systems, including the nervous, vascular, and integumentary systems, are interrelated, and disorders of one of these systems may also affect the musculoskeletal system and complicate diagnosis.

Diseases of the musculoskeletal system most often involve motion deficits, functional disorders, and lameness. The degree of impairment depends on the specific problem and its severity. Skeletal and articular disorders are by far the most common and have the greatest economic impact. In horses and dogs, musculoskeletal injuries are a major source of debilitating pain, economic loss, and loss of athleticism.

Degenerative joint disease is much more common and has a greater economic importance than acute traumatic injuries or respiratory diseases in performance horses. Several studies estimate that problems involving the fetlock and carpal joints account for 25 per cent-28 per cent of horses lost from training. In addition, tendon injury is a common debilitating injury in performance horses. The healing response is prolonged, and the resultant repair tissue is usually of inferior mechanical strength. Consequently, the prognosis for return to previous levels of performance is poor. In dogs, cranial cruciate ligament injury with resulting osteoarthritis is the most common musculoskeletal injury resulting in lameness. Although perhaps less common, primary muscular diseases, neurologic deficits, toxins, endocrine aberrations, metabolic disorders, infectious diseases, blood and vascular disorders, nutritional imbalances or deficits, and occasionally congenital defects are diagnosed as well.

FLUID TRANSPORT IN BODY

The bodies of living humans contain many different types of fluids that play an important role in their function. Blood plasma is the liquid part of blood that carries blood cells, hormones, proteins, and other substances throughout the body. Lymphatic fluid and mucus both play a role in protecting the body from disease. The process of digestion is aided by saliva and gastric juice. Other fluids found in the human body include cerebrospinal fluid, sweat, tears, the aqueous and vitreous humors of the eye, and body fluids related to human reproduction, such as semen and vaginal secretions.

Blood cells are suspended in a fluid called plasma, which is mainly composed of water and a mixture of other dissolved substances, or solutes. Plasma is an important transport mechanism within the human body, as it carries substances like hormones, vitamins, amino acids, and antibodies to where they can be stored or put to use. The plasma also contains proteins called clotting factors that help the blood to coagulate, slowing down the rate of blood loss when a person has an injury that causes blood to hemorrhage. When these clotting factors are removed from the blood plasma, it is known as blood serum.

One of the fluids that directly contributes to the body's defense is lymphatic fluid, a fluid that is very similar in composition to blood plasma. This fluid originates in the circulatory system, but passes out of the network of veins and arteries into a space between cells known as the interstitial space. While in the interstitial space, the fluid is known as interstitial fluid, which "bathes" the body's cells and takes microbes and pathogens away with it. The small percentage that enters the lymphatic system is called lymphatic fluid. Mucus is a viscous fluid that also aids in the body's defense by trapping foreign particles that try to enter the body through the respiratory system.

Some body fluids help break down food that is consumed so the body can absorb nutrients and gain energy. Saliva is secreted by the salivary glands found under the tongue. It contains enzymes that begin the digestive process by breaking down starches and fats in food while it is still in the mouth. After this partially digested food is swallowed, it enters the stomach, where the highly acidic gastric juice continues the process of digestion. Cerebrospinal fluid provides a protective cushion for the brain. Sweat, or perspiration, helps humans maintain a comfortable body temperature. Tears are secreted by the lacrimal glands and help to clean and lubricate the surface of the human eye. Fluids in the inner and outer portions of the eye that maintain pressure in the eye and provide nutrients and immune defense to that organ are called the vitreous and aqueous humors, respectively. Human males produce a fluid called semen that functions as a delivery system for sperm cells, while human females produce vaginal secretions that facilitate sexual intercourse by lubricating the vagina. We may begin with the exchange of gases, which in our own case we call breathing. In simple animals like jellyfish and many worms there are no special organs for this purpose. Dissolved oxygen soaks through their skins from the water in which they live, and dissolved carbon dioxide soaks out. In somewhat more complicated creatures like the earth-worm there is a special fluid, the blood, one of whose functions is to carry oxygen from the skin to the internal organs, and carbon dioxide back.

In the most advanced water-dwellers we find special tufts of thin skin, the gills, into which blood is pumped by a heart or hearts, so as to expose it to water with which it may exchange gases. Gills may be naked, as in the young tadpole, but usually, as they are very delicate, they are protected by lids or pouches, as in fish or lobsters, where they lie behind the head on each side. In air-breathing animals there are two quite different kinds of breathing organ. In insects and spiders, air is carried to every part of the body by tiny branching tubes called tracheae, which open by numerous pores, mainly on the sides of the abdomen.

In air-breathing vertebrates and molluscs the blood is exposed in the lungs to air which is continually renewed by the act of breathing. Some animals combine several methods. Thus a frog can use its skin alone for breathing so long as it does not need much oxygen, but it normally employs its lungs as well. The human lungs are elastic organs of a spongy texture, consisting of millions of very small cavities which open into stiff tubes called bronchi. These in turn open into the windpipe in the front of the neck. Since air cannot enter the space between the lung and the chest-wall, the lungs expand when the chest is expanded. This can happen in two different ways. In the first place the diaphragm, a sheet of muscle separating the chest and belly, and bulging upwards into the former, may contract and force the contents of the belly downwards and outwards.

This pulls the bases of the lungs down, and draws air into them. Or the muscles which lie between the ribs may contract so as to bring the ribs, which normally slope downwards, into a more horizontal position. The breast-bone is thus pushed away from the vertebral column, while at the same time the diameter of the chest from side to side is increased, and the lungs expand to fill the extra volume.

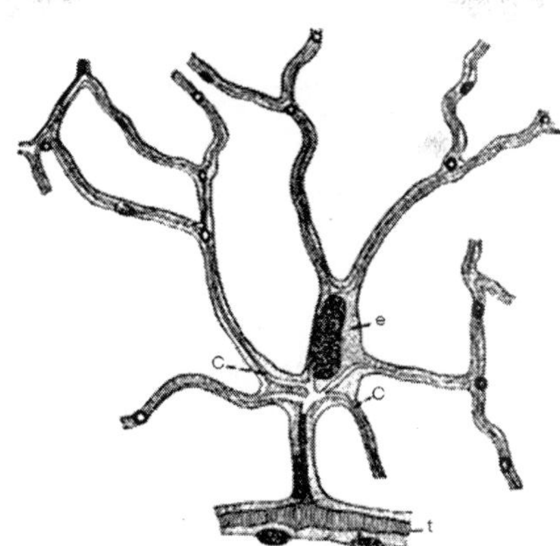

Fig. Final Ramifications of Tracheae in a Caterpillar.

Muscles acting in the opposite direction force the air out again if necessary; generally the elasticity of the lungs is sufficient. Thus the air to which the blood in the lungs is exposed is constantly being changed.

The inspired air contains 21 per cent. of O_2 and only 0.03 per cent. of CO_2, whilst the expired air (after being dried) contains about 17 per cent. of O_2 and 3 per cent. of CO_2. To understand how this change occurs we must study the circulation of the blood. The blood flows to and from the heart, as we have seen, through a closed system of tubes known as arteries, veins, and capillaries. It leaves the heart by the arteries, which are comparatively thick-walled, and seldom near the surface, and returns by the veins, which have thinner walls, and often lie just below the skin.

It passes from the arteries to the veins by the capillaries, which are too small to be seen with the naked eye, but are found in almost every tissue. The most easily felt arteries in man are those of the wrist and temple, the most easily seen veins those on the back of the hand and foot. Finally, the heart, which pumps the blood round, is a hollow muscle with four chambers, lying between the lungs, and about as large as the two fists together. The blood from all parts of the body except the lungs enters the heart from behind, near the right-hand top corner, and flows into a chamber called the right auricle.

This contracts rhythmically (the average rate in a grown man at rest is about seventy times a minute) and forces its contents into a thicker-walled chamber lying below it, the right ventricle. As soon as this is full it contracts in its turn. The blood is prevented from returning into the auricle by a valve, called the tricuspid. It therefore finds its way out through the pulmonary artery, which leads it to the lungs. The semilunar valves at the base of the artery prevent it from flowing back into the ventricle when this relaxes at the end of its stroke. In the lungs it has to pass through capillaries in the walls of the air-sacs, so that it is only separated from the air by a very fine membrane, and can easily lose its carbon dioxide and take up oxygen.

It returns from the lungs by the pulmonary vein, this time to the left auricle, which contracts at the same time as the right auricle, and fills the left ventricle. The left ventricle, which is assisted by valves not unlike those on the right side of the heart, forces the blood into the largest artery, an elastic tube called the aorta, from which it is distributed all over the body by the other arteries.

One way of forcing it round through the narrow capillaries would be to have a cistern at the top of the head from which it flowed down again, but this arrangement would clearly not work when its owner lay down. In reality, a fairly steady pressure is kept up by the fact that the walls of the aorta and the arteries are always stretched, and continue to squeeze the blood along between the strokes of the ventricles.

The pressure in man is about that of a column of blood 1.7 metres high, i.e. equal to the head of blood which would be obtained from a cistern 1.7 metres above the heart. The heart of a grown man at rest delivers about 8 litres per minute, or just over 100 cubic centimetres per beat.

During exercise the heart may deliver three or four times as much per minute, mostly as the result of an increased number of beats per minute. The beat of the heart which is felt below the fifth rib on the left side is due to the left ventricle striking the wall of the chest each time it contracts and stiffens. The blood is squirted along the arteries at a rate which may be as high as 50 centimetres a second, and each fresh wave causes a pulse in the artery.

If an artery is cut, the blood comes in a series of spurts from the side nearest the heart, and can be stopped by pressure on the heart side of the cut. It is easy (and safe) to stop the pulse in the wrist by pressing on the same artery higher up, either inside the elbow or inside the upper arm just below the armpit, where it can be felt. The blood flows through the capillaries very slowly, at about half a millimetre per second. Their average length is about a millimetre, while their diameter may be less than 0.01 millimetre. Their very thin walls allow water, gases, and dissolved substances to be exchanged between the blood and the tissues with great ease. From the capillaries the blood oozes gently into the veins.

They have no pulse, and a comparatively small pressure and rate of flow. A cut vein bleeds steadily and the flow can be stopped by compressing the side away from the heart. The flow of blood in the veins is assisted by the presence of valves in them, which only allow it to move towards the heart. If the finger-tip be run along one of the veins of the forearm away from the heart, the vein will dilate on the heart side of each valve.

When therefore the contraction of various muscles squeezes the veins, the blood can only flow towards the heart. If a man stands quite still the blood tends to accumulate in the veins of his legs, and he is liable to faint from failure of the supply to his brain. When he starts walking the blood is at once squeezed out of these veins. The only veins in man which do not lead straight back to the heart are those from the digestive canal and some other abdominal organs, which pass into the liver.

Here the food absorbed by the blood from the gut is dealt with. As the liver needs oxygen, it has also a supply of fresh arterial blood. In most other animals the circulation is somewhat different. Thus in a fish the blood only goes once through the heart in a complete journey, instead of twice, and it all passes through the gills before going on to the tissues. In the frog, in keeping with its two ways of breathing, we have a condition almost half-way between that found in fish and men. The blood entering the right side of the heart by the main vein flows into *R.A.*, the right auricle; thence, through a valve, into *R.V.*, the right ventricle, which pumps it, through a valve, down *P.A.*, the pulmonary artery, to the lungs, *Lg.*

The blood here flows in capillaries, and is then gathered up into the pulmonary vein, *P.V.*, and taken to the left side of the heart, entering the left auricle, *L.A.*, then (through a valve) the left ventricle, *L.V.*, and by this being pumped out (again through a valve) into the aorta, *Ao.* Some of the blood (A^1) goes to the head and anterior extremities, whence it is returned by the anterior venae cavae (V^1), into which discharges the main trunk of the lymphatic system, the thoracic duct (*Th.D.*). The rest (A^2) goes to the trunk and hind limbs.

That which supplies the digestive tube (*Al.*) passes to the liver (*Lr.*) by the hepatic portal vein (*V.P.*); the liver also receives arterial blood direct by *H.A.*, the hepatic artery. The hepatic vein, *H.V.*, joins the veins from the other posterior regions, V^2, and flows to the heart in the inferior vena cava, *V.C.I.* *Lct.* denotes the lacteal lymphatic vessels from the intestinal wall, *Ly.* ordinary lymphatics. We must now consider how the blood acts as a carrier of oxygen and carbon dioxide.

Water at body-temperature will only take up one two-hundredth of its volume of oxygen from air; if the blood were no better than this we should need a heart working forty times as fast as the one we have. Actually the oxygen is carried round in loose chemical combination with a body called haemoglobin. This is a protein, but contains iron as well as the usual carbon, hydrogen, oxygen, nitrogen, and sulphur. It is of a purple colour, but becomes red on combining with oxygen, which it readily takes up from the air.

Thus the blood in the veins is purplish, but if exposed to air either in the lungs or by opening a vein, it at once becomes red. The haemoglobin which it contains enables blood to hold 18 volumes of oxygen per cent., which is 6/7; of the amount contained in the same volume of air, and about 40 times what the blood could carry without haemoglobin. Since blood carries dissolved solids as well as gases, a single set of capillaries supplies the tissues with all that they need for activity, growth, and repair, besides removing most of the waste products. The carbon dioxide produced in the tissues is mainly carried, not in solution as such (CO_2), but in combination as sodium bicarbonate ($NaHCO_3$).

If we look at a drop of blood under a microscope we see that it consists of a clear fluid full of little reddish-yellow biscuit-shaped bodies about 0.007 millimetre in diameter. They can just be seen with a powerful hand-lens. A cubic millimetre of blood contains about five million, and as a man has about 4 litres of blood the total number in his body is about 20 million million, or far more than the number of men who have lived since history began, or probably at all. Their total surface is about 1,500 times the surface of the body.

All the haemoglobin of the blood is contained in them, and they therefore carry round the oxygen from the tissues. Their huge surface area renders this exchange easy. They are cells which have lost their nucleus and are therefore not fully alive, but act as passive carriers of oxygen. They are always being produced in large numbers in the bone-marrow, and destroyed in the spleen and liver when worn out.

For every 500 or so of these red corpuscles there is one white corpuscle. They are true cells with nuclei, and some of them are capable of active movements. There are at least six different kinds with different functions, mostly of a protective character.

Thus one kind eat up parasites found in the blood, another kind burrow through the walls of capillaries in inflamed areas, and remove dead or injured tissue and disease-germs, often forming collections of 'matter' or pus. Others produce substances which kill disease-germs, and so on. The blood also contains non-cellular bodies called platelets, which are smaller than the corpuscles and are concerned in clotting and in immunity; there may also be tiny drops of oil after a fatty meal. Besides the blood-vessels, all vertebrates possess another system of vessels which open into the veins, but contain clear fluid called lymph.

The lymphatic vessels slowly drain away fluid from the spaces between the cells. On the course of the vessels the fluid passes through small lymph-nodes or glands, which may be felt under the skin in the neck, armpit, or groin, before entering the blood. The lymph contains white corpuscles which are largely produced in these glands, and abnormal bodies from the tissues are dealt with in them. Thus if the arm is inflamed, the lymph-nodes of the armpit are generally enlarged, as they are busy destroying poisons or bacteria from the inflamed tissue.

The lymphatics also play a part in digestion, which we shall study later. We must now see how the cells obtain the food-stuffs which they require. In simple animals such as polyps every cell is so close to the digestive cavity that it can obtain food thence directly. In most higher animals, however, the cells which line the alimentary canal and its glands are highly specialized for the purpose of breaking up the food-stuffs into soluble forms and passing them rapidly into the blood or other body-fluids.

This process is called digestion. A few internal parasites like the tapeworm have no gut, but absorb their food through their skin, relying on their host to break it up for them. The course of digestion in man is as follows. The food is chewed in the mouth, where it is also moistened by saliva, a fluid secreted mainly by three neighbouring pairs of glands. Two pairs of these lie between the tongue and the lower jaw, the third pair (whose inflammation causes mumps) lie below the external ear, mainly inside the lower jaw-bone.

Besides moistening the food, saliva contains an enzyme, ptyalin, which breaks up starch into an easily soluble sugar called maltose. Enzymes play a much larger part in digestion than do mechanical processes. Each digestive enzyme is a definite substance with the property of bringing about, or enormously speeding up, a particular chemical reaction.

Pepsin from the stomach will split up half a million times its weight of protein, but will not alter starch or fat. So delicately is an enzyme adjusted to the substrate on which it acts, that as most food molecules are asymmetrical (as we know from their rotation of the plane of polarized light and their asymmetrical crystals) so are the enzymes that act on them.

Enzymes have been compared to keys which open certain locks only. But they are like 'Yale' rather than ordinary keys. For we can make in the laboratory a sugar or peptide (part of a protein molecule) which only differs from the natural variety in that its molecules are related to the natural molecules as a left hand to a right or an object to its image in a mirror. Enzymes will not act on these artificial substances, though they digest their mirror-images which occur in nature. So Alice, who went through the looking-glass in the story, could not have digested the looking-glass proteins and carbohydrates.

She would have had to get her energy from fat and alcohol, whose molecules are symmetrical, and would finally have died of protein starvation. Enzymes are not alive, and can still work when removed from the body; but they are generally destroyed by boiling. The action of ptyalin can easily be shown. A solution of boiled starch gives a blue colour with iodine.

If saliva is allowed to act on it for a few minutes at body-temperature or a few hours in the cold, the starch is broken down to sugar and loses this property. If the saliva is first boiled no change occurs. When the food is swallowed, it is passed into the gullet or oesophagus. To get there it must pass over the mouth of the wind-pipe, and when any falls down this we choke.

To prevent this, the breathing is stopped while we swallow, and the cartilages at the top of the wind-pipe which are concerned in voice-production are brought together so as to close the top of the larynx. It is further protected by a cartilaginous lid at the back of the tongue called the epiglottis, which is pressed backwards over it by the food during swallowing. The movements of the laryngeal cartilages can easily be felt. As the food leaves the mouth it passes out of the control of consciousness and will. The movements of our digestive canal, except at the two ends, are carried out by smooth or involuntary muscle and are controlled by a special part of the nervous system over which the mind does not preside. The food or drink on leaving the mouth is seized by the smooth muscle of the oesophagus, which contracts behind it and relaxes in front, thus passing it rapidly down into the stomach. Owing to this gripping action one can eat or drink while standing on one's head.

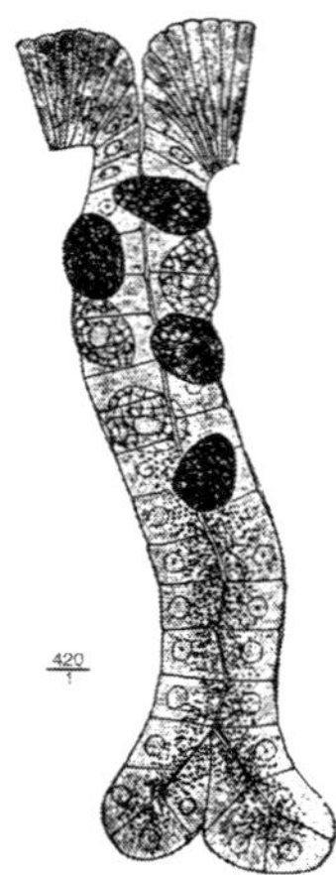

Fig. A Simple Gland From The Stomach of a Bat.

The narrow duct opens above into the cavity of the stomach, among columnar cells. The main part of the gland is a simple tube, formed of a single layer of cells; these secrete pepsin. A few darker-stained cells are seen near the outer side of the tube; these probably secrete hydrochloric acid.

The human stomach is a bag of smooth muscle lined with a membrane consisting mainly of microscopic glands. When expanded it will generally hold about 2 litres. The gastric juice is a clear fluid containing about ½ per cent. free HCl, and several enzymes, of which the most important is pepsin. In presence of acid (though not in a neutral or alkaline fluid), pepsin causes proteins to break up into bodies called peptones and proteoses, which have very much smaller molecules than the proteins from which they are derived, and are more soluble.

Some carbohydrates are attacked by the hydrochloric acid. Thus each molecule of cane-sugar is split into one of glucose and one of fructose, and inulin, a starch-like body found in many plants, is broken up into fructose. Fats are less affected in the stomach. A meal remains in the stomach for a time—generally between one and four hours—which depends on the nature and quantity of the food taken. All this time the muscular walls of the organ are contracting in such a way as to mix the food thoroughly with the gastric juice. Hardly any absorption occurs in the stomach.

When its contents are fully mixed the muscular ring surrounding the lower orifice of the stomach, the pylorus, opens, and a jet of its contents is squirted into the duodenum, the top portion of the small intestine. After a heavy meal the stomach may take several hours in emptying itself.

The human small intestine is a tube about 6 metres long and 3 cm. in diameter when relaxed. It is lined by fine projections of the mucous membrane, the villi, which give it a velvety texture, and increase tenfold the surface available for absorption. Between the bases of the villi are the mouths of numerous microscopic glands, and just beyond the pylorus open the ducts of two large glands, the liver and pancreas.

The liver, among its other functions, secretes bile. This contains substances which have the property, possessed in a less degree by soap, of lowering the surface-tension of water in which they are dissolved. Drops of oil or melted fat tend to join up so as to have as small a surface as possible. This tendency of the surface to shrink is prevented by the bile in the intestine, so when fat-drops are broken up there they do not coalesce again, but form a milky emulsion. Hence the fat-splitting enzyme made in the pancreas can act on a vastly greater surface of fat than would otherwise be available. A man with jaundice from a blocked bile-duct can digest milk, whose fat is already broken up, but not suet or butter, which form big drops.

The bile also contains pigments formed from the haemoglobin of worn-out red corpuscles. These are excreted in the faeces and give them their yellow colour. In jaundice the bile-duct is blocked, and accordingly the skin becomes yellow and the faeces white. Bile is stored in the gall-bladder till required.

The pancreas secretes a juice containing a number of enzymes. One of these, like ptyalin, breaks down starch into maltose. Others break down maltose to glucose, and lactose (milk-sugar) into glucose and galactose, a very similar substance. Another breaks down fat into glycerol and fatty acids, which partly combine with alkali to form soap.

In every case the molecules formed will pass more easily through a membrane than those of the food. If the juice contained a protein-splitting enzyme it would probably digest the pancreas itself and its duct. However, it contains a substance which, on mixing with the secretions of the intestinal glands, yields trypsin, an enzyme which attacks proteins and the products of peptic digestion, breaking them down into amino-acids. These enzymes will not act in an acid fluid, so the bile and pancreatic and intestinal juices contain enough sodium bicarbonate to neutralize the acid of the gastric juice. The secretion of the intestinal glands, besides the substance which helps to form trypsin, contains an enzyme which will break down peptones, though not whole protein molecules, into amino-acids.

There are also enzymes which break down milk-sugar and cane-sugar to sugars containing only six carbon atoms. So far as we know, no animal more complicated than a snail produces an enzyme which will break up cellulose. But grass consists very largely of cellulose, and to digest it hoofed animals and other plant-eaters employ bacteria which grow in their digestive canal. In cud-chewers like the cow and sheep these bacteria live in special compartments of the stomach; in the horse in the large intestine, which may have a capacity of 200 litres. The bacteria can get very little oxygen, so they cannot oxidize the cellulose, but they turn a good deal of it into methane, which is wasted, and leave much undigested. The rest, however, is broken up into small molecules which the animal can absorb. In man, cellulose is not digested, but it is useful in giving bulk to the faeces and preventing constipation, which easily occurs when the food leaves no indigestible residue. The food is thus broken up into easily soluble constituents, and is ready to be absorbed. This is done by the epithelium of the small intestine. The passage through is not a mere filtration. For example, the blood contains one part of sugar per thousand, and if sugar merely filtered across from gut to blood, it could never quite disappear from the gut as it in fact does.

Actually, during the absorption of food, the absorptive cells perform work, for which they need an extra supply of oxygen. The fats are, in part at least, put together again from glycerine and soap, and passed as a fine milky emulsion into the lacteals, as the lymphatics of the small gut are called. These join together to form the thoracic duct, which runs up through the chest and empties into the jugular vein at the base of the neck.

The blood may be noticeably milky after a heavy meal of fat. The rest of the products of digestion are passed into the capillaries, and dissolved in the blood. All the veins from the gut run to the liver, and here the food is further dealt with. Thus sugar, if not needed immediately for oxidation, is stored as a starchy body called glycogen, discovered by Claude Bernard, and gradually liberated as required later on.

Some of the sugar and most of the fat are stored elsewhere. Part of the sugar is stored as glycogen in muscles, but much of it is made into fat and stored under the skin and round some of the internal organs, along with fat from the food. In the frog fat is stored in special fat-bodies. The stored glycogen is later split up into glucose for use in the body by an enzyme, which continues to work after death, and the sugar thus liberated gives liver its well-known sweet taste. Absolutely fresh liver is not sweet. Again, ammonia, which is formed in the digestion of many proteins, is, in the liver, mostly combined with carbon dioxide to form urea ($2\ NH_3 + CO_2 = CON_2H_4 + H_2O$).

Urea is a very innocuous body, but ammonia rather poisonous if it gets to the brain, so that if the blood from the gut is short-circuited into the vena cava instead of going into the liver, a heavy meal of meat may cause convulsions. The liver also deals on the same sort of lines with any excess of amino-acids in the blood and with various poisons; its most important function is thus the regulation of the blood's composition, and not the secretion of bile. During starvation the body lives on its stores of fat, and the liver takes on the new duty of converting the stable fats such as those of suet into oils like that of linseed, which are very easily oxidized. The unabsorbed residue of the food from the small intestine passes into the large intestine, where it remains in man for a day or so, and is acted on by bacteria.

These are of little or no value to man, though very valuable to some animals. In man little but water is absorbed there. By this removal of water the bulk of the waste food is reduced by about nine-tenths. The large intestine also excretes poorly soluble salts, such as calcium phosphate, from the blood. These would clog up the urinary passages if they were excreted by the kidneys. The active tissues take oxygen, sugar, fat, and aminoacids from the blood, and use them for oxidation, growth, and repair. Into the blood they empty waste-products, of which the most important are water, carbon dioxide, and urea, but other soluble waste-products of protein metabolism include sulphuric and phosphoric acids, creatinine, and uric acid.

The last two contain C, H, O, and N. They are all excreted by the kidney except the carbon dioxide and some of the water, which go out by the lungs, and, in the case of water, the skin. The kidneys consist of a mass of tubules (about a million on each side in man) each beginning in a capsule containing a tuft of capillaries, and ending, after a winding course, in the central cavity of the kidney.

The capillary tuft seems to act as a filter, and the fluid that soaks through it is blood minus corpuscles and minus a few of the large molecules, such as the proteins concerned in clotting. As this filtrate runs down the tubules, the cells lining them reabsorb valuable constituents of the blood, such as sugar, and probably add unwanted ones such as urea, ammonia, uric acid, creatinine, and sulphates. The urine trickles down the ureters into the bladder, whence it is emptied from time to time.

An adult man produces on an average about 1.5 litres of urine per day, containing 30 grams of urea, 15 of sodium chloride, and 10 of other soluble waste-products. The blood is thus the medium of exchange between the different parts of the body. The heart keeps it moving, the lungs and gut supply it with fresh oxygen and foodstuffs, other organs get rid of waste products, and all the tissues of the body take from it according to their needs. The life of every part of the organism therefore depends on an adequate supply of blood of proper composition.

BODY TEMPERATURE

In humans and other mammals, temperature regulation represents the balance between heat production from metabolic sources and heat loss from evaporation (perspiration) and the processes of radiation, convection, and conduction. In a cold environment, body heat is conserved first by constriction of blood vessels near the body surface and later by waves of muscle contractions, or shivering, which serve to increase metabolism. Shivering can result in a maximum fivefold increase in metabolism. Below about 40°F (4°C) a naked person cannot sufficiently increase the metabolic rate to replace heat lost to the environment. Another heat-conserving mechanism, goose bumps, or piloerection, raises the body hairs; although not especially effective in humans, in animals it increases the thickness of the insulating fur or feather layer.

In a warm environment, heat must be dissipated to maintain body temperature. In humans, increased surface blood flow, especially to the limbs, acts to dissipate heat at the surface. At environmental temperatures above 93°F (34°C), or at lower temperatures when metabolism has been increased by work, heat must be lost through the evaporation of the water in sweat. People in active work may lose as much as 4 quarts per hour for short periods. However, when the temperature and humidity are both high, evaporation is slowed, and sweating is not effective. Most mammals do not have sweat glands but keep cool by panting (evaporation through the respiratory tract) and by increased salivation and skin and fur licking.

Temperature regulatory mechanisms act through the autonomic nervous system and are largely controlled by the hypothalamus of the brain, which responds to stimuli from nerve receptors in the skin. Continued exposure to heat or cold results in some slow acclimatization, e.g., more active sweating in response to continued heat and an increase in subcutaneous fat deposits in response to continued cold.

Environmental extremes may result in failure to maintain normal body temperature. In both increased body temperature, or hyperthermia, and decreased body temperature, or hypothermia, death may result. Controlled hypothermia is used in some types of surgery to temporarily decrease the metabolic rate. Fever, caused by a resetting of the temperature regulatory mechanism, is a response to fever-causing, or pyrogenic, substances, such as bacterial endotoxins or leucocyte extracts. The upper limit of body temperature compatible with survival is about 107°F (42°C), while the lower limit varies.

In humans the inner body temperature alternates in daily activity cycles; it is usually lowest in early morning and is slightly higher at the late afternoon peak. In human females there is also a monthly temperature variation related to the ovulatory cycle. In many mammals and birds the body temperature shows more pronounced cyclic variations than in humans. For example, in hibernators the body temperature may lower to only a few degrees above the environmental temperature during the dormant periods; mammalian hibernators reawake spontaneously and in their active period are homeothermic.

The body must be kept at a constant temperature, within a small range, in order for all of the systems to work properly. This is the normal body temperature. A change in the temperature of the body is a sign of ill health.

All mammals are endothermic—they maintain and regulate their own body temperature. Living in widespread environments around the world, mammals face daily and seasonal fluctuations in temperatures and some—for example those living in harsh arctic or tropical habitats—face extreme cold or heat. To maintain their correct body temperature, mammals must be able to produce and conserve body heat in colder temperatures as well as dissipate exess body heat in warmer temperatures.

In a healthy individual, body temperature is kept constant in a very small range despite of big differences in temperature of the surroundings and also those in physical activity. Very perfect regulation of body temperature, necessary for optimal progress of enzymatic reactions, is developed in all homoiotermic animals. It doesn't apply to poikilothermic animals. During the most variable changes in human organism, the body temperature may increase. Fever is a natural reaction during a number of illnesses. In several cases, absence of the natural reaction is more alarming sign than the presence of fever itself. Fever is usually accompanied by different general symptoms, such as sweating, chills, sensation of cold, and other subjective sensations. Missing of these symptoms during high temperature may be a sign of a serious illness.

The main task in heat production has thermogenesis caused by the effect of thyroid hormones. Hormones of thyroid gland stimulate Na^{+}–$^{+}$ATP-ase found in cytoplasmic membranes. Increased production of heat is achieved by increasing the metabolic processes in which energy is released in the form of heat. The greatest importance is splitting of ATP when 54kJ are released from one mol of ATP. Skeletal muscles, liver, splanchnic organs, and brain are the biggest producers of heat in an organism. In the heat production the muscles have especially important role. Because of their weight, they are able to produce very large amount of heat very quickly. Increased production of heat takes place in skeletal muscles during increased physical activity.

During the digestion, an increased production of heat occurs also in the GIT. Constant body temperature is achieved by perfect nervous regulation. Nervous system maintains the optimal intensity of metabolism and at the same time regulates the amount of heat loss. In early postnatal development, the thermoregulation is inadequate because of immature CNS. Fever is always achieved by reset the centre of thermoregulation to higher values. Hyperthermia means overheating of an organism caused only by exogenic causes (*e.g*. hot environment, hot bath). In this case the centre of thermoregulation doesn't change its setting up.

Heat is lost from an organism in several ways. The biggest loss is by conduction. It depends on the gradient between the body temperature and the temperature of the surrounding environment. The second way is by radiation. The third way is by evaporation. It is used especially during increased production of heat. Distribution of heat is done by blood circulation. Heat goes from each cell to the surrounding liquid and afterwards to the circulated blood. Modulating factor of heat loss is the amount of blood that circulates through the body surface.

The big flow through the subcutaneous area and the skin secures the income of heat that may be given to the environment through the body surface.

Sweating helps delivering the heat. Sweat glands are controlled by cholinergic impulses through the sympathetic fibres. During intensive sweating, up to one litre of sweat may be formed. When the humidity of the environment is higher, a loss of heat by sweating is easier. When it is necessary to accumulate the heat in an organism, adrenergic stimuli cause reduction of the blood flow through the skin. The skin becomes an isolator decreasing the heat loss to minimum. Control mechanisms regulate the production of heat and its loss. Production and handover (loss) of heat are controlled from the centre in the hypothalamus.

It works on the principle of negative feedback control and includes:

- Receptors registrating central temperature
- Effector mechanisms composed of vasomotors, metabolic effectors, and controls of sweat glands
- Structures recording whether the actual temperature is not too high or too low

Increased central temperature activates mechanisms enabling the heat loss. Low central temperature activates mechanisms enabling the accumulation of heat. These mechanisms work as the thermostat. In healthy individuals, the body temperature (oral temperature) is somewhere between 36.5°C and 37.5°C. It slightly increases during the day since the morning (from 6:00 a.m.). The peak is reached at 6:00 to 10:00 p.m. The lowest temperature is between 2:00 and 4:00 a.m. Diurnal variation depends on the activity throughout the day.

Diurnal variations don't change in persons that work at night and sleep during the day. Such a diurnal variation is also kept when fever occurs. Fever reaches the peak in the evening, and in the morning even a very sick patient may have almost normal temperature. Body temperature changes are more intensive in young person than in old people. The temperature may slightly or temporarily increase in hot environment. Physical activity may also increase the body temperature. In extreme effort, the increase may be very high. The temperature in marathon runners may increase to 39°C to 41°C. The temperature may increase slightly if vasodilatation, hyperventilation, and other compensation mechanisms fail. Small increase in temperature may occur if the surrounding temperature is lower or the jogging is done early in the morning.

Organism uses simple mechanism for temperature regulation. It is the blood flow through the skin and subcutaneous area. Vasoconstriction allows the increased accumulation of heat, and vasodilation secures its quick loss. Changes in temperature up to 3°C don't cause an interuption of physiological functions. Spasms may occur during high fever in children. If the body temperature is increased over 42.2°C, irreversible changes in the brain occur. In humans the temperature usually doesn't overcome 41.1°C. Uncontrolled decrease in temperature below 32.8°C is accompanied by confusions and gradual loss of consciousness. If the decrease continues under 30°C, the fibrilation of ventricles occur that is the sign of fatal termination of this condition.

Brown fat that differs from the white one in structure and sites of location has an important function in thermogenesis in newborns and children. It is found between scapulas, on the neck, in axils, around the aorta and the kidneys. It is highly vascularized, and it has large mitochondria in its cells.

One could say that while the white fat acts as feather-bed, the brown one is an electrical pillow. Receptors of cold conduct the information to the centre of thermoregulation. From this centre the impulses run in the sympathetic nerve fibres and lead to the release of norepinephrine in the brown fat. Norepinephrine activates the enzyme lipase. Activated lipase splits the fat to glycerol and free fatty acids (FFA) and the heat is released. Glycerol and FFA remain in the cell and can perform the resynthesis after some time. An adult person has little brown fat.

HEAT PRODUCTION

The mechanisms mammals have for producing heat include shivering, cellular metabolism, and circulatory adaptations. At some point in our lives, we've all shivered. Shivering generates heat as muscles quickly contract and shake. Cellular metabolism is the chemical breakdown process that occurs within cells.

This process releases heat and warms the body. Circulatory adaptations, such as countercurrent heat exchange introduced above, transfer heat from the core of the animal's body to the periphery by specially designed blood flow paths. Warmer blood from the interior of the animal flows to cold extremities, thereby moderating the temperature of the more exposed limb.

Warmth is one of the necessities of life. Vital activities are possible only between certain narrowly defined limits of temperature. Cold inhibits and excessive heat suspends them. Body heat is energy. It is employed not just in resisting cold, but also in accelerating cellular activities. Temperature, within certain narrow limits, is so absolutely essential to life that all functions are excited by any attempt at its variation. Animals are roughly divided into two major classes: warm-blooded and cold-blooded.

This is according to whether they have means of producing and maintaining their own temperature or are dependent upon the surrounding medium (water or air) to provide it. The invertebrates, although they breathe oxygen and circulate fluids throughout their bodies, have no red blood corpuscles and are cold-blooded animals. Fishes and reptiles, vertebrates with red blood cells, are also called cold-blooded animals, although they are able to maintain an internal temperature above that of the surrounding water or air. Invertebrates have no heat of their own, but receive their temperature from the surrounding media and adapt to it. Except for fishes and reptiles, whose heat-producing and heat-regulating powers are very limited, we may say that all vertebrates are warm-blooded, having red corpuscles, while the reverse is true of the invertebrates which have no red corpuscles.

It may be suggested that since animals can live without red corpuscles and exist without internal heat, the primary office of respiration is more universal than to provide for the production of animal heat. Using a popular phrase in biology, heat production is only a "secondary adaptation." If we look at a large number of lower animals, we find them to be small and living in water. This medium directly and powerfully reduces them to its own temperature, and they are surrounded and permeated with water. In the radiata water actually mingles in large quantities with their digested food, so that they must of necessity remain at or very near water temperature.

Even if they possessed sources of heat within themselves, it becomes evident that heat production cannot be the great end of respiration in these animals. Its primary function must be something very different from this. If we take a second look at these animals, we discover that large numbers of them, especially those that live in fresh water, vary in temperature with the medium in which they live. Often they vary to a great extent, being sometimes near the freezing point and at other times fifty to one hundred degrees above it. Although a particular temperature may be best for each of them, still, many of them can live an active life in temperatures seventy, sixty, fifty and even forty degrees less.

It is obvious that to a small extent they could raise the temperature of their bodies above that of the water, when it is forty or fifty degrees, would be of no great importance. In their case at least, there must be some more important end for respiration than production of heat. Heat supplies a necessary condition of vital activity.

The activities of cold-blooded animals rise and fall as the temperature goes up or down. The higher the temperature, providing it does not go so high so as to destroy life, the greater the activity. If it becomes very cold, they suspend activity. It is not in inorganic chemistry alone that heat promotes the energy and intensity of action.

In "vital chemistry," that is, in living functions, the same phenomenon is observed. An elevation of temperature accelerates all vital functions, both in the cold-blooded and in the warm-blooded animals. A similar thing is seen in plants.

Acceleration of activity increases with the rise in temperature until the temperature reaches a certain variable optimum, after which any added increase in temperature reduces activity. The rate of activity for some of the lower forms may become so great as the temperature rises that they "live too fast" and wear themselves out. When temperature is lowered, vital activities are lowered.

In the cold-blooded animals, some of which may be frozen for long periods and then revived, all activity ceases after the temperature is reduced below a certain variable minimum. Most of the warm-blooded animals die when frozen, their vital activities ceasing before they reach the state of freezing. Higher animals are not so dependent upon the surround-ing temperature.

They are not only equipped with internal sources of heat and mechanisms to control its production and radiation, but they also in most instances have outer coats of hair, feathers or wool to protect them from the cold. They possess means of lowering heat production and increasing heat radiation if the external temperature or their own internal heat due to activity is increased. (By the operation of the same internal heat-regulating mechanism they produce fever when needed.)

Thus, while the very form and habits of the lower orders of life are determined by external surroundings, the forms and habits of life of the higher animals are very largely determined by powers within them. These often prevail over powerful antagonistic forces.

The lower animals are more or less slaves to the external world; the higher animals make the external world serve them. It should be noted that this independence of the higher animals, this internal energy, is in great measure due to a capacity for maintaining their normal temperatures amid the changes in that of the surrounding water and air. The uniform temperatures maintained by higher animals promote and secure a constancy, precision and energy in the nutrition of their tissues, and in the vital functions that supply the animal with resources to carry on active life in the face of opposing influences in the world. A brief glance at the method of maintaining body temperature may be helpful. In respiration we learned of the office of oxidation in the production of heat.

It is necessary that we understand that the body is capable of both increasing and decreasing its rate of heat production as the external temperature falls or rises. These processes are rigidly controlled by the nervous system and fail only in greatly enervated and diseased organisms. But the body also increases and decreases the radiation of heat from the body as need arises. While oxidation warms the body, evaporation (as in sweating) cools it. These physiological processes are carried on in relation to vital wants.

The human body, to narrow our considera-tions at this point, is based upon a system of self-regulation and equipoise, and its temperature relations are beautifully provided for. In a cool atmosphere less heat is lost by evaporation and more produced within the body, while a reverse process is seen in a warm temperature. In all changes of temperature outside the body, some compensatory effort is required. But if our other relations are correct, the internal heat-regulating capacity of the body will be efficient.

The maintenance of the heat-making mechanism of the body is an indispensable condition of health. Feeble and sick individuals who find it difficult or impossible to maintain normal temperature in a cold climate need to be kept warm. Chilling inhibits all functions of life and reduces their already greatly reduced stock of energy. The escape to a warm climate is no mere luxury for such persons. Warmth of some degree is certainly a normal requisite of life. But experience and experiment have shown that when the temperature of the surroundings is out of all proportion to the needs of the body and to its capacity to adjust itself, the body must and does suffer. There is not only discomfort, which normally causes us to seek relief from extremes of heat or cold, but there is some expenditure of energy in resisting extreme temperature.

In lands where fogs, frost and darkness cramp the energies of man, as well as in regions where excessive and long-continued heat depresses his vital activities, life is handicapped. By means of clothing, housing and artificial heating arrangements, we are able to live in cold climates. By means of cooling systems and a reduction of clothing, we live more comfortably in hot regions and seasons. But none of these arrangements are ideal. A warm climate serves man best; first-class habits of living enable him to live better in whatever climate he resides.

DISIPATING HEAT

In warmer climates, excess body heat can accumulate and cause life-threatening problems for a mammal. Circulation near the skin's surface releases heat into the environment. Moisture from sweat glands or respiratory surfaces evaporates and cools the animal. Unfortunately, evaporative cooling is less effective in dry climates where water loss is also costly for mammals. In such situations, mammals often seek cover during the hotter daylight hours and resume active at night.

MUSCLE DISORDERS

The structural and functional unit of skeletal muscle is the motor unit. It consists of a ventral motor neuron with its cell body in the central horn of the spinal cord and its peripheral axon, the neuromuscular junction, and the muscle fibres innervated by the neuron. Each of these components must be functionally intact for the muscle to contract properly. The ventral motor neuron is the final common pathway conducting neural impulses from the CNS to the muscle.

The transmission of a nerve impulse at the neuromuscular junction involves massive release of acetylcholine from small synaptic vessels, where it is stored. The acetylcholine fills the synaptic cleft between the nerve terminal and the muscle fibre membrane, where most of it is destroyed by cholinesterase within a fraction of a second. This short period of activity is sufficient to excite the muscle fibre membrane, which results in a significant increase in membrane permeability to sodium ions and allows rapid influx of sodium into the muscle fibre.

The sodium ion increases the endplate potential, which elicits electrical currents that spread to the interior of the fibres, where they cause a release of calcium ions from the sarcoplasmic reticulum. The calcium ions initiate, in turn, the chemical events of the contractile process. When this occurs in all the muscle fibres innervated by each motor neuron (possibly thousands), muscle contraction results.

Normal muscle, comprising many motor units, is dynamic, and its function and structure can be influenced by many diseases. Complete paralysis, paresis, or ataxia may be caused by primary muscular dysfunctions of infectious, toxic, or congenital origin.

However, in most instances the primary disorder can be attributed to the nervous system (eg, tetanus, rhinopneumonitis, canine distemper, protozoal myelitis), with the muscular system merely representing the effector organ. Disorders that affect the neuromuscular junction (eg, myasthenia gravis, hypocalcemia, hypermagnesemia) can result in muscle fatigue, weakness, and paralysis.

The neuromuscular junction can also be affected by muscle-relaxing drugs (eg, curare, succinylcholine, M99), certain antibiotics, and toxins (eg, botulism, tetanus, venoms).

Disorders primarily of the muscle membrane and, to some extent, of the actual muscle fibres are called myopathies. Muscle membrane disorders may be hereditary (eg, myotonia congenita in goats) or acquired (eg, vitamin E and selenium deficiencies, hypothyroidism, and hypokalemia). Myopathies involving the actual muscle fibre components include muscular dystrophy, polymyositis, eosinophilic myositis, white muscle disease, and exertional rhabdomyolysis.

Various laboratory tests, eg, histopathologic examination, determination of serum enzyme levels, electromyographic studies, thermography, and determinations of conduction velocity, are very useful in confirmation of a specific diagnosis.

MUSCULOSKELETAL SYSTEM, SKIN AND KIDNEYS

This profile line is distinguished by a number of specific research projects: The Small Animal Clinic, in cooperation with various institutions of the Department of Medicine - Charité - University Medicine Berlin and the Institute of Immunology and Molecular Biology, the Institute of Veterinary Biochemistry, and the Institute of Veterinary Pathology, conducts biochemical, immunological, and histopathological analyses of joint disorders in dogs.

The operation of a high-performance multilayer computer tomography system at the Small Animal Clinic, which is part of a cooperative arrangement with the Leibniz-Institute for Zoo and Wild Animal Research (IZW), offers outstanding possibilities for research into joint diseases and disorders. In addition, studies of other diseases and disorders of the musculoskeletal system (examples: healing of fractures, osteoarthritis) are the focus of research both at the Equine Clinic: Surgery, and Radiology and at the Small Animal Clinic, in cooperation with the Institutes of Veterinary Pathology and Veterinary Biochemistry. The search for new diagnostic markers for diseases such as osteoarthritis in animals including dogs and horses is another important goal of the research conducted in this area. In addition, the Institute of Veterinary Anatomy, the Institute of Veterinary Pathology, and the Small Animal Clinic all examine and analyze how various tumors are caused in domestic animals.

MEAT ON THE BONES

Many advanced animals have muscular systems. You know you do. Did you know that your muscular system is made up of three different types of muscular tissue? You have smooth, cardiac, and voluntary muscle tissue in your body. Smooth muscle is muscle you rarely control such as the muscle in your intestinal tract.

Cardiac muscle is very specific tissue found in your heart. Voluntary muscle is the muscle that helps you move. All of those tissues add up to a muscular system that is found through your body. There is more to the muscular system than the muscles that help you move.

WHAT DOES THIS SYSTEM DO?

The big purpose of the muscles found in your body is movement. We could be talking about the movement of your legs while you walk. We could be talking about the beating of your heart. We could also be talking about the contraction of a very small blood vessel in your brain.

You have no control over most of the muscular system. You do control the voluntary muscle in your arms, legs, neck, and torso. You have little or no control over the heart or smooth muscle. Those other muscles are under the control of the autonomic nervous system (ANS).

INTERACTING WITH OTHER SYSTEMS

We just teased the fact that your muscular system is closely connected to the nervous system. That makes sense since you usually have to think before you can move. Even though thinking is not always involved, the neurons of the nervous system are connected to most of the cells in your muscular system. You have smooth muscles that line your digestive system and help move food through your intestines. Smooth muscle also surrounds your circulatory system and lymph system. Those muscle tissues are spread throughout your body and are even involved in controlling the temperature of your body.

MUSCLES HELP YOU MOVE

The main parts of your voluntary muscular system include the muscles, and tendons. The muscle is called the meatus. It happens to be the meat you eat from cows, sheep, and includes the muscle in your biceps. So your bicep it the meat, that meat needs to connect to the bones so that you can move. Tendons connect your muscles to your bone at insertion points.

When the actin and myosin contract in the muscles, the muscle shortens and the bones are pulled closer together. Muscles called flexors force your joints to bend. Muscles called extensors cause your limbs to straighten. A bicep is a flexor and the triceps are extensors. You may have also heard of ligaments. They are batches of connective tissue that bind bones to each other. Muscles, tendons, and ligaments can been found working together in almost all of your joints.

8

Functions of the Nervous System

NERVOUS SYSTEM

Animals are the only living things on Earth with complex nervous systems that first receive and interpret sensory signals from the environment and then send out messages to direct the animal's response.

The complexity of an animal's nervous system depends on its lifestyle and body plan:

- Animals whose bodies don't have a defined head or tail have nerve nets,which are weblike arrangements of nerve cells that extend throughout the body.
- Animals with a defined head possess a two-part nervous system:
- The central nervous system (CNS) consists of the animal's brain and central neurons. It's housed in the head and may continue along the back.
- The peripheral nervous system (PNS) consists of all the nerves that travel from the CNS to the rest of the animal's body.

In all animals with a backbone, including you, the CNS consists of a brain and a spinal cord. The brain contains centers that process information from the sense organs, centers that control emotions and intelligence, and centers that regulate the physiological balance of the body (homeostasis). The spinal cordcontrols the flow of information to and from the brain.

Both the brain and the spinal cord are highly protected. First of all, they sit within a liquid called cerebrospinal fluid that guards the CNS against shocks caused by movement and they're protected by the bones of the skull and vertebrae. CNS also supports the brain and spinal cord by supplying nutrients and helping to remove wastes.

The blood-brain barrier, which is created by the capillaries surrounding the brain, provides yet another layer of protection because the capillaries are highly selective about what they allow to enter the brain or cerebrospinal fluid. A final layer of protection is the meninges, two layers of connective tissue that surround the brain and spinal cord.

The nervous system has three basic functions:

1. *Sensory Function:* To sense changes (known as stimuli) both outside and within the body. For example the eyes sense changes in light and the ear responds to sound waves. Inside the body, stretch receptors in the stomach indicate when it is full and chemical receptors in the blood vessels monitor the acidity of the blood.
2. *Integrative Function:* Processing the information received from the sense organs. The impulses from these organs are analysed and stored as memory. The many different impulses from different sources are sorted, synchronised and co-ordinated and the appropriate response initiated. The power to integrate, remember and apply experience gives higher animals much of their superiority.
3. *Motor Function:* The third function is the response to the stimuli that causes muscles to contract or glands to secrete.

All nervous tissue is made up of nerve cells or neurons. These transmit high-speed signals called nerve impulses. Nerve impulses can be thought of as being similar to an electric current.

THE NEURON

Neurons are cells that have been adapted to carry nerve impulses. A typical neuron has a cell body containing a nucleus, one or more branching filaments called dendriteswhich conduct nerve impulses towards the cell body and one long fibre, an axon, that carries the impulses away from it. Many axons have a sheath of fatty material calledmyelin surrounding them. This speeds up the rate at which the nerve impulses travel along the nerve.

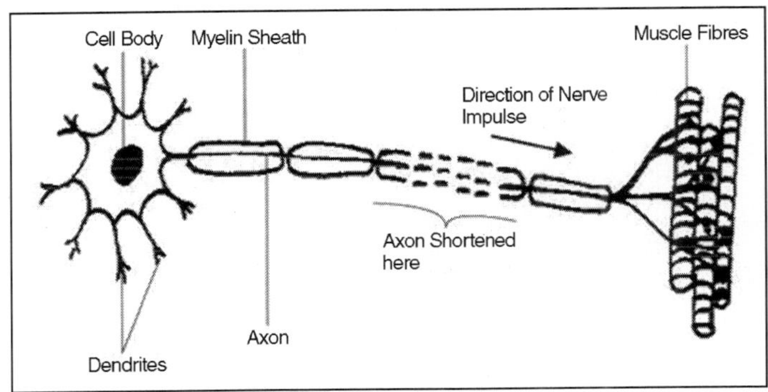

Fig. A Motor Neuron.

The cell body of neurons is usually located in the brain or spinal cord while the axon extends the whole distance to the organ that it supplies. The neuron carrying impulses from the spinal cord to the hind leg or tail of a horse, for example, can be several feet long. A nerve is a bundle of axons.

A sensory neuron is a nerve cell that transmits impulses from a sense receptor such as those in the eye or ear to the brain or spinal cord. A motor neuron is a nerve cell that transmits impulses from the brain or spinal cord to a muscle or gland. A relay neuron connects sensory and motor neurons and is found in the brain or spinal cord.

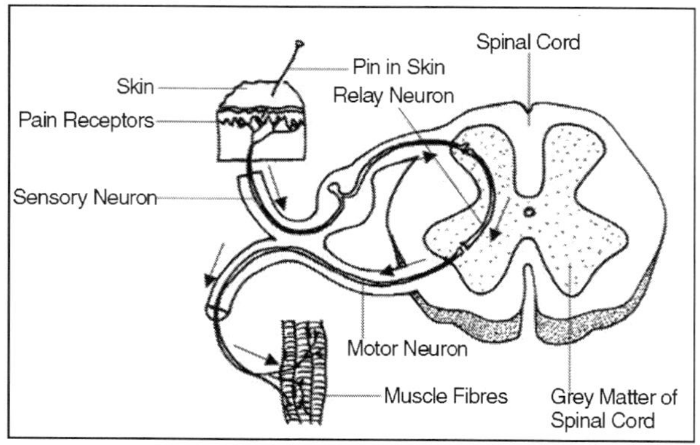

Fig. The Relationship between Sensory, Relay and Motor Neurons.

CONNECTIONS BETWEEN NEURONS

The connection between adjacent neurons is called a synapse. The two nerve cells do not actually touch here for there is a microscopic space between them. The electrical impulse in the neurone before the synapse stimulates the production of chemicals called neurotransmitters (such as acetylcholine), which are secreted into the gap. The neurotransmitter chemicals diffuse across the gap and when they contact the membrane of the next nerve cell they stimulate a new nervous impulse. After the impulse has passed the chemical is destroyed and the synapse is ready to receive the next nerve impulse.

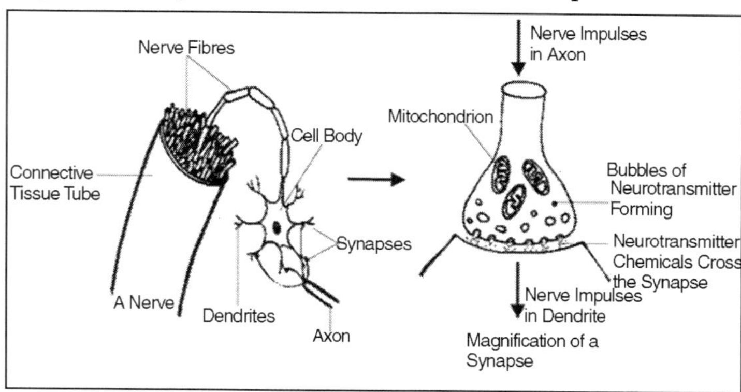

Fig. A Nerve and Magnification of a Synapse.

NERVE NETS IN THE VETERINARY

Cnidarians are radially symmetrical and have the simplest nervous system Nerve network conducts signals from sensory cells to muscle cells. There is no centralization of the nervous system.

CEPHALIZATION AND BILATERAL SYMMETRY

The anterior end of bilaterally symmetrical animals contains most of the sense organs because this end of the animal moves through the environment first. As evolution proceeded, the anterior end of the central nervous system became larger to accommodate these sense organs.

The larger, anterior end of the central nervous system is called the brain. The development of the brain is called *cephalization*; highly cephalized animals have a large brain.

Flatworms

Bilateral symmetry has led to paired structures (nerves, muscles, sense organs, brain). Some flatworms have a nerve net like Cnidarians but others show more organization including a brain and nerve cords.

Planarians

The nervous system of planarians resembles a ladder. It has two nerve cords with ganglia ("a brain") at the anterior end. Sensory receptors are located in the auricles.

The eyespots contain photoreceptors. Transverse nerves that connect the two cords keep movements of the two sides coordinated.

Mollusks

Mollusks show a great diversity of nervous systems. Some mollusks such as bivalves have no cephalization. Slow-moving animals have some cephalization, enabling sensory reception as the animal moves through the environment. The active predatory lifestyle of cephalopods require complex sense organs; they are highly cephalized.

Annelids, Arthropods

Annelids and arthropods have repeating segments and an anterior brain. Each segment contains a ganglion; the nerve cord extends through all of the segments. The ganglion in each segment controls the muscles of that segment. The brain exerts overall control to coordinate the animal.

Echinoderms

Sea stars have a central nerve ring and a nerve that extends from the ring into each arm. Each arm also contains a nerve net.

Vertebrates

Vertebrates have complex sense organs and exhibit complex behaviours. These require a complex nervous system. The vertebrate nervous system is extremely cephalized.

Divisions of the Vertebrate Nervous System

The central nervous system (CNS) is the brain and spinal cord. The peripheral nervous system (PNS) is composed of the nerves and ganglia. Ganglia are clusters of nerve cell bodies outside the CNS.

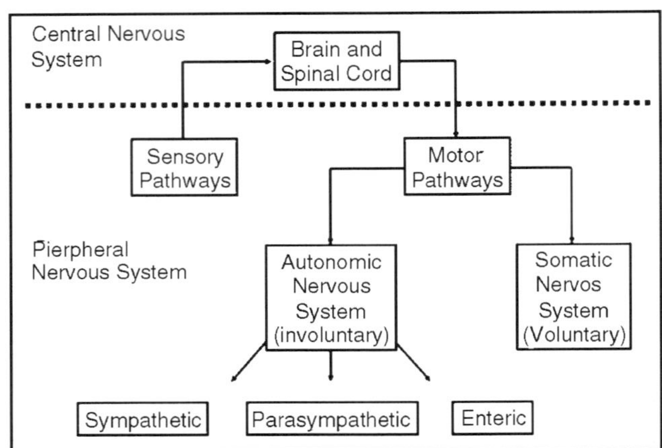

Peripheral Nervous System

Nerves

Nerves are bundles of neurons; either long dendrites and/or long axons. There are no cell bodies in nerves. The cell bodies are in the ganglia (PNS) or nuclei (in gray matter of the CNS). Most nerves contain both kinds of neurons (sensory and motor). The sensory neurons conduct information to the CNS, the motor neurons conduct away from the CNS. All of the neurons in some nerves conduct in the same direction. These nerves contain either sensory or motor neurons.

Cranial Nerves and Spinal Nerves

Cranial nerves are sensory, motor, or mixed, and all but the vagus are involved with the head and neck region; the vagus nerve manages the internal organs. Spinal nerves are all mixed nerves. Their regular arrangement reflects the segmentation of the human body. Spinal nerves are connected to the spinal cord by two branches called roots. The dorsal root contains sensory neurons.

The dorsal root ganglion contains the cell bodies of sensory neurons. Sensory neurons therefore have long dendrites. The ventral root contains motor neurons. Motor neurons have short dendrites and long axons.

Somatic Nervous System

The somatic nervous system provides conscious, voluntary control. It includes all of the nerves that serve the skeletal muscles and the exterior sense organs. It also includes reflexes.

Reflex Arcs

Reflexes are simple, stereotyped and repeatable motor actions (example: movements) brought about by a specific sensory stimulus. The reflex is involuntary but may involve the use of voluntary (skeletal) muscle and nerves.

Reflexes are quick and produce behaviours that are typically beneficial. For example, when you fall, reflex arcs immediately act to extend your arm so that your arm prevents your head and body from hitting the ground.

Some reflexes involve the brain, others do not. A whole series of responses may occur since some sensory neurons stimulate several interneurons which, in turn send impulses to other parts of the CNS. If you were to fall forward, interneurons would use information from the ears to determine the direction of the fall and extend the arms in a forward direction. If you were to fall towards the left side, interneurons would select neurons that activate muscles to extend your arm to the left side.

Example: The stretch reflex

The stretch reflex is involved in helping the body maintain its position without having to consciously think about it. Stretch-sensitive receptors in the muscles contain stretch-gated channels. When the muscle is stretched, the channels open, causing the neuron to depolarize. Action potentials are conducted to the spinal cord. The axon terminals synapse with motor neurons leading right back to the muscles. This causes the muscle to contract to its original position.

Autonomic Nervous System

This part of the nervous system sends signals to the heart, smooth muscle, glands, and all internal organs. It is generally without conscious control. The autonomic nervous system uses two or more motor neurons: The cell body of one of the motor neurons is in the CNS. The cell body of the other one is in a ganglion.

Sympathetic Division

The sympathetic nervous system stimulates the body. For example, it helps prepare the body to deal with emergency situations. This is often called the "fight or flight" response. Stimulation from sympathetic nerves dilates the pupils, accelerates the heartbeat, increases the breathing rate, and inhibits the digestive tract. The neurotransmitter is *norepinephrine*. Sympathetic nerves arise from the middle portion of the spinal cord.

Parasympathetic Division

When there is little stress, the parasympathetic system tends to slow down the overall activity of the body. It causes the pupils to contract, it promotes digestion, and it slows the rate of heartbeat. The neurotransmitter is acetylcholine.

The actual rate of stimulus to each organ is determined by the sum of opposing signals from the sympathetic and parasympathetic systems. Parasympathetic nerves arise from the brain and sacral (near the legs) portion of the cord.

Enteric Division

The enteric division contains neurons that control the digestive tract, pancreas, and gallbladder. Activity of the enteric division is usually regulated by the sympathetic and parasympathetic divisions.

Vertebrate Central Nervous Systems

The central nervous system evolved in vertebrates by adding on to what was there. The oldest parts of the human nervous system deal with reflexes. Newer layers are associated with memory, learning, and thinking. The central nervous system is the brain and spinal cord. It is wrapped in 3 layers of membranes called meninges. Meningitis is an infection of these coverings. The brain contains fluid-filled ventricles that are continuous with the central canal of the cord.

Fluid within the ventricles and central canal originates from the blood. It slowly circulates, carrying nutrients and wastes from cells. The fluid eventually returns to the circulatory system and is replaced by fresh fluid.

Divisions of the Brain

Generally, many body functions involve cells in several areas of the brain. However, certain areas of the brain tend to be more important in some functions while other areas dominate the control of other functions.

Some major parts of the brain are listed below:

- *Hindbrain*: medulla oblongata, cerebellum, pons, Midbrain
- *Forebrain*: thalamus, hypothalamus, cerebrum

Hindbrain

Medulla Oblongata

The medulla controls vital functions such as breathing, heart rate, and blood pressure. It also contains reflexes such as vomiting, coughing, sneezing, hiccupping, swallowing, and digestion. Information that passes between the spinal cord and the rest of the brain must pass through the medulla. In the medulla, sensory and motor axons on the right side cross to the left side and axons on the left side cross to the right side.

As a result, stimuli passing through from the left side of the body are sent to the right side of the brain and signals passing through from the right side of the brain stimulate the left side of the body.

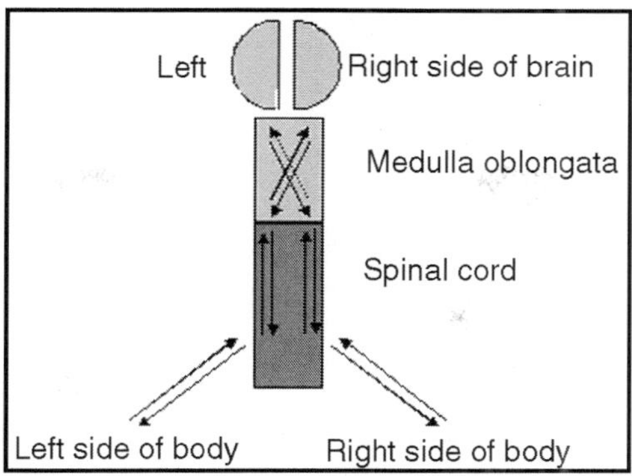

Cerebellum

The cerebellum coordinates and refines complex muscle movements. Movement information that is initiated in higher brain centres (the cerebral cortex) is compared to the actual position of the limbs. The cerebellum then adjusts and refines the movement. It is large in birds because flight requires considerable coordination.

Pons

The pons is involved in some of the same activities as the medulla. For example, it assists the medulla in controlling breathing. The pons functions as a connection between higher brain regions, the cerebellum, and the spinal cord.

Midbrain

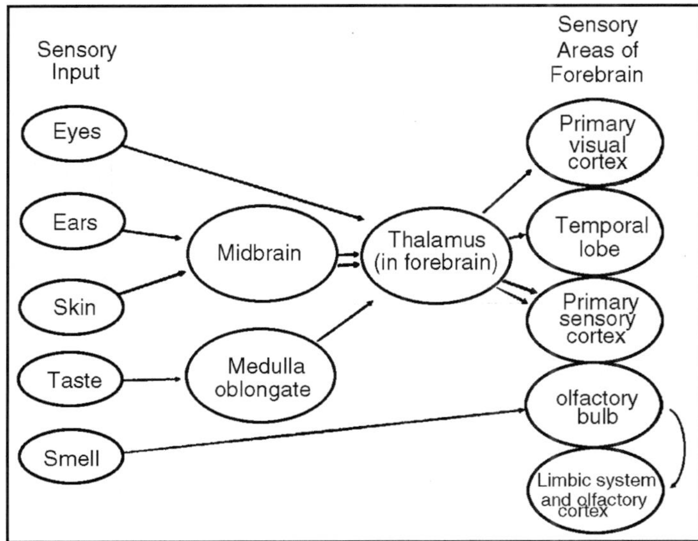

The midbrain receives some sensory information and sends it to the appropriate part of the forebrain. The midbrain originally functioned for reflexes associated with visual input. It is the most prominent part of the brain in fishes and amphibians and has major control of the body. The midbrain of reptiles, birds, and mammals controls visual reflexes such as the pupil response to light intensity but the forebrain of these vertebrates processes the visual information. The midbrain also controls some auditory reflexes and helps control posture.

Brainstem

The medulla oblongata, pons, and midbrain look like the spinal cord and appear to connect the rest of the brain to the spinal cord. They are collectively referred to as the brainstem.

Forebrain

Thalamus

Like the midbrain of mammals, the thalamus serves as a relay area to the cerebrum from other parts of the spinal cord and brain. For example, it receives sensory input (except smell) and sends to appropriate areas of the cerebral cortex. The Thalamus contains part of the reticular formation.

Reticular Formation

The reticular formation is a net of nerve cells extending from the thalamus through the brain stem (midbrain, pons and medulla oblongata) to the spinal cord. It acts as a filter to incoming stimuli and discriminates important from unimportant. Hundreds of millions of sensory receptors flood the brain; the brain does not have the capacity to deal with even a small fraction of this information, so much of it must be ignored.

Examples: You may be unaware of conversation in a crowded room but the system alerts you when you hear your name. You can sleep in the presence of some kinds of sounds but others will wake you. The reticular activating system (RAS) is the part of the reticular formation that controls wakefulness. Sleep centres are located in the reticular formation. Neurons in one sleep centre secrete serotonin, a chemical that inhibits the RAS and thus causes drowsiness and sleep.

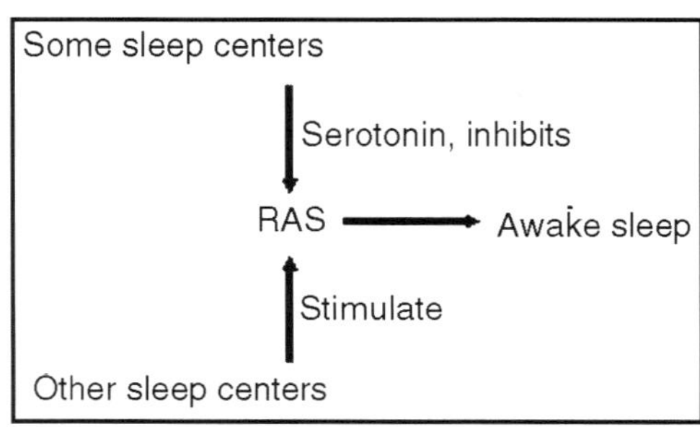

Another sleep centre secretes factors that counteract serotonin and bring about wakefulness. Damage to these centres can lead to unconsciousness or coma.

Hypothalamus

The hypothalamus regulates the endocrine system by controlling the secretions of the pituitary gland or by producing some of the hormones that are secreted by the pituitary. These hormones affect the body or affect other glands in the body.

Their overall affect is to maintain homeostasis. The hypothalamus also contains neurons associated with the limbic system.

Limbic System

The limbic system contains neural pathways that connect portions of the cortex, thalamus, hypothalamus, and basal nuclei (several areas deep within the cerebrum). It causes pleasant or unpleasant feelings about experiences (rage, pain, pleasure, sorrow). This helps guide the individual into appropriate behaviour that is more likely to be beneficial.

Cerebrum

The cerebrum became greatly enlarged as evolution progressed from the earliest vertebrates to mammals. In reptiles, birds, and mammals, it receives sensory information and coordinates motor responses.

Motor responses to the skeletal muscles originate in the cerebrum but are refined and coordinated by the cerebellum. In humans, the cerebrum is the largest part of the brain. Characteristics such as thinking, intelligence, and emotion are controlled here. Olfactory Bulbs- The anterior parts of the cerebral hemispheres are called the olfactory bulbs.

It receives input from the olfactory nerves (smell). The olfactory bulbs of primitive vertebrates comprise a large proportion of the cerebrum.

Cerebral Cortex- Over evolutionary time, gray matter developed over the cerebrum. This is the cerebral cortex and it is an information-processing centre. It increases in size more rapidly than the skull so that it has become folded (convoluted) in order to fit in the skull.

The human cerebral cortex is thin (1.5-4 mm thick) and is highly folded to increase its surface area. Intelligence, emotion, creativity, learning, and memory are localized in the cerebral cortex.

Lobes of the Cerebral Cortex

The cerebral cortex is divided into four lobes, each receives information from particular senses and processes the information into higher levels of consciousness.

Lobe	Function
Frontal	Motor functions; permits conscious control of skeletal muscles; contains the primary motor cortex conscious thought
Parietal	Sensory areas from the skin; contains the primary sensory cortex
Occipital	The primary visual cortex is located within the occipital lobe.
Temporal	Hearing and smell

Primary Sensory and Primary Motor Cortex- The primary sensory cortex is a narrow band of cortex tissue that extends from one side of the cortex near the ear over the top of the brain to the other side. Information from sensory receptors in the skin arrive at this area.

The motor cortex is a band of cortex tissue directly anterior (in front) of the primary sensory cortex. Signals that control the skeletal muscles originate in this area.

Corpus Callosum

The corpus callosum contains neurons that cross from one side of the brain to the other, allowing each half to communicate with each other.

Summary of Brain Structure

Brain Structure	Function
Medulla oblongata	Vital functions such as breathing, heart rate, and blood pressure. Reflexes such as vomiting, coughing, sneezing, hiccupping, swallowing, and digestion Neurons cross.
Pons	Breathing, connects spinal cord, cerebellum and higher brain centres.
Cerebellum	Motor coordination.
Midbrain	Receives visual, auditory, and tactile information. In mammals, this information is sent to the thalamus and higher brain centers. In lower vertebrates, the information is further processed in the midbrain.
Thalamus	Relays sensory information to the cerebral cortex. Contains part of the reticular formation (controls arousal).
Hypothalamus	Maintains homeostasis, regulates the endocrine system Contains part of the Limbic system (controls emotion).
Cerebrum	Processes sensory information and produces signals that move the skeletal muscles.
Cerebral Cortex	This is the outer layer of the cerebrum. Thinking, intelligence, and cognitive functions are located here. Processing of sensory information and motor responses.

Memory

The limbic system is involved in memory formation. The hippocampus, a structure that is deep in the cerebrum and a part of limbic system, is necessary to form new memories. People with a damaged hippocampus cannot remember things since the time the damage occurred but can remember from before that time.

Short-term memory is probably stored as electrical differences because they can be removed by the application of an electrical shock. Long-term memory is probably stored as new or different synapses. Research on snails shows that learning is associated with an increased number of synapses. Forgetting is associated with a decreased number. Disuse can cause a synapse to wither and sever the connection between two neurons. Intensively stimulated synapses form stronger connections, grow, or sprout buds to form more connections. Memory appears to be stored in sensory areas of the cerebrum.

The Spinal Cord

The vertebrae surround and protect the spinal cord. Cerebrospinal fluid within the central canal functions to cushion the spinal cord. Many sensory - motor reflex connections are in the spinal cord. Interneurons often lie between sensory and motor neurons.

ACTIVITY OF NERVOUS SYSTEM

The activities so far described may almost all be found in machines, but a complicated machine needs human control if the parts are to work harmoniously. The body to a large extent runs itself. The diaphragm and heart contract with the appropriate force and rhythm, the pancreas begins to secrete as food reaches the duodenum, and so on. Many of its activities are unconscious: consciousness and will only play a part where our past experience is likely to be of value in influencing our behaviour.

The unconscious responses of the nervous system are called reflex actions, or reflexes; though of course it is also responsible for voluntary actions. The nervous system controls striped muscle, heart muscle, smooth muscle, and glands, but with very few exceptions it is only the striped muscles that the will can influence, and even they are often moved by reflexes.

In every reflex or voluntary action three organs are always concerned, first a receptor organ which is appropriately stimulated, then a longer or shorter path in the nervous system, and finally an effector organ. The latter is always a muscle or gland in man, though other animals have electric and luminous organs under nervous control.

In the case of voluntary action the delay in the central nervous system may be very long, but there is always some external motive for a voluntary action. The nature of reflex and voluntary action will be made clearer by a few examples.

	Action.	*Receptor.*	*Effector.*
1.	Speeding up of the heart on increasing its supply of blood.	Nerve-endings in right auricle.	Heart muscle.
2.	Contraction of pupil in strong light.	Retina of eye.	Smooth muscle of iris.
3.	Reddening of skin after a scratch.	Pain spots of skin.	Smooth muscle of small vessels which open.
4.	Secretion of saliva on smelling food.	Olfactory organ in nose.	Salivary glands.
5.	Knee jerk.	Nerve-endings in tendon.	Extensor muscles of thigh.
6.	Blinking on eye being struck at.	Retina of eye.	Eyelid muscles.
7.	Breathing.	Respiratory centres in brain.	Muscles of chest and diaphragm.
8.	Sneezing.	Nerve-endings in nose.	Muscles of chest and diaphragm.
9.	Answering a bell.	Organ of Corti in ear.	Leg muscles.

All but the last are reflexes. The first three are entirely independent of will or consciousness. They are performed by smooth muscle. The fourth involves consciousness but not will. It can, however, be influenced by voluntary attention. The next four are performed by striped muscle, and are partly under voluntary control. The last is a very simple voluntary action. The line between reflex and voluntary action is not sharp. Only an experienced schoolmaster can tell voluntary from reflex coughing.

It will be seen that the receptor organs are generally, but not always, sense-organs, that is to say, their stimulation produces consciousness as well as reflex action. We can learn a great deal about the properties of nerve by taking a muscle with its motor nerve out of a recently killed animal. If we stimulate the nerve by electrical or chemical means, or mechanically (e. g. by pinching), the muscle will contract. This irritability continues for many hours, though the muscle is very easily fatigued unless it has a proper oxygen supply. The muscle may be made to work a lever which writes on a moving sheet of paper, and the effects of different stimuli can thus be compared.

We can also measure the heat or electrical changes produced. By such means we learn the following facts about nervous conduction. Each fibre conducts independently of the others. It conducts not a steady stream, but a series of nervous impulses. An impulse is not an electric current, but an activity of the nerve-fibre producing an electrical effect and a little heat as it goes along. It travels at about 30 metres per second or 70 miles per hour in man.

Thus a man, hit by a car going at 80 miles per hour, will probably feel nothing because his brain is destroyed before any nervous impulses from his skin reach it. After the passage of an impulse the fibre needs a rest of one-thousandth of a second or more before it can transmit another. All impulses in the same fibre are normally of the same intensity. Thus, from this point of view, we may compare a nerve to a bundle of telegraph wires, down which electrical waves of the same intensity pass at varying intervals, but not to a bundle of telephone wires, in which the intensity of the waves is variable. Finally, the energy of a nervous impulse is so small that about four million impulses (which would take several hours to pass) would be needed to heat a nerve 1° C. A voluntary muscle responds to one nervous impulse by a twitch, to a rapid series by a steady contraction.

A contracting human muscle is getting about forty-five impulses per second. The energy liberated in a gram of contracting muscle is several hundred thousand times greater than that in a gram of the nerve which supplies it. This ratio is about the same as that of the energy developed by a thirty H.P. motor-car running for twelve hours, to that used by the man who turns the starting-handle for a minute.

Muscles can be made to contract by weak artificial electric currents as easily as by those produced by the nerve. We are not yet sure of the details of how a muscle contracts, though it seems that the lactic acid formed causes microscopic fibrils to contract, as many proteins do when placed in weak acid.

A muscle is not a heat engine, for it has a very high efficiency such as is only found in heat engines one part of which is very much hotter than the other. Its chemical energy is converted directly into work without first passing into heat. The actual process of contraction may have an efficiency of 90 to 100 per cent., but an amount of energy greater than the work done in contraction is wasted as heat during the re-synthesis of the lactic and phosphoric acids, so that the whole process has an efficiency of only about 40 per cent.

Moreover, a good deal of energy is needed for the extra breathing and heart action during exercise, besides the basal metabolism which goes on all the time. So, considered as a machine, a man never has an efficiency of more than 25 per cent. At best, he turns three times as much energy into heat as into work. Moreover, a muscle heats up while keeping up a steady contraction, as in standing, supporting a weight, or pushing at a closed door. Striped muscles become quite flabby when their nerves are cut, but heart muscle and smooth muscle remain active.

Striped muscles have probably only one set of motor nerves which make them contract. Involuntary muscles have two sets: stimulation of one set causes increased activity, of the other set rest or lessened activity. The effects of stimulating a nerve-fibre depend mainly on its connexions in the body, to some extent on the quantity and rhythm of the stimulus, but not at all on where in its course it is stimulated. These facts were first discovered by Müller in 1826. Thus a blow on the 'funny-bone' or just above it is felt in the ring and little fingers because the nerve from them runs near the surface at this point, and irritation of the nerves in the stump of an amputated leg will give a man pain which he feels in toes that he may have lost forty years ago. Again, when the nerve to the face muscles has been destroyed, the power to move them may sometimes be regained by grafting the nerve supplying certain neck and shoulder muscles into the old track of the facial. But when connexion has been made the patient, in order to move the face, must will to move the shoulder. The most accessible receptor organs are those of the skin.

They can easily be studied in an area where they are scattered, as on the side of the knee. If the skin is shaved we find that only parts round the hair roots are sensitive to gentle touch with a bristle.

Each root is surrounded by a network of nerve-fibres which are easily stimulated. The small hairs act as levers, and render the 'touch spots' more sensitive. In hairless parts, such as the palm, sole, and lips, there are special receptors for touch. Similarly if we go over the skin with a warm blunt metal point, we find that warmth is only felt at a second set of points (not those sensitive to touch), cold at another set, and pain at a fourth.

Many areas on the thigh are quite insensitive to pain, as they have no pain-spots. It is characteristic of receptor organs to be specially sensitive to one kind of stimulus, which may be physical, as with the skin organs, or chemical as with those of taste and smell.

They will, however, generally respond to inappropriate stimuli, if these are strong enough. Thus mustard will stimulate first the heat and then the pain-spots. A blow or pressure on the eye will make one see stars, and so on. On the other hand each receptor organ, with the paths leading from it to the brain, can generally only give rise to one kind of sensation.

This, however, depends on the part of the brain to which it leads, not on the organ which is stimulated. There is no fundamental difference in the nature of the impulses in different nerves, as there is in their effects.

If we stimulate the optic nerve, even after the loss of the eye, we get visual sensations, and so on. If we put the right hand into hot water, and the left into cold for a minute, and then both into lukewarm water, this feels cold to the right hand and hot to the left.

This is characteristic of the senses. They tell us more about differences of intensity in their stimuli than about their absolute intensity. When we look at a candle in sunlight we find it hard to believe that we can see by it, or even be dazzled by it, at night. We go into a dark room, and see nothing at first, but soon adapt ourselves, and see the things in it instead of a uniform blackness.

After half an hour in a sound-proof room one finds the noise of one's own heart and breathing unpleasantly loud, though normally one cannot hear them. The fineness of discrimination for touch depends mainly on the closeness of touch-spots. Thus, on the palm, where they are very numerous, we can distinguish two points from one if they are 1 centimetre apart. On the back, where there are few touch-spots, this distance must be increased seven times or more. Under the skin are receptors of many kinds. Some respond to deep pressure, and others to pain, but when once the skin is cut through, most healthy tissues are almost insensitive to pain. They become tender, however, when inflamed.

The gut and other hollow organs are insensitive to cutting or burning (stimuli to which they are not normally exposed), but very painful when stretched either by unusually bulky contents or unusually strong contractions of their muscles. There are also receptors in muscles, tendons, and joints. These send impulses to the central nervous system, which inform it of the relative positions and movements of different parts of our body.

Receptors and nerves with this function are called proprioceptive, whilst those whose stimuli come from outside are called exteroceptive. Proprioceptive organs may affect the consciousness. Thus we can tell how much our knee is bent even with our eyes shut, owing to the jointorgans, or how great a weight we are holding, owing to the muscle-organs.

But far more important is the aid they give us without our knowing it, in the co-ordination of muscular movement. If proprioceptive impulses cannot reach the brain from the legs, as happens in a disease of the spinal cord called locomotor ataxy, in which sensation is not lost, the patient cannot co-ordinate the movements or postures of his leg muscles.

In walking he raises his foot too high and brings it down too hard. He cannot stand with his eyes shut. There is no weakness of the muscles, but they cannot be used properly, as the brain gets no information as to what they are doing except through the eyes. The spinal cord consists of a central core of nerve-cells, called the grey matter, surrounded by millions of fibres mostly running lengthways, and called the white matter.

Both include a scaffolding of supporting cells. Between each pair of vertebrae a nerve leaves the spinal canal on each side. It enters the spinal cord by a dorsal and a ventral root. The ventral root fibres go to muscles and glands, and are only traversed by impulses going outwards. The dorsal root consists of fibres carrying impulses from receptor organs to the cord. So if a dorsal root is cut we lose the capacity for feeling with a certain area of the skin, while injury to ventral roots leads to paralysis of muscles. But most nerves contain both sensory and motor fibres, so when a nerve is cut both movement and sensation are lost in the area which it supplies.

The separation of the roots serves to bring all the sensory fibres to one cell-area within the cord, all the motor fibres to another. A nerve's only function is to conduct, but the spinal cord not only conducts impulses to and from the brain with its fibres, but gives rise to reflexes by means of its nerve-cells.

This is shown by what happens when it is divided. If a man breaks his spinal cord in the neck, he dies because his breathing muscles are cut off from the brain, and get no nervous impulses to make them work. If it is broken lower down he may live for some time. He has absolutely no feeling in the parts of his body and no voluntary control over the muscles whose nerve-supply comes from the part of the cord below the break.

But if we examine him six months after the accident we find reflexes occurring in the lower part of his body. If, for instance, we pinch his foot it is drawn upwards without his knowledge or will. If the lower part of the cord is destroyed or the nerves to it cut, all reflexes cease. A great deal has been learnt about nervous activity from the study of spinal reflexes.

They are easily studied on the carcass of a frog whose brain has been destroyed by poking a blunt wire into it from behind. If we irritate its skin its hind leg scratches near the place irritated, but its responses are clumsy, and it does nothing without some fairly violent stimulus. Provided they are in nervous connexion with the brain or spinal cord, the muscles of a limb are never quite flabby. They are mostly in a state of gentle but steady contraction or 'tone', so as to keep the limb in a definite posture.

If then the knee is to be bent, as the flexor (bending) muscles of the thigh contract, its extensor muscles must relax. If they relaxed too little or too slowly there would be a strain and a waste of energy. If they relaxed too quickly or completely the movement would proceed too far, and the kneejoint might be dislocated. Exactly the same applies elsewhere. Almost every muscle in the body, those of the trunk, jaws, and eyes, as well as the limbs, has an antagonist, and arrangements must be made for one to relax as the other contracts.

As there are no inhibitory nerves to striped muscles, this can only be done by inhibiting or switching off the activity of those cells in the central nervous system which are sending impulses to the muscle which has to relax. Figure gives an idea of some of the connexions concerned in a simple spinal reflex. An impulse enters the cord through a fibre in a dorsal root from a pain-spot in the foot.

The fibre divides and its branches end near nerve-cells in the grey matter. One of these cells is represented sending a fibre to a flexor muscle of the knee, another sends a fibre to an extensor. When the pain-spot is stimulated the impulses passing along it cause more nervous impulses to be generated in the cell connected with the flexor muscle, less in that connected with the extensor, so the knee tends to bend, and the foot to be withdrawn. Actually things are far more complicated. Stimulation of a single pain-spot will only cause movement after a long time or never, and, if movement occurs, hundreds of nerve-fibres will be conducting impulses at once.

To get a prompt movement one must stimulate a number of spots or fibres from them at once, as when one treads on a hot coal. Though the type of connexion shown in the figure have actually been observed with the microscope, in most reflexes the excitation has to pass through several neurons before it reaches the cell whose axon is the nerve-fibre to the muscle or other effector.

We must now study the function of the spinal cord in conducting nervous impulses in both directions between the body and brain. In a mixed nerve like the sciatic in the thigh, all sorts of fibres with different functions run together. Some are carrying impulses to the muscles, others from the skin and deep receptors.

As they enter the cord they are sorted out according to which way they conduct, and later on a further sorting process occurs. For example, the impulses which on reaching the brain give rise to sensations of temperature, run up the spinal cord by a different path from those which give rise to sensations of touch.

These paths have been located by several different methods, which have also been applied to the study of the brain itself. First, symptoms are observed in patients, and after their death local injuries of the spinal cord due to splinters of metal or bone, burst blood-vessels, or tumours, are found. When the same symptoms are observed in another patient they can often be relieved by the surgeon owing to the knowledge so gained.

To refuse leave to examine the body in such a case is to condemn some one else to die with those symptoms. Again, after destruction or division of some parts of the nervous system one can observe with the microscope the death and degeneration of groups of nerve-fibres. Now we know that when a fibre is divided, only that part dies which is separated from the cell-body and nucleus of the neuron to which it belongs. So we can discover in which direction the cell-bodies of any bundle of fibres lie. But in the central nervous system the long fibres always conduct nervous impulses away from the nucleus, so we discover the direction in which nervous impulses run in the fibres we have cut.

Finally, we can try the effect on an animal of cutting or stimulating some part of its nervous system. (The lower parts of the system will still work after the animal has been made unconscious by an anaesthetic or by removing its cerebrum). By such methods we can distinguish five main pairs of ascending fibre-tracts in the human spinal cord, besides numerous smaller groups. Two of these go to the cerebellum, and their injury does not affect consciousness, but causes unsatisfactory movements and postures, the brain being without information as to what the muscles are doing.

Two of them send impulses only to parts of the brain concerned in consciousness. One serves both purposes. Before we study the functions of the brain it will be convenient to deal with the special sense-organs in the head which communicate with it directly and not through the cord. The organs of the chemical senses, taste and smell, are found in the mouth and nose. They work together, and much of the sensation we commonly regard as taste includes an element of smell. With the eyes and nose tightly shut, taste will not distinguish an onion from an apple.

The tasteorgans mostly lie in the papillae which roughen the upper surface of the tongue. There are four elementary kinds of taste, namely: salt, sweet, sour, and bitter. Other tastes are combinations of these. Each elementary taste has different end-organs.

Thus, we taste sweet things best with the tip of the tongue, bitter with the back. The end-organs of smell are a little patch of about onequarter of a square inch of yellow epithelium at the top of the internal cavity of the nose. The corresponding area in a dog is ten or more square inches, in a large shark 24 square feet. In man, smell is an unimportant, almost vestigial sense, but in the dog and many other animals it is the most important of all.

So the dog's world is mainly a world of smells. But even in man it is the most delicate of the senses. We can smell mercaptan at a dilution of 1 milligram in 20,000,000 litres of air.

As about 1 cubic centimetre at a time is in the olfactory part of the nose, this means that we are affected by one twenty-thousand-millionth of a milligram, whereas the smallest object we can see with the naked eye is about a million times as large. In ordinary breathing most of the air goes past the olfactory cavity. In sniffing, some is sucked into it. No satisfactory classification of smells has yet been made.

BASIC SENSORY AND MOTOR FUNCTIONS OF THE NERVOUS SYSTEM

The nervous system is composed of billions of neurons with long, interconnecting processes that form complex integrated electrochemical circuits. It is through these neuronal circuits that animals experience sensations and respond appropriately.

Neuronal processes that transmit electrical alterations to the neuron cell body are called dendrites. Dendrites have receptor sites that receive stimulation or inhibition from outside sources. If electrical stimulation of the cell body reaches a critical threshold, an electrical discharge called an action potential develops. The action potential spontaneously travels away from the cell body along an outgoing process called an axon.

When the action potential reaches the terminal branches of the axon, chemicals called neurotransmitters are released. Neurotransmitters either stimulate or inhibit receptor sites on other neurons, muscles, or glands. Although neurons may have a variety of shapes, each one has dendrites, a cell body, and an axon and releases neurotransmitters.

The peripheral nervous system (PNS) s formed by neurons of the cranial and spinal nerves. The central nervous system (CNS) is formed by neurons of the spinal cord, brain stem, cerebellum, and cerebrum.

Groups of neuronal cell bodies in the PNS are called ganglia, whereas those in the CNS are called nuclei. Nuclei form the CNS gray matter. Groups of axons in the CNS form the white matter and are arranged into tracts. The tracts are usually named after their site of origin and termination (eg, the spinocerebellar tract begins in the spinal cord and ends in the cerebellum).

PNS sensory or afferent neurons carry information such as nociception, proprioception, touch, temperature, taste, hearing, equilibrium, vision, and olfaction to the spinal cord or brain stem. CNS sensory neurons carry information to the cerebellum, brain stem, and cerebrum for further interpretation. Important spinal cord and brain-stem sensory tracts include several spinocerebellar, spinothalamic, and spinoreticular tract systems. The spinoreticular tracts begin in the spinal cord and terminate in the reticular formation of the medulla. The dorsal fasciculi gracilis and cuneatus of the spinal cord and the medial and lateral lemniscus of the brain stem are also important sensory tracts. In animals, these sensory tracts may carry fibres from many sensory modalities such as proprioception, nociception (pain), and touch. An alteration in sensation may be due to either CNS or PNS disease.

Reactions to sensory inputs are initiated by efferent or motor neurons in the cerebrum and brain stem called upper motor neurons (UMNs). The UMN axons descend to brain-stem and spinal cord segments in tracts named after their site of origination and termination.

The UMNs of the reticulospinal tracts (from midbrain, pons, and medulla oblongata reticular formation) and the rubrospinal tract (from midbrain) are important for voluntary movements of skeletal muscles in domestic animals. The rubrospinal tract mainly functions to facilitate flexors of the limbs, whereas the pontine and medullary reticulospinal tracts have either a facilitative (pontine) or inhibitory (medullary) effect on the extensors. The corticospinal tracts (cell bodies in the cerebral cortex) are most important for voluntary movement in primates. Domestic animals with severe cerebrocortical disease may suffer only transient loss of voluntary movements, because their corticospinal tract has limited influence.

The pontine reticulospinal (from the pons) and vestibulospinal tracts (from vestibular nuclei of the medulla oblongata) facilitate extensor skeletal muscle activity used to support the body. Knowledge of location and function of sensory and motor brain-stem and spinal tracts is essential to localize nervous system lesions and determine their severity. Mild spinal cord compression affects the superficial spinal cord tracts fasciculus gracilus, cuneatus, spinocerebellar, and vestibulospinal tracts, so initial signs include ataxia and extensor weakness. Important voluntary motor tracts are located in the lateral portions of the spinal cord deep to the spinocerebellar tracts, and paresis or paralysis develops with moderate spinal cord compression. Because many tracts are involved, loss of nociception from the periosteum of the toes and tail (deep pain) occurs when spinal cord lesions are bilateral and severe. This loss of nociception is also an indicator of severe cord injury because those fibres that transmit deep pain are typically non-myelinated, slow-transmitting C type fibres, which are very resistant to pressure.

Motor neurons with cell bodies in the brain stem, and spinal cord gray matter and axons that travel in the PNS cranial and spinal nerves, respectively, are referred to as lower motor neurons (LMNs). Injury to either the UMNs or LMNs results in paresis or paralysis. Brain-stem and spinal cord reflexes are the phylogenetically oldest responses of the nervous system. When the eyelid is touched, it closes; when the toe is pinched, the limb withdraws even before conscious perception intervenes. Only a sensory neuron in the PNS, a connector (internuncial) neuron in the CNS, and an LMN are necessary for a reflex to be present. In a monosynaptic reflex (eg, patellar reflex), only a sensory neuron and LMN are present. During the neurologic examination, testing brain-stem and spinal reflexes is helpful to localize CNS and PNS lesions to specific areas. If a reflex is depressed or absent, a lesion must involve the sensory nerve, internuncial neuron, LMN, or muscle at that particular site.

The autonomic nervous system is divided into sympathetic and parasympathetic portions and controls activity in smooth and cardiac muscles and glands. Visceral afferent (sensory) neurons travel in cranial and spinal nerves and sensory spinal cord tracts to the thalamic and hypothalamic regions of the brain stem.

UMNs in the hypothalamus descend to LMN cell bodies of the brain-stem nuclei and sacral segments for parasympathetic control and to the intermediolateral gray matter of the spinal cord for sympathetic control.

LMNs of the sympathetic nervous system exit through thoracolumbar spinal nerves (T1 to L4) to affect smooth muscles associated with the pupils, eyelids, orbits, hair follicles, blood vessels, and thoracic and abdominal viscera. Horner syndrome (ptosis, miosis, and enophthalmos) is a common finding associated with loss of sympathetic innervation to the eye.

LMNs of the parasympathetic nervous system exit via cranial nerve (CN) III to innervate smooth muscle of the pupils and eyelids, CN VII to the lacrimal and salivary glands, CN IX to salivary glands, and CN X to cardiac muscles and glands and to smooth muscles of all the thoracic and abdominal viscera to the level of the transverse colon. LMNs of the parasympathetic nervous system also exit through the sacral segments to all the viscera in the caudal abdomen, including the bladder and colon. Sacral lesions commonly result in loss of the urinary bladder (detruser) reflex.

DIVISIONS AND EFFECTS OF LESIONS

The PNS consists of 26 or more pairs of spinal nerves that correspond to each spinal cord segment and 12 pairs of cranial nerves that correspond to specific brain and brain-stem segments.

The PNS spinal nerves form the brachial plexus to the thoracic limb; the lumbosacral plexus to the pelvic limb; and the cauda equina to the bladder, anus, and tail. Brachial or lumbosacral plexus lesions cause paresis or paralysis of a thoracic or pelvic limb, respectively, with reduced or absent spinal reflexes and reduced or absent sensation of the limb. Cauda equina lesions result in an atonic bladder; a dilated, unresponsive anus; and a flaccid, paralyzed tail.

Lesions of all spinal nerves (eg, acute polyradiculoneuritis) result in paresis or paralysis of all four limbs (quadriparesis or quadriplegia, respectively) with depressed or absent spinal reflexes and altered sensation of the limbs. Lesions restricted to PNS cranial nerves result in deficits associated with dysfunction of that particular nerve and no signs of dysfunction in the limbs or other parts of the nervous system.

The spinal cord of dogs and cats is divided into 8 cervical, 13 thoracic, 7 lumbar, 3 sacral, and 5 or more caudal segments. Horses and cows have 6 lumbar and 5 sacral segments, and pigs have 6-7 lumbar and 4 sacral segments. Spinal cord lesions from L4 to S2 cause pelvic limb ataxia, conscious proprioceptive deficits, and paresis or paralysis with depressed or absent spinal reflexes and muscle tone (LMN signs).

Sensation may also be depressed or absent below the lesion. Lesions from T3 to L3 cause pelvic limb ataxia, conscious proprioceptive deficits, and paresis and paralysis with normal or exaggerated spinal reflexes (UMN signs). Pelvic limb sensation caudal to the lesion may also be depressed or absent. With spinal cord lesions extending from C6 to T2, thoracic limb spinal reflexes may be depressed or absent, and severe lesions may cause quadriplegia. The spinal reflexes remain intact in the pelvic limbs, but sensation may be affected.

Spinal cord lesions from C1 to C5 cause hemiparesis or hemiplegia (paresis or paralysis of the limbs on one side), or quadriparesis. Spinal reflexes in all four limbs are often preserved. Severe lesions may cause respiratory distress or arrest due to involvement of the UMNs to respiratory muscles in the C5 area.

The brain stem is divided from caudal to rostral into four segments: the medulla oblongata (myelencephalon), the pons (metencephalon), the midbrain (mesencephalon), and the thalamus and hypothalamus (diencephalon).

Similar to lesions of the cervical spinal cord, lesions of the medulla oblongata cause conscious proprioceptive deficits and weakness on the same side (ipsilateral) or both sides with normal or hyperactive limb reflexes. However, involvement of CN nuclei IX, X, XI, or XII localizes the lesion to the caudal medulla oblongata. Involvement of CN nuclei VI, VII, or VIII localizes the lesion to the rostral medulla oblongata. It is rare to have a lesion of the medulla oblongata that does not affect one or more of the cranial nerves as well as sensory and motor tracts.

Pontine lesions cause ipsilateral conscious proprioceptive deficits, hemiparesis or quadriparesis with normal or hyperactive limb reflexes, mental depression from involvement of the ascending reticular activating system (ARAS), and CN V and IV deficits.

The cerebellum is part of the metencephalon and is attached to the dorsal surface of the pons and medulla by rostral, middle, and caudal cerebellar peduncles. The cerebellum coordinates all muscle activity and establishes muscle tone. The flocculonodular lobe of the cerebellum has equilibrium functions and is considered part of the vestibular system. Unilateral lesions of the cerebellum cause ipsilateral dysmetria (hypermetria or hypometria) and a contralateral (paradoxical) head tilt. Bilateral lesions of the cerebellum cause generalized incoordination of the head and limbs, head tremors (intention tremors), and generalized dysequilibrium.

Midbrain (mesencephalon) lesions cause contralateral conscious proprioceptive deficits and hemiparesis. CN III nucleus involvement is present on the ipsilateral side and localizes the lesion to the midbrain. In large, midbrain lesions, the ARAS is affected, and the animal will be stuporous or comatose. If the sympathetic UMNs and parasympathetic LMNs are both affected in the midbrain, the pupils will be midrange size and unresponsive to light.

Diencephalic lesions can be difficult to differentiate from cerebral cortical lesions, because many tracts going to and from the cerebrum pass through the diencephalon by way of the internal capsule. The thalamus, hypothalamus, and subthalamus of the diencephalon have many important structures that alter feeding, drinking, breeding, sleeping, and other behaviours, as well as regulate body temperature. The pituitary gland, which controls many hormonal functions of the body, is connected to the hypothalamus. The ARAS projects through the subthalamus area, in which lesions also produce stupor or coma.

The telencephalon, also called the cerebral cortex, is divided into the neo-cortex, paleocortex, and archicortex. The paleocortex and archicortex include the olfactory and limbic regions, which provide smell and emotional reactions to all stimuli.

The neo-cortex is divided into the frontal, parietal, occipital, and temporal lobes. The frontal cortex functions include intelligence and fine motor skills (corticospinal tract).

Lesions in this area cause dementia, lack of recognition of the owner, difficulty in training, compulsive pacing, circling towards the side of the lesion (adversion syndrome), and motor seizures with contralateral involuntary muscle twitching. Contralateral hopping and placing deficits are also found with frontal lobe lesions. Ascending and descending tracts to and from the frontal lobe form the internal capsule through the region of the basal nuclei and diencephalon. Lesions of the internal capsule can produce the same signs as frontal lobe lesions. The parietal lobe (somesthetic cortex) is for interpretation of general perception, nociception, temperature, and pressure; lesions result in proprioceptive deficits on the contralateral side of the body.

Occipital lobe and optic radiation lesions result in blindness with pupils that respond normally to light. Unilateral occipital lobe and optic radiation lesions result in some degree of visual loss in the contralateral eye, depending on the percentage of crossover of the optic nerve fibres in the optic chiasm of the species (65 per cent in cats; 75 per cent in dogs; 80 per cent-90 per cent in cattle, horses, pigs, and sheep). The pupils still respond normally to light.

Blindness with pupils that do not respond to light is associated with lesions of the retina, optic nerve, optic chiasm, or rostral optic tract.

Difficulty in localizing sound is hard to evaluate clinically. It may occur with temporal lobe lesions, as may psychomotor seizures characterized by hysterical running. "Fly-biting" or "star gazing" hallucinations are suspected to occur with lesions in the temporal-occipital region. Aggression occurs when the pyriform area (paleocortex) of the temporal lobe and the underlying amygdaloid nucleus are affected. Aggression can also occur with hypothalamic lesions.

Lesions of the olfactory region may alter feeding or breeding behaviour. Slow-growing lesions of the cerebrum and diencephalon often result in few clinical signs because of the adaptability of functions in these areas in animals.

MECHANISMS OF DISEASE

Disease processes affecting the nervous system may be congenital or familial, infectious or inflammatory, toxic, metabolic, nutritional, traumatic, vascular, degenerative, neo-plastic, or idiopathic.

Congenital disorders may be obvious at birth or shortly after (eg, an enlarged head from hydrocephalus or an uncoordinated gait from an underdeveloped cerebellum). Some familial disorders (eg, lysosomal storage diseases) cause a progressive degeneration of neurons in the first year of life, whereas others (eg, inherited epilepsy) may not manifest for 2-3 yr.

Infections of the nervous system are due to specific viruses, fungi, protozoa, bacteria, rickettsia, prions, and algae. Non-infectious inflammations such as steroid-responsive meningoencephalomyelitis and meningoencephalomyelitis of unknown etiology (MUE), formerly called granulomatous meningoencephalomyelitis, Pug dog encephalitis, and other CNS inflammatory diseases, may be immune-mediated. Until there is a histologic diagnosis, the term MUE is used.

Toxicity of the nervous system is most frequently caused by organophosphates, pyrethrins, carbamates, bromethalin, metaldehyde, ethylene glycol, metronidazole, theobromines, sedatives, and anticonvulsants (eg, phenobarbital, bromide). Botulinum, tetanus, and tick toxins, as well as coral and certain other snake venom intoxications, cause neurologic signs.

Metabolic alterations of nervous system function most commonly result from hypoglycemia, hypoxia or anoxia, hepatic dysfunction, hypocalcemia, hypomagnesemia,hypernatremia,hypokalemia, and uremia. Hypothyroidism, hyperthyroidism, hypoadrenocorticism, and hyperadrenocorticism are endocrine disorders that can cause neurologic dysfunction.

Thiamine deficiency results in ataxia, stupor, and coma or seizures in dogs, cats, and cattle. Deficiency of vitamin B6 may cause seizures.

Trauma to the PNS and CNS causes focal and multifocal neurologic signs from physical damage, hemorrhage, edema, and progressive formation of oxygen-containing free radicals and nervous system destruction that is usually complete in 24-48 hr but lasts as long as 4 days because of the slow influx of inflammatory cells..

Vascular lesions of animals are usually due to septicemia and bacterial embolization of the CNS. Fibrocartilaginous embolization of the spinal cord is common in dogs. Arteriovenous malformations occur occasionally and cause spontaneous hemorrhages. Cerebrovascular disease from arteriosclerosis is rare in domestic animals but has been associated with hypothyroidism caused by hyperlipidemia. Cerebrovascular disease from hypertension is rare but may be seen as multiple cerebral microbleeds with MRI.

Familial degeneration of neurons occurs in lysosomal storage disorders. Degeneration of intervertebral discs that subsequently herniate into the vertebral canal often produces paresis and paralysis in dogs.

Neo-plasms of the CNS and PNS are most common in dogs and cats. Astrocytes, oligodendrocytes, and microglia can all become neo-plastic and form astrocytomas, oligodendrogliomas, and gliomas. Ependymal cells and the choroid plexus, which line the internal cavities of the CNS and produce CSF, also can become neo-plastic and form ependymomas and choroid plexus papillomas.

Meningeal cells of the dura, arachnoid, and pial membranes form meningiomas, which are common in dogs and cats. Neurofibrosarcomas are common tumors of the nerve sheaths of peripheral nerves in dogs. Lymphosarcoma is a common metastatic tumor of the PNS and CNS in dogs, cats, and cattle. Hemangiosarcoma is the most common metastatic tumor of the CNS in dogs. The idiopathic mechanism of disease is reserved for described syndromes with characteristic clinical signs, predictable outcomes, and no known necropsy findings.

SENSES OF NERVOUS SYSTEM

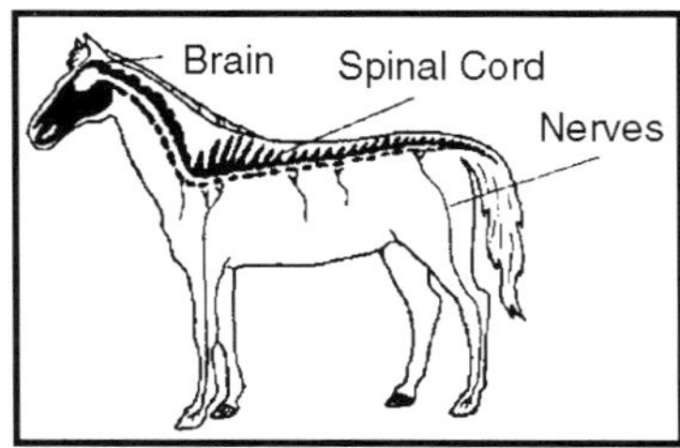

The brain also controls the senses, the sense organs are:

- The eyes for sight
- The ears for hearing

- The nose for smell
- The tongue for taste
- The skin for touch

Multicellular animals must monitor and maintain a constant internal environment as well as monitor and respond to an external environment. In many animals, these two functions are coordinated by two integrated and coordinated organ systems: the nervous system and the endocrine system..

Three basic functions are prformed by nervous systems:

1. Receive sensory input from internal and external environments
2. Integrate the input
3. Respond to stimuli

Sensory Input

Receptors are parts of the nervous system that sense changes in the internal or external environments. Sensory input can be in many forms, including pressure, taste, sound, light, blood pH, or hormone levels, that are converted to a signal and sent to the brain or spinal cord.

Integration and Output

In the sensory centres of the brain or in the spinal cord, the barrage of input is integrated and a response is generated. The response, a motor output, is a signal transmitted to organs than can convert the signal into some form of action, such as movement, changes in heart rate, release of hormones, etc.

Endocrine Systems

Some animals have a second control system, the endocrine system. The nervous system coordinates rapid responses to external stimuli. The endocrine system controls slower, longer lasting responses to internal stimuli. Activity of both systems is integrated.

Divisions of the Nervous System

The nervous system monitors and controls almost every organ system through a series of positive and negative feedback loops.The Central Nervous System (CNS) includes the brain and spinal cord. The Peripheral Nervous System (PNS) connects the CNS to other parts of the body, and is composed of nerves (bundles of neurons).

Not all animals have highly specialized nervous systems. Those with simple systems tend to be either small and very mobile or large and immobile.

Large, mobile animals have highly developed nervous systems: the evolution of nervous systems must have been an important adaptation in the evolution of body size and mobility. Coelenterates, cnidarians, and echinoderms have their neurons organized into a nerve net. These creatures have radial symmetry and lack a head. Although lacking a brain or either nervous system

(CNS or PNS) nerve nets are capable of some complex behaviour.

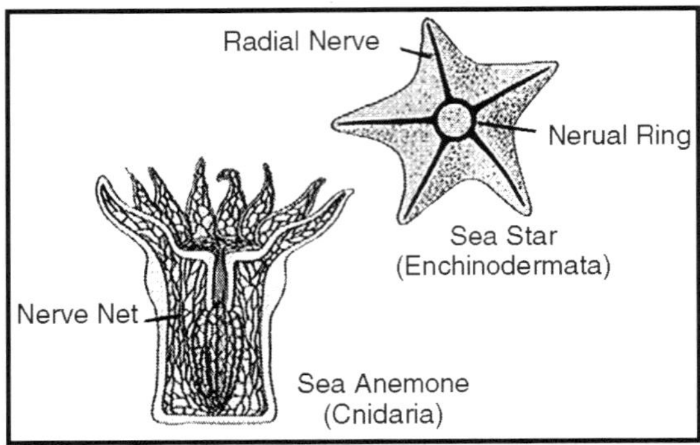

Fig. Nervous Systems in Radially Symmetrical Animals.

Bilaterally symmetrical animals have a body plan that includes a defined head and a tail region. Development of bilateral symmetry is associated with cephalization, the development of a head with the accumulation of sensory organs at the front end of the organism. Flatworms have neurons associated into clusters known as ganglia, which in turn form a small brain. Vertebrates have a spinal cord in addition to a more developed brain.

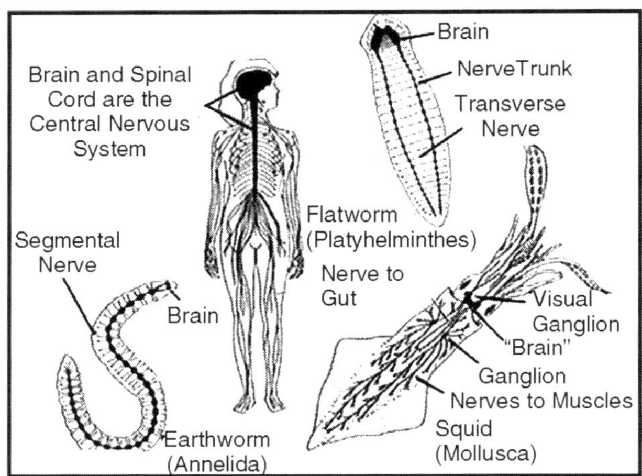

Fig. Some Nervous Systems in Bilaterally Symmetrical Animals.

Chordates have a dorsal rather than ventral nervous system. Several evolutionary trends occur in chordates: spinal cord, continuation of cephalization in the form of larger and more complex brains, and development of a more elaborate nervous system. The vertebrate nervous system is divided into a number of parts. The central nervous system includes the brain and spinal cord. The peripheral nervous system consists of all body nerves. Motor neuron pathways are of two types: somatic (skeletal) and autonomic (smooth muscle, cardiac muscle, and glands). The autonomic system is subdivided into the sympathetic and parasympathetic systems.

Peripheral Nervous System

The Peripheral Nervous System (PNS)contains only nerves and connects the brain and spinal cord (CNS) to the rest of the body. The axons and dendrites are surrounded by a white myelin sheath. Cell bodies are in the central nervous system (CNS) or ganglia. Ganglia are collections of nerve cell bodies. Cranial nerves in the PNS take impulses to and from the brain (CNS). Spinal nerves take impulses to and away from the spinal cord. There are two major subdivisions of the PNS motor pathways: the somatic and the autonomic.

Two main components of the PNS:

1. Sensory (afferent) pathways that provide input from the body into the CNS.
2. Motor (efferent) pathways that carry signals to muscles and glands (effectors).

Most sensory input carried in the PNS remains below the level of conscious awareness. Input that does reach the conscious level contributes to perception of our external environment.

Somatic Nervous System

The Somatic Nervous System (SNS) includes all nerves controlling the muscular system and external sensory receptors. External sense organs (including skin) are receptors. Muscle fibres and gland cells are effectors.

The reflex arc is an automatic, involuntary reaction to a stimulus. When the doctor taps your knee with the rubber hammer, she/he is testing your reflex (or knee-jerk). The reaction to the stimulus is involuntary, with the CNS being informed but not consciously controlling the response. Examples of reflex arcs include balance, the blinking reflex, and the stretch reflex.

Sensory input from the PNS is processed by the CNS and responses are sent by the PNS from the CNS to the organs of the body. Motor neurons of the somatic system are distinct from those of the autonomic system. Inhibitory signals, cannot be sent through the motor neurons of the somatic system.

Autonomic Nervous System

The Autonomic Nervous System is that part of PNS consisting of motor neurons that control internal organs. It has two subsystems. The autonomic system controls muscles in the heart, the smooth muscle in internal organs such as the intestine, bladder, and uterus. The Sympathetic Nervous System is involved in the fight or flight response. The Parasympathetic Nervous System is involved in relaxation. Each of these subsystems operates in the reverse of the other (antagonism). Both systems innervate the same organs and act in opposition to maintain homeostasis.

For example: when you are scared the sympathetic system causes your heart to beat faster; the parasympathetic system reverses this effect. Motor neurons in this system do not reach their targets directly (as do those in the somatic system) but rather connect to a secondary motor neuron which in turn innervates the target organ.

Central Nervous System

The Central Nervous System (CNS) is composed of the brain and spinal cord. The CNS is surrounded by bone-skull and vertebrae. Fluid and tissue also insulate the brain and spinal cord.

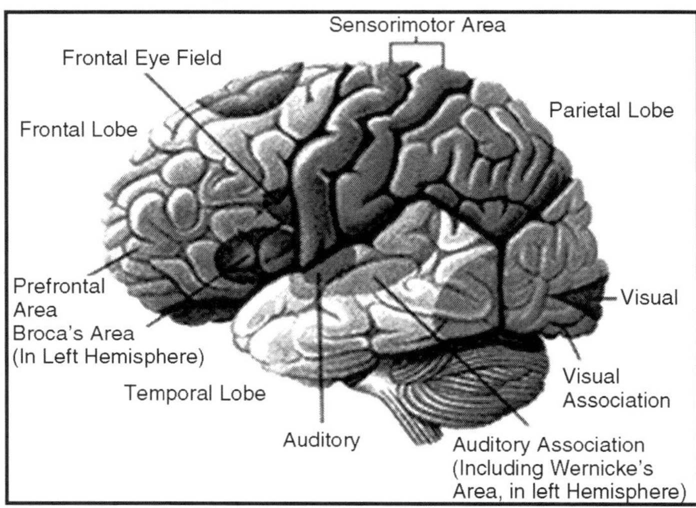

Fig. Areas of the Brain

The brain is composed of three parts: the cerebrum (seat of consciousness), the cerebellum, and the medulla oblongata (these latter two are "part of the unconscious brain"). The medulla oblongata is closest to the spinal cord, and is involved with the regulation of heartbeat, breathing, vasoconstriction (blood pressure), and reflex centres for vomiting, coughing, sneezing, swallowing, and hiccuping. The hypothalamus regulates homeostasis.

It has regulatory areas for thirst, hunger, body temperature, water balance, and blood pressure, and links the Nervous System to the Endocrine System. The midbrain and pons are also part of the unconscious brain. The thalamus serves as a central relay point for incoming nervous messages. The cerebellum is the second largest part of the brain, after the cerebrum. It functions for muscle coordination and maintains normal muscle tone and posture. The cerebellum coordinates balance.

The conscious brain includes the cerebral hemispheres, which are are separated by the corpus callosum. In reptiles, birds, and mammals, the cerebrum coordinates sensory data and motor functions. The cerebrum governs intelligence and reasoning, learning and memory. While the cause of memory is not yet definitely known, studies on slugs indicate learning is accompanied by a synapse decrease. Within the cell, learning involves change in gene regulation and increased ability to secrete transmitters.

The Brain

During embryonic development, the brain first forms as a tube, the anterior end of which enlarges into three hollow swellings that form the brain, and the posterior of which develops into the spinal cord. Some parts of the brain have changed little during vertebrate evolutionary history.

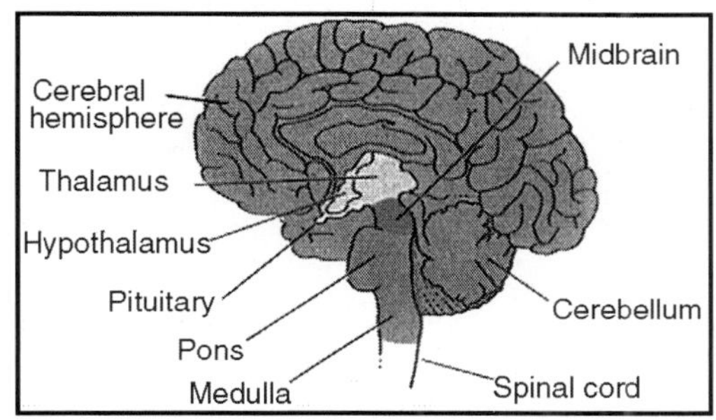

Fig. Parts of the Brain as seen from the Middle of the Brain.

Vertebrate evolutionary trends include:

- Increase in brain size relative to body size.
- Subdivision and increasing specialization of the forebrain, midbrain, and hindbrain.
- Growth in relative size of the forebrain, especially the cerebrum, which is associated with increasingly complex behaviour in mammals.

The Brain Stem and Midbrain

The brain stem is the smallest and from an evolutionary viewpoint, the oldest and most primitive part of the brain. The brain stem is continuous with the spinal cord, and is composed of the parts of the hindbrain and midbrain. The medulla oblongata and pons control heart rate, constriction of blood vessels, digestion and respiration. The midbrain consists of connections between the hindbrain and forebrain. Mammals use this part of the brain only for eye reflexes.

The Cerebellum

The cerebellum is the third part of the hindbrain, but it is not considered part of the brain stem. Functions of the cerebellum include fine motor coordination and body movement, posture, and balance. This region of the brain is enlarged in birds and controls muscle action needed for flight.

The Forebrain

The forebrain consists of the diencephalon and cerebrum. The thalamus and hypothalamus are the parts of the diencephalon. The thalamus acts as a switching centre for nerve messages. The hypothalamus is a major homeostatic centre having both nervous and endocrine functions. The cerebrum, the largest part of the human brain, is divided into left and right hemispheres connected to each other by the corpus callosum. The hemispheres are covered by a thin layer of gray matter known as the cerebral cortex, the most recently evolved region of the vertebrate brain. Fish have no cerebral cortex, amphibians and reptiles have only rudiments of this area. The cortex in each hemisphere of the cerebrum is between 1 and 4 mm thick. Folds divide the cortex into four lobes: occipital, temporal, parietal, and frontal. No region of the brain functions alone, although major functions of various parts of the lobes have been determined.

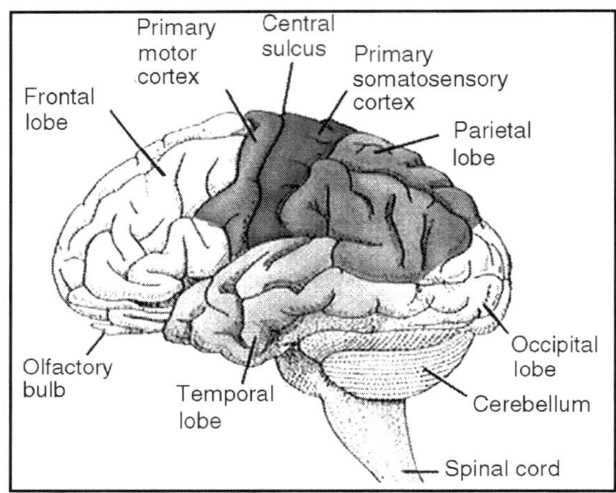

Fig. The Major Brain Areas and Lobes.

The occipital lobe receives and processes visual information. The temporal lobe receives auditory signals, processing language and the meaning of words. The parietal lobe is associated with the sensory cortex and processes information about touch, taste, pressure, pain, and heat and cold.

The frontal lobe conducts three functions:

1. Motor activity and integration of muscle activity
2. Speech
3. Thought processes

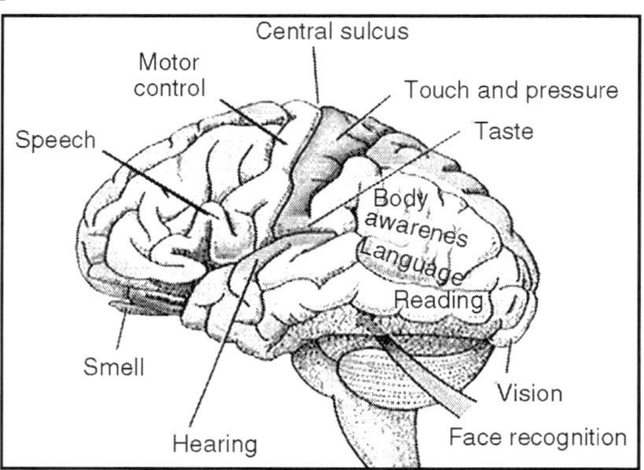

Fig. Functional Areas of the Brain.

Most people who have been studied have their language and speech areas on the left hemisphere of their brain. Language comprehension is found in Wernicke's area. Speaking ability is in Broca's area. Damage to Broca's area causes speech impairment but not impairment of language comprehension. Lesions in Wernicke's area impairs ability to comprehend written and spoken words but not speech. The remaining parts of the cortex are associated with higher thought processes, planning, memory, personality and other human activities.

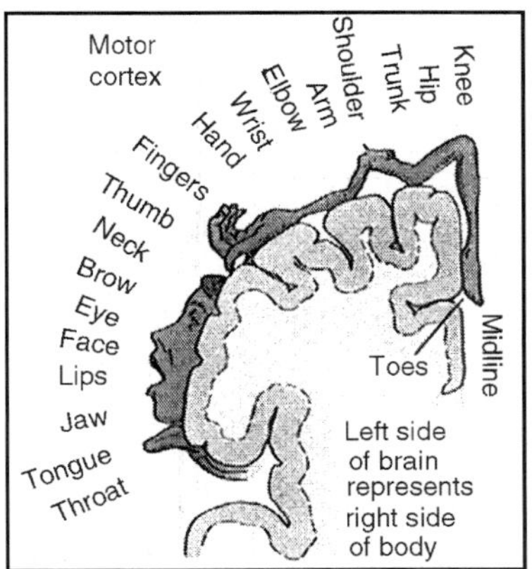

Parts of the cerebral cortex and the relative areas that are devoted to controlling various body regions.

The Spinal Cord

The spinal cord runs along the dorsal side of the body and links the brain to the rest of the body. Vertebrates have their spinal cords encased in a series of (usually) bony vertebrae that comprise the vertebral column.

The gray matter of the spinal cord consists mostly of cell bodies and dendrites. The surrounding white matter is made up of bundles of interneuronal axons (tracts). Some tracts are ascending (carrying messages to the brain), others are descending (carrying messages from the brain). The spinal cord is also involved in reflexes that do not immediately involve the brain.

The Brain and Drugs

Some neurotransmitters are excitory, such as acetylcholine, norepinephrine, serotonin, and dopamine. Some are associated with relaxation, such as dopamine and serotonin. Dopamine release seems related to sensations of pleasure. Endorphins are natural opioids that produce elation and reduction of pain, as do artificial chemicals such as opium and heroin.

Neurological diseases, for example Parkinson's disease and Huntington's disease, are due to imbalances of neurotransmitters. Parkinson's is due to a dopamine deficiency. Huntington's disease is thought to be cause by malfunctioning of an inhibitory neurotransmitter. Alzheimer's disease is associated with protein plaques in the brain.

Drugs are stimulants or depressants that block or enhance certain neurotransmitters. Dopamine is thought involved with all forms of pleasure. Cocaine interferes with uptake of dopamine from the synaptic cleft. Alcohol causes a euphoric "high" followed by a depression. Marijuana, material from the Indian hemp plant (Cannabis sativa), has a potent chemical THC (tetrahydracannibinol) that in low, concentrations causes a euphoric high (if inhaled, the most common form of action is smoke inhalation). High dosages may cause severe effects such as hallucinations, anxiety, depression, and psychotic symptoms.

Cocaine is derives from the plant Erthoxylon coca. Inhaled, smoked or injected. Cocaine users report a "rush" of euphoria following use. Following the rush is a short (5-30 minute) period of arousal followed by a depression. Repeated cycle of use terminate in a "crash" when the cocaine is gone. Prolonged used causes production of less dopamine, causing the user to need more of the drug. Heroin is a derivative of morphine, which in turn is obtained from opium, the milky secretions obtained from the opium poppy, Papaver somniferum. Heroin is usually injected intravenously, although snorting and smoking serve as alternative delivery methods.

Heroin binds to ophioid receptors in the brain, where the natural chemical endorphins are involved in the cessation pain. Heroin is physically addictive, and prolonged use causes less endorphin production. Once this happens, the euphoria is no longer felt, only dependence and delay of withdrawal symptoms.

Senses

Input to the nervous system is in the form of our five senses: pain, vision, taste, smell, and hearing. Vision, taste, smell, and hearing input are the special senses. Pain, temperature, and pressure are known as somatic senses. Sensory input begins with sensors that react to stimuli in the form of energy that is transmitted into an action potential and sent to the CNS.

Sensory Receptors

- Sensory receptors are classified according to the type of energy they can detect and respond to.
- *Mechanoreceptors*: hearing and balance, stretching.
- *Photoreceptors*: light.
- *Chemoreceptors*: smell and taste mainly, as well as internal sensors in the digestive and circulatory systems.
- *Thermoreceptors*: changes in temperature.
- *Electroreceptors*: detect electrical currents in the surrounding environment.

Mechanoreceptors vary greatly in the specific type of stimulus and duration of stimulus/action potentials. The most adaptable vertebrate mechanoreceptor is the hair cell. Hair cells are present in the lateral line of fish. In humans and mammals hair cells are involved with detection of sound and gravity and providing balance.

Hearing

Hearing involves the actions of the external ear, eardrum, ossicles, and cochlea. In hearing, sound waves in air are converted into vibrations of a liquid then into movement of hair cells in the cochlea. Finally they are converted into action potentials in a sensory dendrite connected to the auditory nerve. Very loud sounds can cause violent vibrations in the membrane under hair cells, causing a shearing or permanent distortion to the cells, resulting in permanent hearing loss.

Orientation and Gravity

Orientation and gravity are detected at the semicircular canals. Hair cells along three planes respond to shifts of liquid within the cochlea, providing a three-dimensional sense of equilibrium. Calcium carbonate crystals can shift in response to gravity, providing sensory information about gravity and acceleration.

Photoreceptors Detect Vision and Light Sensitivity

The human eye can detect light in the 400-700 nanometer (nm) range, a small portion of the electromagnetic spectrum, the visible light spectrum. Light with wavelengths shorter than 400 nm is termed ultraviolet (UV) light. Light with wavelengths longer than 700 nm is termed infrared (IR) light.

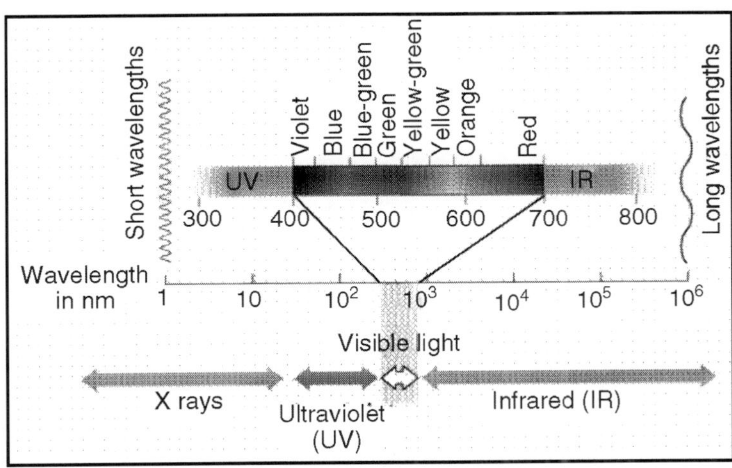

Fig. The Electromagnetic Spectrum.

Eye

In the eye, two types of photoreceptor cells are clustered on the retina, or back portion of the eye. These receptors, rods and cones, apparently evolved from hair cells. Rods detect differences in light intensity; cones detect colour. Rods are more common in a circular zone near the edge of the eye. Cones occur in the centre (or fovea centralis) of the retina. Light reaching a photoreceptor causes the breakdown of the chemical rhodopsin, which in turn causes a membrane potential that is transmitted to an action potential. The action potential transfers to synapsed neurons that connect to the optic nerve. The optic nerve connects to the occipital lobe of the brain. Humans have three types of cones, each sensitive to a different colour of light: red, blue and green. Opsins are chemicals that bind to cone cells and make those cells sensitive to light of a particular wavelength (or colour). Humans have three different form of opsins coded for by three genes on the X chromosome. Defects in one or more of these opsin genes can cause colour blindness, usually in males.

NERVOUS SYSTEM IN ORGANIC REGULATION

The nervous system serves to co-ordinate the activities of the different organs to some extent, but it is not in itself essential for the life of the tissues. A leg will live for years without nerves, but only for an hour or less without blood or some artificial substitute for blood. The cells in a higher animal are like skilled workmen, very efficient at their own job, but not at other jobs.

Thus a single cell in Hydra may serve for protection, be sensitive to external stimuli, contract when stimulated, pass on excitation to its neighbours, and perhaps secrete mucus, but in none of these ways will it act as efficiently as the various cells of a mammal, each of which performs one of these special functions.

The latter are enabled to specialize largely because they have a nearly constant environment, constant in chemical composition and temperature, and do not spend any energy in adapting themselves to change in it.

This environment is supplied by the fluid part of the blood. In this and the next chapter we shall consider some of the factors in the internal environment, and how they are kept steady or adapted to new conditions.

Most of the general symptoms of disease are due to upsets of the internal environment. Each organ must have food, oxygen, and a means of getting rid of waste products. But this is not all. It must have them in the right amounts. Too much oxygen is just as deadly as too little. And it must also have in the right amounts other substances which it does not use for work or repair. An animal dies if we halve or double the amount of potassium salts in its plasma, though it does not turn potassium salts into anything else.

So these too have to be kept steady. Further, an organ may need different amounts of a given substance at different times. If a muscle suddenly starts work, its O_2 -consumption and CO_2 -production increase about fifty times. It was already using most of the oxygen in the blood which passed through it, so it must increase its blood-supply correspondingly. When it is at rest about five out of every six of its capillaries are shut. When it begins to contract these at once open and the others open wider. The small arteries also open wider. In a resting muscle they are kept almost shut by the slight alkalinity of the blood, and also probably by the presence of oxygen.

Now if we cut the leg off a recently killed frog and run fluid through the blood-vessels, they will open up if this fluid is not sufficiently alkaline, or is short of oxygen. Just the same thing happens when a muscle contracts or a gland begins to secrete.

The O_2 flows from the blood and CO_2 is poured into it, making it acid; the blood-vessels relax and widen, and the organ obtains an adequate flow of blood. Other products of activity besides CO_2 probably co-operate in producing this effect. But when any large organ opens up its vessels the arterial pressure would fall unless the heart pumped harder. The other organs would then go short of blood. We must therefore study the working of the heart.

Like other involuntary muscles, it will work without any nervous control. If we take the heart out of a recently dead animal or man, and supply it with warm blood or an appropriate salt solution containing oxygen, it begins to beat again and may go on for many hours. Even an isolated piece of it will beat. In a mammal the beat starts at the entrance of the great veins to the right auricle in a special piece of tissue known as the 'pacemaker', which does not contract but stimulates the neighbouring muscle.

If we warm the pacemaker, the whole heart beats faster; if we destroy it, the heart first stops, then begins to beat at a slower pace of its own. The auricles contract almost instantaneously when stimulated by the pacemaker, but they are only connected with the ventricles by a narrow bridge of conducting tissue in which the wave of excitation is delayed for about one-tenth of a second, and then passed on almost simultaneously to all parts of the ventricles.

If the bridge is damaged, as in some forms of heart-disease, the ventricle may only respond to every second or third beat of the auricles. If it is destroyed they beat at their own rather slow rate, and cannot be speeded up. Now if we take an isolated heart, or a heart whose nerves have been cut, and give it an increased supply of blood, it can increase its output per beat but will not increase its rate at all.

The rate is governed by two pairs of nerves. Of these, the vagi are one; if they are stimulated the heart slows down; if they are cut it speeds up, showing that they are normally acting as a brake on it, mainly through the pacemaker. The other pair, called the accelerators, come through sympathetic ganglia from the spinal cord. Stimulation of them speeds up the heart. Both pairs are governed by the same centres in the medulla oblongata. If the blood-supply to the heart is increased, the great veins and auricles are distended, and receptor organs in their walls send impulses up to the brain which result in the vagus brake being slackened by a reflex action; and if the stimulus is sufficient, the accelerators are set to work.

Hence, when more blood reaches the heart from the open vessels of an active muscle, it increases its rate and force. Another set of reflexes keep the arterial pressure steady. A pair of nerves called the depressors run from receptor organs in the aorta to the medulla oblongata, which they enter with the vagus. If the aorta be distended by an abnormally high blood-pressure, impulses run up them to the medulla. The reflex response to this is a slowing of the heart by the vagus and an opening of small arteries. The opposite occurs if the aortic pressure falls. There is also a pressure-gauge in the brain itself.

If pressure is put on the brain from outside, for example, by a clot of blood under the skull, its vessels will collapse, and the brain will force the heart to raise the arterial pressure till they open up again. In this way the arterial blood-pressure is kept steady, so that any organ can obtain the blood-supply it needs by opening up its bloodvessels. But the brain does not allow an indiscriminate competition between different organs for blood-supply.

The arteries as well as the heart are under nervous control. A series of nerves called vasoconstrictors run in the sympathetic system to the smooth muscle of the arterial walls. The vasoconstrictors come into play in circumstances which affect the body as a whole, such as change of posture, or violent exercise.

When a man gets up after lying down the blood tends to flow into his belly and legs, and this is prevented by the contraction of the arteries of these parts, under impulses from the vasomotor centre, which lies near the heartregulating centre in the brain. If he has been in bed some days the vasomotor centre is out of practice and his brain runs short of blood, so that he becomes *dizzy* and may faint. If there is a great deal of blood in the guts and skin, as when we are sitting before the fire after a heavy meal, this may even happen on getting out of a chair. Again, during muscular exertion the arteries to the guts contract, and digestion has to stop.

The vasoconstrictor nerves are also excited by chemical stimuli to the brain. If we are throttled or breathe very impure air, the CO_2 of the blood goes up and the O_2 down. The vasomotor centre then narrows down all arteries except those to the heart, lungs, and brain, and the blood-pressure rises. These three essential organs must have an adequate supply of oxygen, whatever else goes short. The other organs, if left to themselves, would open up their vessels, but in a general emergency they are not allowed to do so. The heart is also speeded up. There are also vasodilator nerves.

For example, when a dog gets hot the vessels in its tongue are opened up by a special nerve. Moreover, many of the nerve-fibres whose stimulation causes pain send branches to the local blood-vessels. When a pain-spot is stimulated, impulses run up to the spinal cord. They also run directly to the local vessels, which open up, causing reddening of the skin; this is almost the only reflex in higher animals of which the nervous path is entirely outside the central nervous system. The above are cases where an organ gets blood which is not to be used mainly as a gas-carrier. The same occurs in an actively secreting gland. A salivary gland when active uses three times as much oxygen as when at rest.

But it also needs a great deal of water to make saliva, and it is as a source of water rather than of oxygen that it needs blood. Its bloodsupply must go up five times, and as the ordinary chemical call for blood is not effective, a vasodilator nerve is used. As the blood-supply goes up more than the oxygen-consumption, the venous blood of the active gland is actually redder than usual. A much more important case of non-respiratory bloodsupply is the skin's. The human skin excretes energy just as the kidneys excrete matter. All the heat produced in the body has to get out, and seldom does more than a fifth of it get out in the breath.

The remainder goes through the skin, and its loss is regulated in such a way as to keep the temperature of the body very constant. If we go into a hot room the same amount of heat has to be lost in a given time, but it is obviously harder to get rid of it.

If we work hard and produce more heat in our bodies, more heat has to be lost in a given time, though the loss of a given amount is no harder. In each case the skin responds in the same way. Its small arteries open up and it gets red and warm. Heat is thus brought from the inside to the surface in large amounts and rapidly lost, as from the radiator of a motor vehicle. If this means of losing heat is insufficient, we begin to sweat.

The sweat comes from microscopic glands under nervous control. It consists of water containing less salt than the plasma. When this evaporates the skin is greatly cooled, for water has a big latent heat of evaporation. Sweat that does not evaporate does not cool us, and it cannot evaporate if the air is already saturated with water-vapour. So sweating is useless in a hot and damp atmosphere, which is therefore far more oppressive than a dry one of the same temperature. The ordinary thermometer does not tell us whether we shall be able to lose heat or not.

For this purpose we use a 'wetbulb' thermometer. The bulb is wrapped in a wet cloth, so that the drier the air is, the more heat it can lose by evaporation. It is therefore in the same position as a man whose clothes are soaked with sweat. If the air is saturated with water the wet- and dry-bulb thermometers have the same reading, if the air is dry the wet-bulb thermometer may read more than 100° F. lower. Men can stand dry heat far above boiling-point, staying in a room where a steak is cooked in five minutes, and only coming out when their hair begins to singe.

But a wet-bulb temperature above 90° F. is fatal, and above one of 75° F. the capacity for work is lowered. We get an idea of the efficiency of sweating by considering a man in fairly dry air at body-temperature (98·5° F.). He can lose no heat by conduction or convection, so it must all be used in evaporating water.

He has to lose 3,000 kilocalories per day. But the evaporation of 1 litre of water at body-temperature requires 570 kilocalories, so in a day he must sweat 5·3 litres, or 9·3 pints. Actually many men can sweat 1 litre per hour, and the world's sweating record is held by an English coalminer who lost 18 pounds (1·8 gallons, or 8 litres) in 51/2 hours. To make up for the loss of sweat one must drink more water and eat more sodium chloride than usual.

Miners working in great heat are therefore fonder than the average man of bacon, kippers, and salt. Many animals, such as dogs, have very few sweat-glands, but produce a very thin saliva which they evaporate by rapid shallow breathing, panting with open mouth and tongue hanging out.

Several parts of the brain are concerned in heat regulation. They receive nervous impulses from the skin, and also from local organs in the brain which measure the temperature of the blood like thermometers. Thus, if certain parts of an animal's brain, or the blood going to them, are heated, the animal begins to flush and sweat, and the rest of its body is cooled down.

If the brain is cooled the animal shivers and its temperature rises. During adaptation to heat we cannot cut down our heatproduction except by keeping still, but when cold, besides shutting down the skin-vessels, we first tighten up our muscles, then shiver, and finally take exercise. In all these ways more heat is produced. In many diseases the temperature rises.

This is not due to increased heat-production, but to diminished heat-loss owing to perverted function of the temperature centres. A man whose temperature is thus rising feels very cold until it has reached the new level to which he is regulating.

He shivers and complains of the draught, to which he may put down his illness. If his temperature falls quickly he sweats profusely and feels very hot. Mammals and birds have a nearly constant temperature, but other animals have a variable temperature, a fraction of a degree above their surroundings. If we warm a 'cold-blooded' animal through about 5° C. we double its rate of oxygen-consumption, and all its other activities.

For example, it is possible to read the temperature within 1° F. by measuring the distance walked by an ant in a minute! Cold-blooded animals cannot move quickly in winter, and mostly die or rest in holes. The activities of mammals and birds are not slowed down, so they are the dominant animals in temperate and cold climates. But in hot countries, snakes, crocodiles, and so on, are able to compete successfully with warm-blooded animals. A few mammals, such as hedgehogs and dormice, compromise by sleeping through the winter at a low temperature (and therefore a low rate of oxidation), but they never let their temperature fall to that of their surroundings. We must now turn to chemical regulation of the composition of the blood and tissues.

It will be convenient to begin with the gases, the quantity of which in the blood is regulated by breathing. The obvious duties of the lungs are to get rid of CO_2 and let in O_2, and if we go into a room containing say 6 per cent. of CO_2 instead of the normal 0·03 per cent., or 10 per cent. of O_2 instead of the normal 20·9 per cent., the breathing increases greatly. However, a small drop in the O_2 of the air breathed has no visible effect on the breathing, because the haemoglobin is already almost saturated with oxygen at a pressure less than that in the lungs. So want of O_2 cannot be what normally keeps the breathing going.

To find out how the breathing is regulated we must take the samples of air from the very bottom of the lungs, where it is in equilibrium with the blood. This, which is called the alveolar air, can be obtained at the end of a deep breath out. The amount of carbon dioxide in it is very constant, about 51/2 per cent., whereas the amount of oxygen varies a good deal.

If the amount of carbon dioxide increases by only 3 per cent. of its normal value, the breathing is doubled; if it falls by the same amount, as after voluntary over-breathing, the breathing stops.

The main reason why we breathe more during moderate muscular exercise is because more carbon dioxide is being produced, and this stimulates the respiratory centres in the brain to make the breathing muscles do more work. Thus the lungs have the function of keeping the CO_2 pressure in the tissues at the normal level, not merely of excreting it.

Carbonic acid seems merely to act on the respiratory centre in virtue of its being an acid. If another acid, such as hydrochloric, is injected or drunk, the breathing is greatly increased, while it slows down when an alkaline substance such as sodium hydrogen carbonate is taken. The most familiar case, however, is that of very violent exercise.

When the muscles are working so fast that they cannot get enough oxygen for their recovery process, lactic acid accumulates in them and leaks out into the blood, from which it is only gradually removed. So after running a quarter-mile the extra carbon dioxide is got rid of in the few minutes of violent panting which succeed the race, but a small increase of the breathing, due to lactic acid, may persist for half an hour or so.

During this time the alveolar carbon dioxide pressure is kept below normal by the extra breathing, thus compensating for the acidity which would otherwise be produced by the lactic acid. Serious oxygen-want also excites the respiratory centre.

If one goes into air containing only about half the normal 20·9 per cent. of O_2, one at once begins to pant, but after a while the panting dies down, because a lot of CO_2 has been blown out of the body by the increased breathing, and the respiratory centres have no more reason to discharge nervous impulses than before, their normal stimulus, CO_2, being reduced in quantity. So a man who has gone into bad air at first pants enough to keep his blood supplied with oxygen. Then the breathing becomes normal, and he falls unconscious with oxygen-want.

A candle is often a much better measure of oxygen-want than one's own feelings. Another way in which the breathing is affected is by the process of digestive secretion. When the stomach secretes hydrochloric acid the blood would be too alkaline if carbonic acid were not kept back to take its place, so the breathing is slightly slowed down. Later on, the pancreas and intestine begin to remove alkali from the blood for their secretions, and to prevent it getting too acid the breathing has to be increased.

These changes are too small to observe directly, but can easily be measured. We can get some idea of why the alkalinity of the tissues has to be regulated so carefully by experimenting with tissue or enzymes taken from them. If we take a dead organ and preserve it carefully from bacteria it does not putrefy. But if it is kept at body-temperature the tissues gradually soften and are found to be digesting themselves.

This is due to enzymes in them. The dying tissues produce acids, and in a slightly acid medium these enzymes work very much more rapidly than in an alkaline or neutral one. Thus, to prevent an organ from digesting itself it must be kept slightly alkaline. The best known of these enzymes is that in the liver which breaks up its glycogen into sugar. A quite fresh liver, besides being very tough, does not taste sweet. If it is allowed to digest itself for a few days it not only becomes tender, but sweet.

Some other enzymes act more rapidly in a medium more alkaline than the normal, so if the reaction of the tissues is altered the normal balance between the different chemical processes is upset, and death may occur. Just as the lungs regulate the amount of gases in the blood, the kidneys regulate the amount of the soluble bodies.

The blood which passes through these organs is always altered so as to resemble an 'ideal' blood. Thus, if there is more water in the blood-plasma than in this ideal or standard plasma the kidney secretes an unusually watery urine, and the plasma of the blood in the renal vein therefore contains less water than the arterial blood, and resembles the standard plasma more closely.

If, as is more usual, especially in hot weather, there is rather less water in the plasma than in the standard plasma, the kidney secretes a concentrated urine, so the blood leaving the kidney contains more water than that entering it. The substances found in blood and urine can be divided into two classes. The first class includes almost all foreign substances, for example, iodides, dyes, or foreign proteins injected into the blood. These are removed by the kidneys, however little there is in the blood. It also includes some very important waste-products, such as urea, the substance which contains most of the nitrogen resulting from protein oxidation.

The rate at which such substances are excreted is roughly proportional to the amount in a given volume of blood. The second class includes most of the normal constituents of plasma, such as sodium, potassium, calcium, magnesium, chloride, bicarbonate, phosphate, and sugar. These substances are only excreted if the quantity of one of them contained in a given volume of plasma exceeds a certain limit, called the 'threshold'.

For example, the amount of chloride in the plasma is generally a few per cent. above the threshold, and there are, therefore, chlorides. in normal urine. But if we drink a lot of water after violent sweating, the amount of chloride in the plasma falls below the threshold, and it disappears from the urine.

Normal blood contains about 0·10 per cent. of glucose, a simple sugar. If a healthy man takes 100 grams of glucose the amount in the blood rises to about 0·13 per cent., but none appears in the urine.

The threshold value for the kidney is about 0·17 per cent. If, therefore, the arrangements for storing sugar are out of order, as in diabetes, a dose of 100 grams will make the blood-sugar rise above 0·17 per cent., and sugar will appear in the urine. Besides excreting substances found in the blood, the kidney makes a few substances.

For example, sulphuric and phosphoric acids are made throughout the body by the oxidation of the proteins. The kidney has to get rid of these, but its cells and those of the urinary passages are damaged by strong acids. It therefore excretes the sulphuric acid not as such, but as ammonium sulphate, which is neutral in reaction. But there is not enough ammonia in the blood to furnish all that is required for this purpose.

Ammonia and ammonium salts are poisons when injected into the blood-stream, and the liver converts almost all the ammonia reaching it into urea, which is nearly harmless. So the kidney has to make its own ammonia, and the more acids it has to excrete the more ammonia it makes.

The kidney is doing work like a muscle, for work has to be done in concentrating substances, just as in compressing gases. For example, to concentrate the urea in a litre of blood into about 20 cubic centimetres of urine, as the kidney does every 20 minutes or so, requires at least as much work as to compress a litre of gas containing as many molecules as there are urea molecules in the blood, into 20 cubic centimetres.

Actually the number of urea molecules in a litre of blood is the same as that in a litre of gas at a tenth of an atmosphere pressure, so the work needed is that required to compress this gas to a pressure of five atmospheres, i. e. 40 kilogrammetres. In order to do this work the kidney needs oxygen. Its oxygen-consumption can be measured by determining the rate at which blood flows through it and the amount of oxygen lost by this blood. As a matter of fact, the kidney uses a good deal more oxygen per gram per minute than the heart, and like the heart, will increase its oxygen-consumption three or four times if it is given work to do.

But if we inject salt-solution of about the composition of plasma, the kidney needs no more oxygen, although the volume of urine secreted per minute is increased. This is because it has no work to do in concentrating the salt, but it merely acts like a filter. If on the other hand we inject urea or sodium sulphate, its oxygen-consumption increases, as these substances have to be concentrated. Other glands behave in a similar manner, requiring more oxygen when stimulated to do work.

9

Zoonotic Disease

INTRODUCTION

Zoonoses are diseases and infections naturally transmissible from vertebrate animals to man by direct contact with infected animals, insects or animal excreta. While it is possible for anybody to become infected with a zoonotic agent, certain population groups such as the very young, the elderly and immunocompromised are particularly vulnerable and at greater risk of more serious consequences. The eradication of zoonoses in humans and animals is a difficult if not impossible goal to achieve. However, the impact of zoonoses on the health of humans and animals can be limited by monitoring the reservoirs of infectious zoonotic agents with a view to understanding and controlling their modes of transfer, while educating the public about how to avoid or limit the risk of infection.

There are two types of zoonotic diseases that concern pet owners: illnesses that can be transmitted from pets to humans - like leptospirosis - and diseases that infect both people and pets - like Lyme disease. That's why it's important to take precautions to protect both your family and your pets from zoonotic diseases.

DEFINITION OF ZOONOTIC DISEASE

Any disease that is spread from animals to people. There are many known zoonotic diseases, some of them very familiar such as Lyme disease and malaria. Less familiar zoonotic diseases (beginning with the letters "a" and "b") include alveolar hydatid disease (echinococcosis), ancylostoma infection (hookworm), ascariasis (intestinal roundworm infection), babesiosis (babesia infection), and baylisascaris infection (raccoon roundworm).

DESCRIPTION

Although many diseases are species specific, meaning that they can only occur in one animal species, many other diseases can bespread between different animal species. These are infectious diseases, caused by bacteria, viruses, or other disease causingorganisms that can live as well in humans as in other animals.

There are different methods of transmission for different diseases. In some cases, zoonotic diseases are transferred by direct contactwith infected animals, much as being near an infected human can cause the spread of an infectious disease. Other diseases are spreadby drinking water that contains the eggs of parasites.

The eggs enter the water supply from the feces of infected animals. Still others arespread by eating the flesh of infected animals. Tapeworms are spread this way. Other diseases are spread by insect vectors. An insect,such as a flea or tick, feeds on an infected animal, then feeds on a human. In the process, the insect transfers the infecting organism.

The Centers for Disease Control (CDC) in Atlanta have said that most emerging diseases around the world are zoonotic. The director ofthe CDC has said that 11 of the last 12 emerging infections in the world with serious health consequences has probably arisen fromanimal sources.

Wild animal trade occurs across countries and many people take in wild animals as domestic pets. However, pet shopsand food markets are not properly testing for diseases and parasites that can cause harm to humans and other animals.

Some zoonotic diseases are well known, such as rats (plague), deer tick (Lyme disease). Others are not as well known. For example,elephants may develop tuberculosis, and spread it to humans.

CAUSES AND SYMPTOMS

The following is a partial list of animals and the diseases that they may carry.

(Not all animal carriers are listed, nor are all the diseases that the various species may carry).

- Bats are important rabies carriers, and also carry several other viral diseases that can affect humans.
- Cats may carry the causative organisms for plague, anthrax, cowpox, tapeworm, and many bacterial infections.
- Dogs may carry plague, tapeworm, rabies, Rocky Mountain Spotted Fever, and Lyme disease.
- Horses may carry anthrax, rabies, and Salmonella infections.
- Cattle may carry the organisms that cause anthrax, European tick-borne encephalitis, rabies, tapeworm, Salmonella infections andmany bacterial and viral diseases.
- Pigs are best known for carrying tapeworm, but may also carry a large number of other infections including anthrax, influenza, andrabies.

- Sheep and goats may carry rabies, European tick-borne encephalitis, Salmonella infections, and many bacterial and viral diseases.
- Rabbits may carry plague and Q-Fever.
- Birds may carry Campylobacteriosis, Chlamydia psittaci, Pasteurella multocida, Histoplasma capsulatum, Salmonellosis, and others

Zoonotic diseases may be spread in different ways. Tapeworms can often spread to humans when people eat the infected meat of cattle,and swine. Other diseases are transferred by insect vectors, often blood-feeding insects that carry the cause of the disease from oneanimal to another.

Diagnosis

Diagnosis of the disease is made in the usual manner, by identifying the infecting organism. Each disease has established symptomsand tests. Identifying the carrier may be easy, or may be more difficult when the cause is a fairly common infection.

For example, tapeworms are usually species specific. Cattle, pigs, and fish all carry different species of tapeworms, although all can be transmitted tohumans who eat undercooked meat containing live tapeworm eggs. Once the tapeworm has been identified, it is easy to tell whichspecies the tapeworm came from.

Other zoonotic infections may be harder to identify. Sometimes the infection is fairly common among both humans and animals, and it isimpossible to tell. Snakes may carry the bacteria Escherichia coli and Proteus vulgaris, but since these bacteria are already commonamong humans, it would be difficult to trace infections back to snakes.

Because of increased trade between nations, and changes in animal habitats, there are often new zoonotic diseases. These may befound in animals transported from one nation to another, bringing with them new diseases. In some cases, changes in the environmentlead to changes in the migratory habits of animal species, bringing new infections.

Treatment

Treatment is the established treatment for the specific infection.

Prevention

Prevention of zoonotic infections may take different forms, depending on the nature of the carrier and the infection.

Some zoonotic infections can be avoided by immunising the animals that carry the disease. Pets and other domestic animals shouldhave rabies vaccinations, and wild animals are immunised with an oral vaccine that is encased in a suitable bait. In some places, thebait is dropped by airplane over the range of the potential rabies carrier. When the animal eats the bait, they also ingest the oral vaccine,thereby protecting them from rabies, and reducing the risk of spread of the disease. This method has been used to protect foxes, coyotes, and other wild animals.

Many zoonotic diseases that are passed by eating the meat of infected animals can be prevented by proper cooking of the infectedmeat. Tapeworm infestations can be prevented by cooking, and Salmonella infections from chickens and eggs can be prevented bybeing sure that both the meat and the eggs are fully cooked.

ZOONOTIC NEMATODE INFECTIONS

TRICHINELLOSIS

Parasitic nematodes of the genus Trichinella are remarkable as the mature L1 larva occupies two distinct intracellular niches within a single vertebrate host (the intestinal epithelia and the skeletal muscle), whereas the immature L1 larvae are solely extracellular.

After ingestion of infected meat, the L1 larvae are released from muscle tissue by host-digestive enzymes in the stomach. The free L1 larvae then migrate to the small intestine where they penetrate the intestinal mucosa and undergo four successive moults, becoming mature adult worms within little more than 24 h. Mating also occurs within this niche and from this site the newborn larvae migrate via the blood and lymphatic systems to skeletal muscle, where they infect the myofibres and develop into the encysted infective L1 stage.

Human infection occurs following consumption of raw or undercooked meat containing encysted Trichinellalarvae. Symptoms are varied (including nausea, vomiting, diarrhoea, fatigue, fever and abdominal discomfort) and the severity of the disease is dependent on the dose of infective larvae ingested. Infected individuals can also suffer from heart and breathing problems and in severe cases death can occur. The disease is best treated early with a combination of benzimidazoles and anti-inflammatory corticosteroids such as prednisone.

The range of ambiguous and changing symptoms that occur during human infections often leads to misdiagnosis of the disease. The definitive method for diagnosis of trichinellosis is microscopic analysis of muscle biopsies though this has limited use for detection of light and moderate infections. More recent alternatives include detection of antibodies against Trichinella spiralis excretory–secretory (E–S) proteins in human sera by enzyme-linked immunosorbent assay and polymerase chain reaction (PCR)-based identification approaches. The release of the T. spiralis genome sequence draft assembly together with recent advances in proteomics for the identification of individual Trichinella E–S proteins has expanded the panel of Trichinella antigens that may be used to detect trichinellosis earlier post-infection. The current status of nucleotide sequence databases for the major zoonotic helminths.

Summary of the Current Status of Nucleotide Sequence Databases for the Major Zoonotic Helminth Species. CHGCS, Chinese Human Genome Center at Shanghai; NAUM, National Autonomous University of Mexico; NHGRI, National Human Genome Research Institute (USA).

Species	Project Type	Status
Nematodes		
Trichinella spiralis	whole genome draft	complete
Anisakis simplex L3 larvae	1 cDNA library	493 ESTs
cestodes		
Taenia solium adult	1 cDNA library; full genome sequence	16 000 ESTs; planned
Echinococcus granulosus	whole genome shotgun	planned
Echinococcus multilocularis	reference genome	sequencing and assembly
trematodes		
Schistosoma japonicum	full genome sequence	complete
Clonorchis sinensis adult	2 cDNA libraries	2815 ESTs
metacercaria	1 cDNA library	419 ESTs
Opisthorchis viverrini adult	1 cDNA library	5000 ESTs
Paragonimus westermani adult	2 cDNA libraries	1000 ESTs
Fasciola hepatica adult	4 cDNA libraries	11 066 ESTs

In recent years, trichinellosis has been considered to be a truly emerging (or re-emerging) zoonosis owing to increased infection rates as a direct result of changing human dietary trends and the breakdown of veterinary management practices in several developing countries. Indeed, human cases of the disease have been documented in 55 (27.8 per cent) countries around the world. By far, the major causative agent of trichinellosis is *T. spiralis* although cases of human infection caused by other *Trichinella species*, including *Trichinella pseudospiralis*, *Trichinella nativa*, *Trichinella murrelli* and *Trichinella britovi* have been reported. The major reservoir host for *T. spiralis* is the domestic pig which has been responsible for a growing number of outbreaks of trichinellosis in eastern European countries since the break-up of the USSR in the early 1990s. The European countries most affected by human Trichinella infection include Poland where there have been a number of outbreaks within the last 8 years, the Slovak Republic and the Baltic states of Lithuania, Latvia and Estonia. Consumption of raw horsemeat has led to cases of human trichinellosis in Italy and France and even the practice of hunting and eating wild animals (including wild boar and bears) has contributed to a number of human infections worldwide.

ANISAKIASIS

Anisakiasis results from infection with the larvae of the nematodes Anisakis simplex and *Pseudoterranova decipiens*. In humans, infection occurs following ingestion of marine fish (such as mackerel, cod and herring) containing the infective L3 nematode larvae. The disease occurs worldwide but is particularly prevalent in those countries where fish is eaten raw, smoked or is undercooked such as in parts of northern Asia, The Netherlands and Scandinavia. Of the 20 000 or so cases of human anisakiasis that were diagnosed by 2005, around 90 per cent came from Japan where about 2000 individual cases are reported annually. The clinical manifestations of anisakiasis can be varied and depend on the location of the larvae in the gastrointestinal tract, although the majority of cases (97 per cent) manifest as acute gastric anisakiasis where the nematode larvae reside within the gastric mucosa. Confirmation of the condition and removal of the parasite(s) can be readily carried out by endoscopy following which the epigastric pain suffered by the patient is quickly resolved.

The occurrence of human anisakiasis has risen dramatically since it was first described almost 50 years ago with a number of human and environmental factors likely contributing to the rise. The advent of the endoscope has undoubtedly led to the detection of more cases of human anisakiasis and this, together with advances in the immunological diagnosis of the disease, should see that this trend will continue.

Changing dietary trends may also have contributed to the spread of human anisakiasis. Eating raw fish such as sushi (a practice that has been ongoing in Japan for many centuries) has become highly fashionable in many western societies and has led to an increased risk of infection of populations that would not usually be exposed. It has also been suggested that greater numbers of the natural definitive hosts of anisakid nematodes (large marine mammals such as whales, dolphins, sea-lions and seals) brought about by increased regulatory controls over hunting has resulted in greater levels of contamination of fish used for human consumption.

These trends have clear implications for human health given the severe hypersensitivity reactions that can occur against anisakid antigens. At least seven different protein allergens have been identified from A. simplex, some of which are known to be heat-stable. In fact, cooking or freezing of fish containing A. simplex antigens may not be sufficient to prevent allergic reactions to the parasite in humans. Moreover, it has been reported that ingestion of chickens that were fed on fishmeal contaminated with A. simplex antigens caused hypersensitivity reactions in anisakid-sensitised individuals. At present, there is no genome-sequencing project for Anisakis. However, a small-scale expressed sequence tag (EST) project identified 493 sequences that provide a useful first look at the transcriptome of the infectious A. simplex L3 stage larva. The continued use of molecular biology approaches to identify and characterise anisakid allergens is central to our understanding of anisakiasis and will aid the diagnosis and treatment of the disease in the future.

ROLE OF WILDLIFE IN ZOONOSIS

The significance of wild life as animal reservoir for zoonotic viruses has been traced long back with two important ancient diseases such as rabies and West Nile virus and represent as large spectrum of transmission mode. Of the total emerging diseases, 75 per cent are considered zoonotic with wild life as a major source of reservoir.

Recent emerging viral diseases which moved into new species such as AIDS, SARS and avian influenza have a strong evidence of wild life origin due to human encroachment and changed international trade and travel patterns. Commonly the pattern of moving of viral agents from wild animal species to human occurs either as actual transmission being rare (HIV, Influenza A, Ebola and SARS) but will be maintained and has potential of man to man transmission or direct/indirect manner through animal bite and arthropod vectors (rabies, Nipah, West Nile virus and hantavirus). Many zoonoses with a wildlife origin are spread through insect vectors (Rift Valley fever, equine encephalitis and Japanese encephalitis), whereas, rabies by animal bite and hantaviruses by contact with rodent excreta is common.

The outcome in the form of clinical manifestation in humans depends on the transmission pattern of the agent causing the disease. Direct contact and vector bite lead to the formation of rashes and ulcers, whereas, intake of contaminated meat/water lead to digestive tract problems and diseases transmitted by inhalation of infected foci of dust cause pneumonia like illness. Wild life are basically involved in epidemiology of the disease which is influenced by other factors such as change in agro-climatic conditions, host abundance, movement of pathogens/vector/animal host including migratory birds and anthropogenic factors. For example, increase in transmission and subsequent spread of Sin Nombre Hantavirus causing Hantavirus Pulmonary Syndrome (HPS) to humans is due to increase in heavy rainfall and host abundance in USA. Increase in the emergence of some wild life diseases result in high potential of emergence of human pathogens as in the case of West Nile virus spread in USA. A potential threat to human health, animal welfare and species conservation from domesticated and wild life is presented equally by emergence of human and wild life pathogens.

MANIFESTATIONS OF VIRAL ZOONOSES

Zoonotic infections are broadly grouped in to:

- Diseases causing no illness,
- Non-specific viral syndrome and
- Severe illness.

The third category of infections is further classified in to:

- Hemorrhagic fever,
- Encephalitis and/or rash arthralgia,
- Emerging and reemerging and
- Rare zoonotic infections.

Encephalitis

The major viral zoonoses, which are associated with encephalitis. They are arthropod borne and belong mostly to five viral families (Rhabdoviridae, Flaviviridae, Togaviridae, Reoviridae and Bunyaviridae). Most of them are transmitted through mosquito or tick bites, except a few which are transmitted through bite of an infected host (rabies). Mosquitoes and ticks are major vectors for this category of infections.

They cause symptoms like fever, vomition, encephalitis, headache and neurological disorders. Some of these infections are confined to a particular country (Colorado tick fever), while others are distributed worldwide (rabies). Prophylactic/therapeutic measures are available for some of the infections, while for others vector elimination is the only means of control.

Intense research is required towards the development of vaccines including conventional as well as recombinant. Specific diagnosis of this group of infections is done employing serological tests like Hemagglutination-Inhibition (HI), Complement Fixation (CF) and Virus Neutralisation (VN).

Hemorrhagic Fevers

Most of the viral zoonoses causing haemorrhagic fevers are reported to be of emerging and reemerging in nature. There are more than 16 zoonotic infections in this category belong mainly to four viral families (Arenaviridae, Bunyaviridae, Flaviviridae, Filoviridae). These infections are often associated with extensive bleeding in human. Most of them are transmitted upon vector bite. The common vectors are mosquitoes and ticks. Vaccines are not available for majority of the infections and therefore, control relies on supportive treatment. Control of vector is the main means of control. Chemotherapy is available for some of the infections (Crimean-Congo haemorrhagic fever) with a limited success.

Rashes and Arthralgia

A very few viruses are associated with local rashes and arthralgia and almost all belong to *Togaviridae* family. Most of them are transmitted to humans through infected mosquito bites. These vectors are mainly from *Aedes* and *Culex* families. No specific treatment is available and control depends on the elimination of vectors. EU countries appear to be free, while other continents are endemic for these infections.

WILD ANIMALS IN URBAN/PERI-URBAN AREAS

According to McKinney, urbanisation is one of the leading causes of species extinction. The decline in species richness is explained by the inability of many native species to cope with the environmental alterations associated with urbanisation, eventually leading to extinction in the urban core. However, the impact of urbanisation on biodiversity depends on the ecological structure of the urban and peri-urban areas: replacement of natural ecosystems by densely populated uniform settlements in resource-poor countries has a clearly different effect than the spread of suburban landscapes into agricultural land in the industrialised world. Urban and peri-urban environments can be very attractive for adaptable wild animals. The biodiversity of plants and animals in these areas frequently exceeds the biodiversity in more natural environments due to the close proximity and variation of different habitat types (*e.g.* gardens and forest remnants). Additionally, the supply of food resources (waste food, pet food or garden produce) of urban and periurban areas in industrialised countries is far higher than in natural or rural environments. Urban and periurban areas are therefore very attractive for adaptable species, which may reach far higher population densities than in more natural or rural landscapes. These species are typically food generalists. Shochat et al. (2006) discriminate between 1. synanthropic generalist species, able to tolerate a wide range of urban conditions; 2. urban adapters, able to adapt to urban habitats but also utilising natural resources; and 3. urban exploiters which are dependent on urban resources.

Species range and density of wild animals in urban areas are determined by the type of urban habitats. According to researchers anthropogenic disturbances of various nature (noise, traffic, presence of humans and pet animals) vary in intensity between different urban, peri-urban or rural environments, which will select for the adaptability of individual species to these conditions. Observations in rapidly expanding urban areas have revealed that some wild animals not only cope well with urbanisation but are actually attracted to urban environments.

Therefore, urbanisation is a very dynamic process and changes in the composition of wildlife communities in urban and peri-urban areas are also very important for zoonotic vector-borne infections, because many of these highly adaptable species are important reservoir hosts for vector-transmitted pathogens. Therefore, changes in the abundance of certain wild animals will affect vector populations as well. Recently, abundant tick populations have been detected in peri-urban and urban areas worldwide, increasing the risk of zoonotic infections of humans and domestic animals. An increasing number of studies have been initiated to understand the complex processes involved in these developments.

ZOONOTIC PARASITES AND URBAN/PERI-URBAN AREAS

As a result of established wildlife populations in and around human settlements, zoonotic diseases (including such that are caused by parasites) can be transmitted in the immediate environment of humans. The range of pathogens transmitted not only depends on the species and abundance of individual host species, but, especially with parasites, on the host communities as a whole. Considering the complexity of parasitic life cycles (especially zoonotic vector-transmitted infections) which often include several different hosts, it is obvious that urbanisation may be beneficial for the transmission of some parasites, but not for others to the point that the parasite's life cycle is inhibited completely. Therefore, the importance, transmission and prevalence of a parasite in a given host cannot be simply extrapolated from the natural (or rural) to the urban situation.

Factors influencing the transmission of zoonotic parasites in urban areas are not well understood. As an example, rich food resources may increase the birth and litter survival rates of urban-adapted species, thus intensifying the parasite transmission due to the abundance of highly susceptible juvenile hosts. On the other hand, decreased hunting pressure may change the age pyramid in favour of older animals, which causes the opposite effect.

Pet animals may be involved in the transmission cycles of these parasites in urban areas, and the presence and frequency of pets may have a significant effect on disease pressure to humans. In urban and peri-urban areas, the frequency of contact between wildlife and humans changes from sporadic encounters to permanently sharing the environment, thus greatly increasing the chance of parasite transmission to humans. More than 75 per cent of human diseases are of zoonotic origin and are related to wildlife and domestic animals. Therefore, more information is required to better understand the dynamics between wildlife species, humans and domestic animals in urbanised areas.

The state (most often, the lack) of knowledge on various helminths and ticks whose zoonotic potential in urban and peri-urban environments has been recognised. We review examples from contrasting types of urbanised areas in central Europe and Australia, respectively.

ECHINOCOCCUS MULTILOCULARIS

Background on Transmission Factors

Alveolar echinococcosis (AE), caused by the larval stage of the cestode *Echinococcus multilocularis*, is a zoonotic disease of increasing importance in the northern hemisphere. Incidence and prevalence of human AE vary widely across the expansive range of *E. multilocularis* for reasons, which are only partly understood.

The wide geographical spread results from the ability of the parasite to use a large variety of local predatorprey systems for its transmission. Thus, the parasite is endemic in natural ecosystems like arctic tundra or Tibetan high-altitude grassland, as well as in highly anthropogenic central European farming landscapes or Japanese city parks.

In the far north, *E. multilocularis* cycles between arctic foxes (*Vulpes lagopus*) and northern voles (*Microtus oeconomus*). In the temperate parts of Eurasia, red foxes (*V. vulpes*) are the principal definitive hosts, although other canids may regionally also contribute to the life cycle, *e.g.* Tibetan foxes (V. ferrilata), raccoon dogs (Nyctereutes procyonoides), golden jackals (*Canis aureus*), coyotes (*C. latrans*), wolves (*C. lupus*) or domestic dogs. Concerning intermediate hosts, the situation is even more complex. In most of Europe, Microtus arvalis seems to be the most important species, while *e.g.* in central

Asia, other grassland-adapted rodents are principal intermediate hosts. In contrast, *Myodes* spp., living in dense forest undergrowth, maintain the life cycle in northern Japan

Therefore, factors that drive the transmission of this parasite and risk factors for human disease are necessarily different across geographical regions, and possibly even between different ecosystems of the same area:

Definitive hosts: wild and domestic canids as competent hosts are widespread and occur in all endemic regions. However, canid species differ in their capacities to support worm populations, and their infection risk differs due to habitat and prey preference. Moreover, their population densities vary due to species-specific parameters and available food resources. As the age structure of the canid population is known to be important (juvenile red foxes have far higher worm burdens than adults), hunting pressure or disease mortality has an impact on transmission. Repeated infections with *E. multilocularis* elicit intestinal immune responses, which act as a downregulating factor on parasite egg production in highly endemic areas.

Intermediate hosts: different rodent species differ drastically in their susceptibility to, and tolerance of, the parasite, as well as in their habitat preference on a small spatial scale. Some species maintain rather stable populations (at different densities), while others tend towards cyclic population outbreaks and crashes. The amplitude of the population cycles, again, is determined by the landscape pattern. Varying population densities of the same species not only change the predation rates of the canids, but may also change their predation behaviour with respect to other food sources. Availability (microhabitats, diurnal activity patterns) and attractiveness as prey is different among rodent species.

Environmental conditions: climate and anthropogenic influences determine the vegetation type and, thereby, the species composition and density of host species. Climatic factors (*e.g.* precipitation) and soil parameters act on the survival time of E. multilocularis eggs in the environment. Weather conditions (*e.g.* snow cover in winter) influence the survival of rodents and their availability as prey.

Human behaviour: Attitude to wildlife, hunting pressure and rodent pest control act on host populations. Intentional or accidental introduction of new host species can change life cycle patterns, and the parasite can be introduced into non-endemic areas via travelling dogs or translocated wild animals. Dogs kept for various purposes may complement the life cycle, or may act as a specific risk factor for human AE. The presence or absence of good personal hygiene behaviour are likely to be key factors for the frequency of human disease.

E. Multilocularis in Urban and Peri-urban Areas of Europe

Until the 1990s, AE in central Europe was considered to be a disease associated with rural areas and farming activities. Since then, the annual incidence of human AE has increased at least in parts of the region, a development which seems to be correlated with the general increase of European fox populations beginning in the early 1990s. In addition, human cases are being reported increasingly from urban areas, which appear to be a consequence of the urbanisation of the *E. multilocularis* life cycle.

For most of the 20th century, foxes outside Britain were not known to occur in larger towns and cities, and the principal intermediate hosts, *M. arvalis* and *Arvicola scherman*, are typical rodents of meadows, pastures and orchards in rural landscapes. From that time onwards, however, habitat preferences of some red fox populations have changed. Regular sightings of foxes inside larger human settlements were first reported from the middle of the 1990s, and by the early 2000s several larger cities of central Europe were known to support resident fox populations. The most obvious characteristic of these urban foxes is tolerance of disturbing factors like traffic and the immediate vicinity of humans and pet animals. Initially, this phenomenon was thought to be the result of population pressure from rural areas to less suitable urban habitats in the wake of general fox population increases in the 1990s (probably aided by reduced mortality after successful rabies vaccinations).

Genetic studies, however, showed that populations of urban foxes are self-sustaining and show reduced gene flow to and from surrounding rural populations. Typically, these synanthropic foxes live in higher population densities than their rural counterparts, aided by sufficient and seasonally stable food from anthropogenic sources. For urban and suburban areas in Switzerland and southern Germany, radio-tracking data suggest densities of >10 resident adult foxes per km^2, compared with <3 per km^2 in rural areas.

Relatively few studies have been conducted on the infection of such foxes with E. multilocularis. Reported prevalences in different cities and towns vary drastically, being *e.g.* 4 per cent in Nancy (France) and 44 per cent in Zurich (Switzerland). Urban *E. multilocularis* life cycles are assumed to result from the establishment of these synanthropic fox populations. However, earlier presence of the parasite in urban areas cannot be excluded, since relevant studies were only initiated after the urban fox phenomenon was recognised. At least in the periphery of cities and towns, rural (shy) foxes are known to utilise anthropogenic food sources and might be able to maintain a certain level of transmission inside the settlement area.

The same applies for domestic dogs, whose generally low *E. multilocularis* prevalence is compensated by their extremely large numbers in urban and peri-urban areas. In any case, the prevalence of *E. multilocularis* in synanthropic foxes is the only practically available indicator for presence and frequency of the parasite. Data suggest that, even as fox population densities increase from rural through peri-urban to urban areas, *E. multilocularis* frequency shows the opposite trend, *e.g.* in the cities of Zurich, Geneva, Stuttgart and Nancy.

This is usually explained by decreased availability of suitable intermediate hosts in highly urbanised areas, which either depend on extensively managed grassland which becomes increasingly rare towards city centers (*M. arvalis*), or which are not as easily accessible as prey for foxes due to low density, burrowing habits or sise (*A. scherman*, *M. glareolus*, *Ondatra zibethicus*). Based on population densities of both foxes and rodents, peri-urban areas appear to be focal points for transmission of *E. multilocularis*. Such areas are characterised by:

- Higher population densities of foxes compared to strictly rural landscapes (as foxes are able to supplement their natural food sources with anthropogenic sources like waste or pet food),
- Presence of intermediate host species at sufficient frequency to serve as regular fox prey (even though at reduced densities or with patchy distribution compared to strictly rural landscapes), and
- High density of humans and their pet animals. E. multilocularis prevalence of foxes in such areas is usually lower than in adjacent rural habitats (reflecting the reduced availability of intermediate hosts), but this is counteracted by the larger fox densities.

Such peri-urban areas are a contact zone between humans and infected foxes and therefore hypothetically more important than rural (few humans) or highly urbanised areas (few infected animals). In addition, dogs and cats can complement the life cycle of E. multilocularis when preying on rodents, *e.g.* in the city periphery or in parks and gardens. Although cats are known to be inferior hosts for this parasite, and dogs are generally rarely infected, dogs in particular are thought to be an important conduit for human infection due to their frequent and close contact (compared to foxes) with people. In addition, even at very low prevalences, dogs may also contribute substantially to transmission due to their large number: it has been estimated that, under urban conditions, dogs may contribute 6.818.9 per cent of the total egg output of all definitive hosts combined.

A definition of urban or peri-urban life cycless for *E. multilocularis* is difficult to formulate for a number of reasons. Even within a region like central Europe, the character of urbanisation varies considerably. Size, distribution and management of green areas inside human settlements differ, which has an impact on the suitability of these areas as habitats for host species.

At the periphery of cities, there is necessarily a contact zone between typical synanthropic fox populations and those from surrounding rural areas that also exploit anthropogenic food sources using different strategies. The dependency of urban E. multilocularis life cycles on these periphery foxes (whose home ranges can include both agricultural grassland and urban parts) is not known. Likewise, it is unclear which species of intermediate hosts can maintain the life cycle in urban/peri-urban areas. For open landscapes of central

Europe, stable populations of common voles (M. arvalis) seem to be more important for the parasite than any other rodent species, and some data from France suggest that this may also be the case for cities and towns.

Water voles (*A. sherman*) can be frequently infected in city parks and gardens, although their role in transmission is less clear. Likewise, 15.2 per cent of 46 muskrats (*O. zibethicus*) were found to be infected at a recreational lake within the city of Stuttgart, Germany , but their impact on transmission may be marginal due to localised occurrence and low predation by foxes.

There are considerable gaps of knowledge concerning such basic epidemiological parameters. Better understanding of urban/periurban life cycles and their link with the surrounding rural landscape, however, is crucial for the development of countermeasures against the parasite which have been specifically recommended for peri-urban areas with increased fox-human contact. Various deworming schemes using anthelmintic fox baits have been described from Europe and Japan.

In urban areas, they were conducted with different degrees of success, and comparative data from two French studies indicate that failure in one area is linked to parasite infection pressure from surrounding landscapes. In conclusion, it is apparent that even within Europe, there is no uniform pattern of urban/peri-urban transmission of *E. multilocularis*, and even less so when comparing areas (*e.g.* in Japan or North America) where other host species with different ecological requirements occur.

BAYLISASCARIS PROCYONIS IN EUROPE

Raccoons are opportunistic carnivores native to North and Central America. They are highly adaptable to various environments and settle in rural, as well as peri-urban and urban areas. Raccoons have been introduced to Europe in the early 20th century and are now known to occur in at least 20 European countries. Stable populations are presently developing in Spain and France and a few raccoons appear occasionally in Denmark and other Scandinavian countries.

Raccoons have been released deliberately for hunting purposes (in Russia and Poland), escaped from fur farms or set free by pet owners. High population densities are recorded in Germany and it is estimated that at least 500,000 raccoons are living there. In 2012, the hunting index increased up to 67,000 individuals. In some urban areas in Germany, raccoons may reach a population density of up to 100 individuals/km^2 due to their adaptable behaviour, their omnivorous feeding habits, their high reproductive potential and the lack of natural predators. The high population density of raccoons in some European urban settlements greatly exceeds the known density of other wild carnivores in these environments. Raccoons are competent hosts for various pathogens, but only *Baylisascaris procyonis*, the common raccoon roundworm, poses a serious threat to humans in Europe. Apart from raccoons, this nematode can also develop into the mature stage in dogs (but not cats). Larvae, however, may start their body migration in a wide range of hosts (birds, reptiles and mammals including humans).

The eggs of *B. procyonis* remain infectious for months in humid soil or water. Raccoons apparently aquire the infection by the uptake of embryonated eggs from contaminated environments, but especially adult raccoons may also become infected by the consumption of third-stage larvae in intermediate hosts. Raccoons defecate at latrines close to their resting and sleeping places, and in case of raccoons adapted to peri-urban and urban areas these can be located in barns, lofts, attics, chimneys and garages. The surroundings of such latrines may become heavily contaminated with B. procyonis eggs, increasing the risk of human infections.

In humans, the larval stages may cause ocular and visceral larva migrans, which may become fatal when larvae invade the central nervous system. The prevalences of *B. procyonis* in European raccoon populations vary considerably, as high as 70 per cent in parts of Germany (Hesse) and as low as 3 per cent in adjacent countries. Although the prevalence of *B. procyonis* may be very high in urban raccoons, human cases of baylisascariosis are rare both in Europe and elsewhere. Infection is usually restricted to patients who had close contact with raccoons, *i.e.* pet owners. The results of serological studies indicated, however, that many more individuals showed increased antibody levels against B. procyonis, although clinical symptoms were lacking.

PARASITIC ZOONOSES OF PERI-URBAN WILDLIFE CARNIVORES

The wildlife hosts of parasitic zoonoses occurring in peri-urban areas of Australia comprise wild dogs (dingoes - *Canis lupus dingo* - and dingo/domestic dog hybrids), foxes (*Vulpes vulpes*) and feral cats (*Felis catus*).

Origin of wild Dogs, Foxes and Feral Cats in Australia

Dingoes, foxes and cats were all introduced into Australia at various times. Dingoes by south-east Asian seafarers somewhere between 4000 and 5000 years ago. Over time, they out-competed the indigenous Australian marsupial predators, Thylacines (*Thylacinus cynocephalus*) and *Tasmanian Devils* (*Sarcophilus harrisii*), and established themselves as a new Australian top-order predator. From 1788, European settlers with dogs began arriving in Australia and it soon became evident that dingoes and domestic dogs could hybridise and produce fertile young.

The result has been that currently in much of the suitable dingo habitat in Australia, the top-order predators consist no longer of pure-bred dingoes but dingo/domestic dog hybrids together with a few pure-bred dingoes. These populations of wild canids are commonly referred to as wild dogs, but importantly dingoes and their hybrids are readily susceptable to infection with all parasitic zoonoses associated with domestic dogs.

Foxes arrived in Australia much more recently than dingoes, having been introduced by the early settlers for sport and to control rabbits (*Oryctolagus cuniculus*) (also introduced). However, within a few decades foxes themselves had become a major agricultural pest. It is generally accepted that the first successful introduction of foxes occurred in 1871 in southern Victoria; they spread rapidly, reaching Western Australia in the 1920s.

Foxes are now found in all parts of Australia except the tropical north. They were also recently illegally introduced into Tasmania and there followed an intense eradication campaign, but the current status of foxes in Tasmania is unclear. Foxes, like dingoes and their hybrids, can act as definitive host for the same suite of potential helminth zoonoses found infecting dogs, including *E. granulosus*.

Cats were introduced into Australia in the early 1800s by settlers intending to have them as companion animals, but some soon became feral. Feral cats are now widespread, in almost all environments of Australia, and a major environmental pest. Cats share a number of the zoonotic helminths found in wild dogs and foxes, but importantly they do not act as a definitive host for E. granulosus.

The most important zoonotic helminth parasite recorded infecting wild dogs and foxes living in peri-urban and urban environments is *Echinococcus granulosus*. However, a number of other zoonotic helminths including *Dipylidium caninum*, *Spirometra erinacei*, *Toxocara canis* and *Toxascaris leonina*, Ancylostoma caninum, A. ceylanicum and A. braziliensie also occur. Zoonotic helminths of feral cats include *Toxocara* cati, *T. canis* and *T. leonina* and Ancylostoma tubaeforme, but they can also become infected with *S. erinacei* and *D. caninum*. Although *S. erinacei* and *D. caninum* are zoonotic parasites, their transmission to humans is indirect, requiring ingestion of parasite stages residing in intermediate hosts, not a parasite stage emanating from the definitive host. Therefore, *S. erinacei* and *D. caninum* will not be included in this review of parasitic zoonoses of peri-urban wildlife carnivores in Australia.

Echinococcus granulosus in Peri-urban wild Dogs (Dingoes) and Foxes

Humans are accidental intermediate hosts for *E. granulosus* becoming infected through ingestion of eggs passed into the environment in the faeces of infected carnivores. Infection (cystic echinococcosis, or hydatid disease) manifests as large fluid-filled cysts developing mainly in the liver and/or lungs, causing morbidity and occasionally death.

Infection with *E. granulosus* is common and it is often present in large numbers in the small intestine, not only in the wild dogs living in the bush, but also in those encroaching into peri-urban and urban areas. Reports of wild dogs encroaching into peri-urban and urban areas are increasing. In a recent study, satellite tracking collars were attached to a number of urban wild dogs that were released back into their territories and followed for varying periods of time. It was clear from the data that these animals were including urban, peri-urban and adjacent bushland in their home range, moving freely between all three habitats.

The few published reports containing data on *E. granulosus* in wild dogs encroaching into peri-urban and urban areas have all originated from studies in Queensland. However, the migration of wild dogs into urban and peri-urban areas is not restricted to Queensland; it is also happening in and around urban centres in New South Wales. The prevalence of *E. granulosus* in a study of wild dogs moving between adjacent bushland and peri-urban and urban habitat in Townsville (North Queensland) was 22.2 per cent.

The prevalence of *E. granulosus* in 108 wild dogs caught around Maroochydore (south-eastern Queensland) was 46.3 per cent, with individual worm burdens in excess of 100,000 worms in some animals. Of particular importance is that at least some of these animals are moving close to, and in some cases, entering the gardens of residents and defecating. It is of interest to note that in their study of the intestines and scats from wild dogs collected in bushland adjacent to northern and southern Cairns in northern tropical Queensland, researchers found no evidence of *E. granulosus* either in scats or in wild dogs examined *post mortem*.

The prevalence of *E. granulosus* in foxes in rural areas in Australia can be as high as 45.8 per cent, but the worm burdens of infected foxes are always low, usually less than 50 tapeworms. However, more commonly the prevalence of E. granulosus in foxes in rural areas and in peri-urban areas is lower, with worm burdens also less than 50 worms.

The contribution of Australian foxes in contaminating the environment with eggs of *E. granulosus*, particulually in the bush, is small by virtue of their small worm burdens and the generally low prevalence of infected animals. However, their importance may increase in peri-urban and urban areas, particularly around areas such as popular barbecue or picnic sites. These locations attract foxes to come and scavenge rubbish bins looking for food scraps left by visitors. If several foxes visit one of these barbecue or picnic sites, the area can become heavily contaminated with fox faeces, and if one or more of these animals is infected with *E. granulosus*, this may present an important potential public health risk.

An important consideration in respect of the epidemiology of *E. granulosus* in peri-urban and urban environments infiltrated by *E. granulosus*-infected wild dogs and/or foxes is the role of coprophagous flies in egg dispersal. A study demonstrated the capacity of several species of coprophagous flies for the dispersal of eggs of taeniid cestodes. They showed that individual flies can ingest more than 800 eggs, over 80 per cent of the eggs were excreted within 24 hours and that eggs ingested by flies remained infective to sheep. These data suggest that the potential role of coprophagous flies in the transmission of *E. granulosus* in peri-urban and urban environments also inhabited by wild dogs and foxes infected with *E. granulosus* could be more important than is currently realised.

Ancylostoma Species and Uncinaria Stenocephala

Human infection with hookworm species commonly causes cutaneous larval migrans, with painful, itchy eruptions along the path of migrating larvae. Lesions occur most commonly in the skin on the feet, legs, buttocks and hands, but lesions can occur anywhere on the body. Lesions from *A. braziliense* and *U. stenocephala* may persist for many weeks to a year before the larvae die, while lesions caused by *A. caninum* are small and transient. Complications may be secondary bacterial infection following scratching lesions with dirty hands. *A. caninum* has also been implicated in causing eosinoplilic enteritis in humans. Until the cause of this eosinophilic enteritis was revealed, patients had large sections of intestine resected.

The prevalences of hookworm infections in wild dogs and foxes from peri-urban and urban environments are high. *U. stenocephala* is a cold adapted species and is found almost exclusively in domestic and wild dogs and foxes inhabiting the cooler areas of southeastern Australia, especially areas associated with the Great Dividing Range where cold winters with severe frosts occur.

Whereas *A. caninum* occurs along the warmer coastal fringe of eastern Australia, becoming more widespread in the damper, warmer areas of tropical Australia. *A ceylanicum* and *A. braziliense* also occur mainly in more tropical areas. *A. ceylanicum* is able to cause patent enteric infection in humans and patent infections have been identified in dingoes in the Cairns district in Queensland.

Zoonotic Hookworm Species Recovered from Australian Peri-Urban wild Dogs and Foxes.

Location	Definitive host(n)	Parasite species	Prevalence %(n)
Townsville	Wild dogs(27)	*A. caninum*	74 (20)
Maroochy Shire	Wild dogs(108)	*A. caninum*	37 (40)
Fraser Island	Wild dogs(18)	*A. caninum*	83.3 (15)
Cairns	Wild dog scats(38)	*A.caninum*	78.9 (30)
		A.ceylanicum	55.3 (21)
		A.braziliense	2.6 (1)
Canberra	Foxes(45)	*U. stenocephala*	80 (36)
Maroochy Shire	Foxes(7)	*A. caninum*	42.8 (3)

Toxocara Species and Toxascaris Leonina

The most important of these parasites is *T. canis* because of its impact on human hosts. Accidental ingestion of embryonated *T. canis* eggs, usually by children, results in visceral larval migrans and in some cases larvae migrate to the eyes, leading to blindness, commonly unilateral. *T. cati* and *T. leonina* have not been definitely implicated as causes of visceral larval migrans in humans, but *T. cati* has been shown to produce a similar impact in pigs.

T. canis occurs in wild dogs and foxes encroaching into peri-urban and urban areas; however, the prevalence of infection is commonly low, but can be unexpectedly high. In wild dogs from the Maroochy Shire, 5/108 (4.6 per cent) of the animals examined were infected, but none of 7 foxes examined was infected.

Hovever, in the same study, 5/18 (27.8 per cent) wild dogs from Fraser Island were infected, a likely reflection of the close proximity of the Fraser Island wild dogs with human habitation. In the Townsville study, researchers did not recover *T. canis* in any of the 27 wild dogs examined in contrast to who reported a prevalence of 46 per cent in their study in Townsville. Data from a survey of 25 road-killed urban foxes and 43 shot peri-urban foxes in and around Canberra, revealed prevalences of *T. canis* of 12 per cent and 0 per cent, respectively.

Feral Cats

Domestic cats also accompanied some settlers to Australia and the progeny of these animals soon established feral populations in the bush. Cats in Australia do not act as definitive host for *E. granulosus*. There are a few data available regarding the zoonotic parasites of peri-urban feral cats. However, cats living in and around urban rubbish dumps and cats from council shelters have been found infected with *Ancylostoma tubaeforme*, *Toxocara cati*, *T. leonina*, *D. caninum*, *S. erinacei*, *Cryptosporidium*, *Giardia*, and *Toxoplasma*. However, the habit of cats to bury their faeces may reduce the transmission of potential zooneses.

In a study of 54 cats trapped over three rubbish dumps around Canberra, the average prevalence of A. tubaeforme was 3.8 per cent (range 07 per cent), and in the study of the mean prevalence of hookworm was reported as 2.9 per cent (range 1.44.4 per cent) but the species present were not reported.

IXODES SPECIES AND THE TRANSMISSION OF PARASITES/ PATHOGENS IN PERI-URBAN/URBAN AREAS

Ticks, mosquitoes and fleas are important arthropod vectors in the transmission of parasites and other pathogens, some of which are zoonotic. In the northern hemisphere, the majority of vector-borne infections are transmitted by ticks, especially Ixodes species that are highly competent vectors for a variety of different pathogens including parasites, bacteria and viruses. In general, the eco-epidemiology of zoonotic vector-borne diseases is still little understood, as it depends on the interaction of a vector with (often several) reservoir hosts and a pathogen which is transferred from the reservoir to the human host. *Ixodes* species have a three-host life cycle with larvae feeding predominantly on small mammals whereas adults prefer larger mammals. Nymphs tend to feed on small as well as large mammals. The most abundant tick in central Europe, Ixodes ricinus, has the capacity to feed on more than 300 different vertebrate host, including small rodents, lizards, hares, hedgehogs as well as larger animals like deer, red foxes or wild boar. *I. ricinus* populations are usually associated with deciduous and mixed forests, but recent studies show that this tick species can also be highly abundant in peri-urban and urban areas.

The urbanisation changes the local wildlife composition drastically. This has important consequences for tick densities, because the local composition of host species and their abundance affects the capacity of the environment to support tick populations. Roe deer (*Capreolus capreolus*), red foxes (*Vulpes vulpes*) and wild boar (*Sus scrofa*) are particularly important for the maintenance and the geographical distribution of *I. ricinus*, because they host all three different developmental stages of *I. ricinus*, can carry a large number of ticks and may migrate over long distances.

Importantly, they are often attracted by peri-urban and urban areas. Roe deer and other cervids as well as foxes or wild boar are important reservoir hosts of numerous pathogens which may be transmitted by ticks to humans, so their high abundances in peri-urban and urban areas increase zoonotic infection risks.

Researchers collected *I. ricinus* in several parks within different cities in southern Germany, which were found to contain Babesia and several bacterial pathogens. Interestingly, the composition of pathogens in urban ticks revealed differences when compared to woodlands. They collected more than 10000I. ricinus ticks from four different urban parks, a pasture and a natural area in Bavaria, Germany.

The prevalence of *Babesia* spp. was generally higher in the pasture and the natural area compared to the urban parks. Three species, *Babesia microti*, *B. venatorum* and *B. capreoli*, were detected in ticks collected in the natural area, whereas in the pasture and the urban habitats only one species, *B. venatorum*, was frequent.

It is important to note that *B. venatorum* may infect humans and that roe deer are reservoir hosts of this parasite. Researchers pointed out that tick abundance is positively correlated with deer abundance, and those habitats with high densities of deer or cervids in general are therefore areas with a higher risk of infection. Habitat fragmentation and landscape conversion may also favour high population densities of small mammals, mainly rodents, which are crucial as hosts for tick larvae and nymphs as well as important reservoirs for many tick transmitted pathogens. The most prevalent tick-borne infection in the northern hemisphere is Lyme borreliosis. In northeastern North America, extensive studies were conducted on the interactions between *Borrelia burgdorferi* and the different hosts which are involved in the transmission of this pathogen from wild animals to humans. Adult Ixodes scapularis, as the most important vector, feeds on white-tailed deer (*Odocoileus virginianus*), which is important for the maintenance of the tick population and reaches high population densities in peri-urban areas. I. scapularis becomes infected with *B. burgdorferi* when feeding on *Peromyscus leucopus*, the white-footed mouse which is the most competent reservoir host for the pathogen and reaches high population densities due to habitat fragmentation in the vicinity of humans settlements. An infected *I. scapularis* transmits the pathogen to humans.

The importance of rodents and other small mammals as bridge hosts is more and more recognised, because some species are well adapted to urban environments, are competent reservoir host of many pathogens and may introduce the parasites or pathogens to new habitats. In addition, small mammals are maintenance hosts for different tick species, which means that pathogens can be exchanged between the different ticks. This host switch may be important because the behaviour and the habitat requirements of tick species differ concerning biotic and abiotic parameters.

European hedgehogs (*Erinaceus europaeus*) can serve as an example for such a host switch. They are common animals, well adapted to urban areas and are frequently infested with two different tick species (*I. ricinus* and *I. hexagonus*), both competent vectors for many pathogens. *I. ricinus* is a generalist, whereas *I. hexagonus* feeds almost exclusively on hedgehogs. *I. hexagonus* was shown to maintain a high infection rate of pathogens within hedgehog populations, whereas *I. ricinus*, becoming infected when feeding on hedgehogs, can transmit these pathogens to various other hosts due to their low host specificity. These so-called subcycles are important for maintaining stable pathogen populations in urban areas.

CLASSIFICATION OF ZOONOTIC DISEASE

All classes of disease agents cause zoonotic disease, including bacteria, viruses, parasites, and fungi. Although zoonotic diseases can be classified according to their infectious agents, they also can be subdivided into those diseases that are transmitted from non-human animals to humans or from humans to non-human animals. Examples of the complex pathways of transmission among zoonotic diseases include the spread of Mycobacterium tuberculosis from humans to cattle and elephants and the transmission of methacillin-resistant *Staphylococcus aureus* (MRSA) from humans to horses and back to humans. Some diseases are considered to be zoonotic even though they are rarely transmitted between non-human animals and humans; an example is foot-and-mouth disease in cattle.

Zoonotic diseases also can be classified according to their life cycle. Diseases that are transmitted directly (*e.g.*, through direct contact or a mechanical vector) and that are maintained in nature in a single vertebrate host species are known asorthozoonoses; an example is rabies, which is maintained by canids.

Cyclozoonoses, such as echinococcosis, require more than one vertebrate host for development.Metazoonoses require both a vertebrate host and an invertebrate host; an example istrypanosomiasis. Zoonotic diseases that require a vertebrate host and another type of environmental reservoir (*e.g.*, food or soil) are known as saprozoonoses. Listeriosisand histoplasmosis are examples of saprozoonoses.

CLASSES OF ZOONOSES

VIRAL ZOONOSES: RABIES

A viral disease associated with mammals, including dogs, cats, horses, and wildlife. Rabies can be transmitted through bites, scratches, aerosolised respiratory secretions, and saliva. It may take several weeks or even a few years for people to show symptoms after getting infected with rabies, but usually people start to show signs of the disease 1 to 3 months after the virus infects them.

The early signs of rabies can be fever or headache, but this changes quickly to nervous system signs, such as confusion, sleepiness, or agitation. Once someone with rabies infection starts having these symptoms, that person usually does not survive. For this reason, all animal health care workers should be vaccinated against rabies and should have their titers checked every other year.

Many kinds of animal can pass rabies to people. Wild animals are much more likely to carry rabies, especially raccoons, skunks, bats, foxes, and coyotes. However, dogs, cats, cattle, or any warm-blooded animal can pass rabies to people.

West Nile Virus

A viral disease spread by mosquitoes which can affect birds, horses, and other mammals. Mosquitoes become infected when they feed on infected birds. Infected mosquitoes can then spread WNV to humans and other animals when they bite. About one in 150 people infected with WNV will develop severe illness. The severe symptoms can include high fever, headache, neck stiffness, stupor, disorientation, coma, tremors, convulsions, muscle weakness, vision loss, numbness and paralysis. These symptoms may last several weeks, and neurological effects may be permanent.

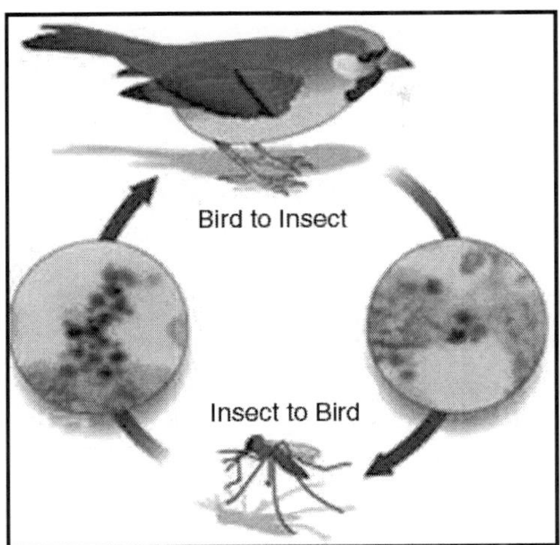

Fig. Typical cycle of West Nile Virus.

Up to 20 per cent of the people who become infected have symptoms such as fever, headache, and body aches, nausea, vomiting, and sometimes swollen lymph glands or a skin rash on the chest, stomach and back. Symptoms can last for as short as a few days, though even healthy people have become sick for several weeks. Approximately 80 per cent of people (about 4 out of 5) who are infected with WNV will not show any symptoms at all. People typically develop symptoms between 3 and 14 days after they are bitten by the infected mosquito.

There is no specific treatment for WNV infection. In cases with milder symptoms, symptoms pass on their own. In more severe cases, people usually need to go to the hospital where they can receive supportive treatment including intravenous fluids, help with breathing, and nursing care.

Personal protective measures are the primary way to avoid contracting the virus.

Equine Encephalitis

A mosquito borne infection normally maintained in nature by a cycle from an arthropod vector to a vertebrate reservoir host. Although some people experience it only as a mild illness, eastern equine encephalitis is fatal in about one-third of the cases.

Symptoms of eastern equine encephalitis usually appear three to 10 days after a bite by an infected mosquito. A vaccine exists for horses but not for humans. Personal protective measures are the primary way to avoid contracting the virus.

A. Diagnostic Tests/Lab Tests/Lab Values:

1. ELISA (Enzyme Lined Immuno-Sorbent Assay)- detects the actual disease. May not be sensitive enough to detect infection in the asymptomatic carrier.

2. PCR (Polymerase Chain Reaction)- amplifies minute quantites of microbial DNA or RNA allowing for recognition of latent phases of viral diseases. May yield false positive result for the disease but give a true positive for infection within the agent.
3. Serology (Indirect Fluorescent Antibody Testing)- used to detect Rickettsial organisms which cause Ehrlichiosis and Rickettsia

ZOONOTIC DISEASES

Zoonoses are infections or diseases that can be transmitted directly or indirectly between animals and humans, for instance by consuming contaminated foodstuffs or through contact with infected animals. The severity of these diseases in humans varies from mild symptoms to life-threatening conditions.

Research indicates that between one third and one half of all human infectious diseases have a zoonotic origin, that is, are transmitted from animals. About 75 per cent of the new diseases that have affected humans over the past 10 years (such as the West Nile Virus) have originated from animals or products of animal origin. Zoonoses are transmissible between animals and humans in a variety of ways and an infection can also often be transmitted through multiple ways:

Food-borne Zoonotic Diseases

- Food-borne zoonotic pathogens are transmitted through consumption of contaminated food or drinking water. Infectious agents in foodstuffs include bacteria such as *Salmonella* and *Campylobacter*, viruses such as norovirus or hepatitis A virus, and parasites such as *Trichinella*.
- The infectious agent which causes Bovine Spongiform Encephalopathy (BSE) in cattle can also be transmitted to humans through consumption of contaminated meat causing variant Creuzfeldt-Jakob disease. Unlike other food-borne diseases which are spread by microorganisms, BSE is caused by a prion, which is an abnormal form of a protein (known as PrP^{c}).

Non-Food-Borne Zoonotic Diseases

- By vectors, *i.e.* living organisms that transmit infectious agents from an infected animal to a human or another animal. Vectors are frequently arthropods, such as mosquitoes, ticks, flies, fleas and lice and can transmit diseases such as malaria, West-Nile virus and Lyme disease.
- Through direct contact or close proximity with infected animals. Diseases that are mainly transmissible to other animals or humans in this way include:
- Avian influenza, which is a viral disease occurring in poultry and other birds. Pigs can also be carriers of this virus as well as of other

influenza viruses. Avian influenza primarily affects birds, but there have been cases of viruses being transmitted to humans and other animals through close contact with infected birds.

- Q fever is a disease, caused by the Coxiela burnetti bacterium, affecting animals and humans. It has been reported to be present in a wide range of species, including cattle, sheep and goats as well as birds and arthropods. Human infection mainly results from the inhalation of dust contaminated with bacteria from the placenta and birth fluids or faeces from infected animals. Other modes of transmission, such as through contaminated water or the feces of infected arthropods are rare.
- A specific strain of the Meticillin-resistant *Staphylococcus aureus* (MRSA) bacterium (CC398) which can be transmitted through contact with live animals.
- *Salmonella* infections can originate from contact with infected reptiles and amphibians such as pet snakes, iguanas and frogs or their environment.
- Verotoxin-producing *Escherichia coli (E. coli)* can be acquired through contact with infected farm animals.
- These diseases can also be transmitted through the environment, *e.g.* Verotoxin-producing *E. coli* in contaminated swimming water.

CAUSES OF SWINE FLU

Swine flu is contagious, and it spreads in the same way as the seasonalflu. When people who have it cough or sneeze, they spray tiny drops of the virus into the air. If you come in contact with these drops or touch a surface (such as a doorknob or sink) that an infected person has recently touched, you can catch H1N1 swine flu. Despite the name, you can't catch swine flu from eating bacon, ham, or any other pork product.

SWINE FLU SYMPTOMS

People who have swine flu can be contagious one day before they have any symptoms, and as many as 7 days after they get sick. Kids can be contagious for as long as 10 days.

Most symptoms are the same as seasonal flu. They can include:

- Cough
- Fever
- Sore throat
- Stuffy or runny nose
- Body aches
- Headache
- Chills
- Fatigue

Like seasonal flu, swine flu can lead to more serious complications, including pneumonia and respiratory failure. And it can make conditions like diabetes or asthma worse. If you have symptoms like shortness of breath, severe vomiting, abdominal pain, dizziness, or confusion, call your doctor or 911 right away.

Tests for Swine Flu

It's hard to tell whether you have swine flu or seasonal flu, because most symptoms are the same. People with swine flu may be more likely to feel nauseous and throw up than people who have seasonal flu. But a lab test is the only way to know for sure. Even a rapid flu test you can get in your doctor's office won't tell you for sure.

To test for swine flu, your doctor takes a sample from your nose or throat. You may not need to be tested.

The CDC says the people who need to be tested are those in the hospital or those at high risk for getting life-threatening problems from the flu, such as:

- Children under 5 years old
- People 65 or older
- Children and teens (under age 18) who are getting long-term aspirintherapy, and who might be at risk for Reye's syndrome after being infected with swine flu. Reye's syndrome is a life-threatening illness linked to aspirin use in children.
- Pregnant women
- Adults and children who have chronic lung, heart, liver, blood,nervous system, neuromuscular, or metabolic problems
- Adults and children who have suppressed immune systems (including those who take medications to suppress their immune systems or who have HIV)
- People in nursing homes and other long-term care facilities

Treatment of Swine Flu

Some of the same antiviral drugs that are used to treat seasonal flu also work against H1N1 swine flu. Oseltamivir (Tamiflu), peramivir (Rapivab), and zanamivir (Relenza) seem to work best, although some kinds of swine flu are resistant to oseltamivir. These drugs can help you get over swine flu faster. They can also help keep it from being too severe. They work best when taken within 48 hours of the first flu symptoms, but they can help when taken later.

Antibiotics won't help, because flu is caused by a virus, not bacteria.

Over-the-counter pain remedies and cold and flu medications can help relieve aches, pains, and fever. Don't give aspirin to children under age 18 because of the risk for Reye's syndrome. Check to make sure that over-the-counter cold medications do not have aspirin before giving them to children.

Vaccine for Swine Flu

The same flu vaccine that protects against seasonal flu also protects against the H1N1 swine flu strain. You can get it as a shot or as a nasal spray. Either way, it "teaches" your immune system to attack the real virus.

H1N1 VIRUS PANDEMIC HISTORY

The phylogenetic origin of the flu virus that caused the 2009 pandemics can be traced before 1918. Around 1918, the ancestral virus, of avian origin, crossed the species boundaries and infected humans as human H1N1. The same phenomenon took place soon after in America, where the human virus was infecting pigs; it led to the emergence of the H1N1 swine strain, which later became the classic swine flu.

New events of reassortment were not reported until 1968, when the avian strain H1N1 infected humans again; this time the virus met the strain H2N2, and the reassortment originated the strain H3N2. This strain has remained as a stable flu strain until now.

The mid-1970s were important for the evolution of flu strains. First, the re-emergence of the human H1N1 strain became a seasonal strain. Then, a small outbreak of swine H1N1 occurred in humans, and finally, the human H2N2 strain apparently became extinct. Around 1979, the avian H1N1 strain infected pigs and gave rise to Euroasiatic swine flu and H1N1 Euroasiatic swine virus, which is still being transmitted in swine populations.

The critical moment for the 2009 outbreak was between 1990 and 1993. A triple reassortment event in a pig host of North American H1N1 swine virus, the human H3N2 virus and avian H1N1 virus generated the swine H1N2 strain. Finally, the last step in S-OIV history was in 2009, when the virus H1N2 co-infected a human host at the same time as the Euroasiatic H1N1 swine strain. This led to the emergence of a new human H1N1 strain, which caused the 2009 pandemic. On June 11, 2009, the World Health Organisation raised the worldwide pandemic alert level to Phase 6 for swine flu, which is the highest alert level. This alert level means that the swine flu had spread worldwide and there were cases of people with the virus in most countries. The pandemic level identifies the spread of the disease or virus and not necessarily the severity of the disease.

Swine flu spread very rapidly worldwide due to its high human-to-human transmission rate and due to the frequency of air travel.

In 2015 the instances of Swine Flu substantially increased to five year highs with over 10000 cases reported and 660 deaths in India. The states reporting the highest number of cases and deaths are Rajasthan, Gujarat, Madhya Pradesh, Maharashtra, Delhi, and Telengana. The circulating strain of influenza being the same, unmutant strain that caused global pandemic in 2009 (A H1N1 pdm 09), the sudden spurt of the cases in the beginning of 2015 left the Indian government unexplained but concerned. Government instructed the affected states to investigate into the epidemiological reasons of such spurt in the states, and had detailed the advisory guidelines to all states.

The guidelines are mainly for:

- Description of A H1N1 for prompt identification, detection, and distinction from the symptoms of other similar infection such as common flu(cold)
- Categorisation of screening of influenza A H1N1 cases,
- Clinical management protocol of Pandemic influenza A H1N1,
- Providing home care,
- Collection of human sample.

Besides, through the National Centre for Diseases Control (NCDC), Directorate General of Health Services (DGHS), Government of India (GoI) had placed a tender to procure 8 kits of Assay sets, 37 kits of one step RT-PCR kit, and 36 kits of viral RNA extraction kits.

TRANSMISSION

Transmission between Pigs

Influenza is quite common in pigs, with about half of breeding pigs having been exposed to the virus in the US. Antibodies to the virus are also common in pigs in other countries. The main route of transmission is through direct contact between infected and uninfected animals. These close contacts are particularly common during animal transport.Intensive farming may also increase the risk of transmission, as the pigs are raised in very close proximity to each other. The direct transfer of the virus probably occurs either by pigs touching noses, or through dried mucus. Airborne transmission through the aerosols produced by pigs coughing or sneezing are also an important means of infection. The virus usually spreads quickly through a herd, infecting all the pigs within just a few days. Transmission may also occur through wild animals, such as wild boar, which can spread the disease between farms.

Transmission to Humans

People who work with poultry and swine, especially those with intense exposures, are at increased risk of zoonotic infection with influenza virus endemic in these animals, and constitute a population of human hosts in which zoonosis and reassortment can co-occur. Vaccination of these workers against influenza and surveillance for new influenza strains among this population may therefore be an important public health measure. Transmission of influenza from swine to humans who work with swine was documented in a small surveillance study performed in 2004 at the University of Iowa. This study, among others, forms the basis of a recommendation that people whose jobs involve handling poultry and swine be the focus of increased public health surveillance. Other professions at particular risk of infection are veterinarians and meat processing workers, although the risk of infection for both of these groups is lower than that of farm workers.

Interaction with Avian H5N1 in Pigs.

Pigs are unusual as they can be infected with influenza strains that usually infect three different species: pigs, birds and humans. This makes pigs a host where influenza viruses might exchange genes, producing new and dangerous strains. Avian influenza virus H3N2 is endemic in pigs in China, and has been detected in pigs in Vietnam, increasing fears of the emergence of new variant strains. H3N2 evolved from H2N2 by antigenic shift. In August 2004, researchers in China found H5N1 in pigs.

These H5N1 infections may be quite common; in a survey of 10 apparently healthy pigs housed near poultry farms in West Java, where avian flu had broken out, five of the pig samples contained the H5N1 virus. The Indonesian government has since found similar results in the same region. Additional tests of 150 pigs outside the area were negative.

SIGNS AND SYMPTOMS

In Swine

In pigs, influenza infection produces fever, lethargy, sneezing, coughing, difficulty breathing and decreased appetite. In some cases the infection can cause abortion. Although mortality is usually low (around 1–4 per cent), the virus can produce weight loss and poor growth, causing economic loss to farmers. Infected pigs can lose up to 12 pounds of body weight over a three- to four-week period.

HEMORRHAGIC FEVER

Hemorrhagic fever, common name for a group of acute viral diseases, the symptoms of which usually begin with fever and muscle aches and progress to dizziness, collapse, swelling, and shock. Depending upon the particular virus, hemorrhagic fevers may progressively produce respiratory problems, internal bleeding, kidney problems, and death. Most hemorrhagic fever viruses have only been recognised within the past 65 years and new hemorrhagic fever viruses are identified each year.

Hemorrhagic fevers are caused by more than 20 known viruses from four different families: Arenaviridae, Bunyaviridae, Flaviviridae, and Filoviridae. The viruses are often named for the region, town, or geographic feature where they were first identified. The Arenaviridae family includes Lassa, Junín (the cause of Argentine hemorrhagic fever), Machupo (the cause of Bolivian hemorrhagic fever), and Guanarito (the cause of Venezuelan hemorrhagic fever) viruses. While these viruses are usually transmitted to humans by rodents, human-to-human transmission can occur, particularly with Lassa fever.

The Bunyaviridae family includes Rift Valley fever virus, a notable mosquito-borne virus in Africa, and the hantaviruses. During the Korean War (1950-1953), thousands of American troops developed mysterious symptoms including high fevers, headaches, internal bleeding, and kidney failure. It was not until 1976 that the viral cause of the disease was identified as Hantaan virus, a hantavirus. The disease is now recognised as one of a group of diseases called hemorrhagic fever with renal syndrome. A related virus, named Sin Nombre, was discovered in the United States in 1993. Sin Nombre was found to cause severe respiratory distress syndrome, which starts with flulike symptoms followed by respiratory failure and often death. The original 1993 outbreak struck New Mexico, Colorado, Arizona, and Utah, killing 58 people. Today, Sin Nombre virus is known to exist in deer mice in more than 30 American states, and similar viruses have been found in South America and Canada.

The Flaviviridae family includes the viruses that cause dengue hemorrhagic fever and yellow fever. These viruses are transmitted by the bites of infected mosquitoes. Dengue hemorrhagic fever occurs mostly in children under the age of ten who live in areas where milder dengue fever is common. Dengue fever resembles the flu with fever, tiredness, and muscle aches from which patients recover in about a week, but dengue hemorrhagic fever is also accompanied by internal hemorrhaging and shock and may cause death. Yellow fever, found mostly in Africa and South America, is spread in urban areas by the bite of the mosquito, Aedes aegypti. In the jungle, yellow fever is carried by various mosquito species and monkeys that live high in the tree canopy, the uppermost layer of spreading branches in the forest.

The Filoviridae family includes Marburg and four strains of Ebola viruses. Ebola hemorrhagic fever was first recognised in Zaire (now the Democratic Republic of the Congo, or DRC) and the Sudan in 1976 where it caused deadly epidemics. The virus reemerged in Kikwit, Zaire, in 1995 and Gabon in 1996, causing additional, frightening epidemics. Persons infected with the Ebola virus experience headache, high fever, muscle pain, vomiting, and internal and external bleeding. The mortality rate of Ebola hemorrhagic fever ranges from 50 to 90 per cent.

HOW INFECTION OCCURS

Viruses that cause hemorrhagic fever are zoonotic-they carry out life cycles within multiple animal reservoir hosts (organisms in which viruses normally live but do not harm) and only infect humans incidentally. When these viruses infect humans, they can replicate well and cause severe, even lethal, disease. In some cases other animals, such as birds, monkeys, sheep, goats, and cattle, are also infected incidentally, like humans. For some viruses, such as the hantaviruses, human exposure occurs by contact with a reservoir host's feces or urine. In the case of Sin Nombre virus, rodent feces containing the virus dry out, turn into dust, become airborne, and are inhaled by humans.

Another means of transmission to humans is by direct contact with infected human blood, urine, feces, or saliva. There is a high risk of infection for health care providers who care for patients suffering from Ebola hemorrhagic fever or Lassa fever. Gloves, gowns, and eye shields are necessary when caring for hemorrhagic fever patients.

Once inside the body, many of the hemorrhagic fever viruses attack white blood cells called macrophages (cells of the immune system that normally protect the body against infection). Macrophages carry these viruses through the bloodstream, distributing them to tissues and organs that are most susceptible to infection.

SYMPTOMS

Once infection occurs, the time it takes symptoms to develop, known as the incubation period, depends upon the virus and its rate of growth in human tissues. For example, humans develop symptoms 3 to 6 days after being bitten by a mosquito carrying yellow fever virus, 5 to 7 days after direct contact exposure to Ebola virus, 10 to 14 days after exposure to dried rodent excretions containing Lassa virus, and 14 to 30 days after exposure to rodent excretions containing Hantaan virus, the cause of hemorrhagic fever with renal syndrome.

In addition to fever and severe muscle pain, persons with hemorrhagic fever often develop bloodshot eyes and redness of the face and upper body. They may experience vomiting, diarrhea, and mild, general edema (swelling caused by accumulation of fluids in tissue spaces). Tiny, pinpoint-sized purple or red spots on the skin, known as petechiae, are also common. As the infection progresses, it often impairs the blood's ability to clot. The walls of the capillaries (smallest blood vessels) may be damaged, permitting blood to escape and causing hemorrhaging (excessive bleeding). The amount of blood circulating through the body is reduced, sometimes producing shock, characterised by pale, cold extremities; a rapid, weak pulse; and falling blood pressure. Arenavirus infections may cause severe encephalopathy (any of various diseases of the brain) with convulsions, deafness, or encephalitis (inflammation or swelling of the brain). Kidney failure and pulmonary edema (accumulation of fluid in the lungs) are characteristics of hantaviral diseases.

TREATMENT AND PREVENTION

There is currently no cure for any of the viral hemorrhagic fevers. Treatment consists of supportive care and prevention and treatment of shock by careful use of intravenous fluids and drugs to combat low blood pressure. Blood dialysis (mechanical process of removing waste products from blood) is used to treat kidney failure in patients with hemorrhagic fever with renal syndrome. In Argentina, patients infected with Junín virus are treated with plasma containing antibodies from persons who have recovered from the infection. A vaccine is used to prevent Junín virus in people at high risk for infection, such as farm workers. An effective vaccine is available to prevent yellow fever, and dengue vaccines are presently under development. The only effective antiviral drug against a hemorrhagic fever virus is ribavirin, which is used for patients suffering from Lassa fever. Rodent control campaigns have been highly effective in preventing Machupo hemorrhagic fever in Bolivian villages.

Despite all these measures, fatality rates from hemorrhagic fevers range from 1 to 5 per cent for Junín infection to as high as 90 per cent for Ebola hemorrhagic fever. In 1998 researchers in the United States developed a vaccine that protects monkeys from the Marburg virus. In the future, scientists hope to develop vaccines to protect humans against Marburg, Ebola, and other viruses that cause hemorrhagic fevers.

Hemorrhagic Fever Outbreaks

In many cases, the rising incidence of hemorrhagic fever outbreaks may be directly related to human activities. The cutting of rain forests in South America is bringing mosquitoes infected with yellow fever virus down from the treetops to where people live and work. Explosive population growth in Latin America, accompanied by poor sanitation and housing, is increasing the habitat for the reservoir hosts of mosquito-borne viruses. The use of broadleaf herbicides in corn fields in Argentina is leading to the dominance of the grass-loving rodent that carries Junín virus and presents a deadly risk to farm workers. The discovery of diamonds in the West African country of Sierra Leone has led to the development of housing compounds for thousands of immigrant workers and their families. The rodent that carries Lassa virus thrives in this habitat with its new source of food and shelter.

DENGUE FEVER PREVENTION

There are no approved vaccines for the dengue virus. Prevention thus depends on control of and protection from the bites of the mosquito that transmits it.

The World Health Organisation recommends an Integrated Vector Control programme consisting of five elements:

- Advocacy, social mobilisation and legislation to ensure that public health bodies and communities are strengthened;
- Collaboration between the health and other sectors (public and private);
- An integrated approach to disease control to maximize use of resources;

- Evidence-based decision making to ensure any interventions are targeted appropriately; and
- Capacity-building to ensure an adequate response to the local situation.

Dengue fever can be prevented by stopping mosquitoes from biting because they are the vectors the dengue viruses require for transfer to humans. *The CDC (2010) has supplied these general rules to prevent transfer of viruses and other pathogens by mosquitoes and other biting vectors:*

- *Avoid outbreaks:* To the extent possible, travelers should avoid known foci of epidemic disease transmission. The CDC Travelers' Health web page provides alerts and information on regional disease transmission patterns and outbreak alerts.
- *Be aware of peak exposure times and places:* Exposure to arthropod bites may be reduced if travelers modify their patterns of activity or behaviour. Although mosquitoes may bite at any time of day, peak biting activity for vectors of some diseases (for example, dengue, chikungunya) is during daylight hours. Vectors of other diseases (for example, malaria) are most active in twilight periods (for example, dawn and dusk) or in the evening after dark. Avoiding the outdoors or focusing preventive actions during peak hours may reduce risk. Place also matters; ticksare often found in grasses and other vegetated areas. Local health officials or guides may be able to point out areas with greater arthropod activity.
- *Wear appropriate clothing:* Travelers can minimize areas of exposed skin by wearing long-sleeved shirts, long pants, boots, and hats. Tucking in shirts and wearing socks and closed shoes instead of sandals may reduce risk. Repellents or insecticides such as permethrin (Elimite) can be applied to clothing and gear for added protection.
- *Bed nets:* When accommodations are not adequately screened or air conditioned, bed nets are essential to provide protection and to reduce discomfort caused by biting insects. If bed nets do not reach the floor, they should be tucked under mattresses. Bed nets are most effective when they are treated with an insecticide or repellent such as permethrin. Pretreated, long-lasting bed nets can be purchased prior to traveling, or nets can be treated after purchase. The permethrin will be effective for several months if the bed net is not washed. (Long-lasting pretreated nets may be effective for much longer.)
- *Insecticides:* Aerosol insecticides, vaporising mats, and mosquito coils can help to clear rooms or areas of mosquitoes; however, some products available internationally may contain pesticides that are not registered in the United States. Insecticides should always be used with caution, avoiding direct inhalation of spray or smoke.
- Optimum protection can be provided by applying repellents.

The CDC recommends insect repellent should contain up to 50 per cent DEET (N,N-diethyl-m-toluamide) which is the most effective mosquito repellent for adults and children over 2 months of age. There are no vaccines currently available commercially for dengue virus serovars. However, researchers are actively trying to produce vaccines that will protect people from all dengue viral serovars.

TREATMENT FOR DENGUE

There are actually no known antiviral drugs or injections available for the cure of dengue. However, the disease can be treated with plenty of supportive care and treatment that would eventually help save the patient's life. Dengue is characterised by fever and intense body ache. The fever can be treated with antipyretic drugs such as paracetamol and the body ache can be treated with analgesics that help relieve the pain.

Drugs such as aspirin and ibuprofen should be avoided as they may increase the risk of hemorrhage. The patient can also be treated with natural home remedies such as papaya leaves, kiwi and other food items that have been proven to help in the increase of platelet count, which gets affected during dengue.

In the case of more severe forms of dengue, such as dengue hemorrhagic disease or dengue shock syndrome, it a must for the patient to be admitted to a hospital and given proper care. The mortality rate of a dengue patient without hospitalisation increases about 50 per cent.

Treatments such as intra-venous fluid replacements should be administered to these patients to prevent shock. Patients should drink plenty of fluids, as dehydration is prevalent among those affected with Dengue. Vaccines for all of the serotypes are being developed, which will be the most effective way to cure the disease.

10

Animal Diseases

DIAGNOSIS OF SKIN DISEASES

Definitive diagnosis of the causes of various skin diseases requires a detailed history, physical examination, and appropriate diagnostic tests. Many skin diseases look alike, and a definitive diagnosis is made over time by including or excluding possible causes, evaluating responses to therapy, and/or process of elimination.

HISTORY

A careful dermatologic history is critical to interpret the physical examination findings and choose appropriate diagnostic tests. A complete general history should be obtained, including information about prior illnesses, vaccinations, husbandry (housing, feeding practices, etc), changes in attitude and food consumption, elimination practices, exposure to other animals, and travel within the past 6-12 mo. This should be followed by a detailed dermatologic history. Use of a preprinted history form can be very useful for chronic or complicated cases. A good history is important, because many skin diseases that look similar are differentiated based on interpreting clinical signs and historical patterns.

The following information should be obtained: 1) the primary complaint; 2) length of time the problem has been present; 3) age at which the skin disease started (distinct age predilections are seen in many diseases, eg, demodicosis and dermatophytosis in pediatric animals and signs of atopic dermatitis in animals 1-3 yr old); 4) breed (breed predilections include a predisposition of Cocker Spaniels to primary disorders of keratinization, and of terriers to atopic dermatitis); 5) presence and severity of pruritus (including licking, rubbing, scratching, or chewing behaviours-owners often do not realize licking may be a sign of pruritus); 6) how the disease started and its progression (diseases that begin with pruritus may lead to self-trauma and subsequent development of secondary skin lesions [alopecia, seborrhea] or infections [bacterial or yeast pyoderma]); 7) type and progression of lesions noted by the owner; 8) evidence of seasonality (suggesting fleas, allergic skin disease, or weather-related diseases); 9) area on the body the problem was first noticed (ie, regional patterns seen in atopic dermatitis [typically the face and feet], cheyletiellosis [primarily dorsal], scabies [primarily ventral], and endocrine hair loss [usually involves the trunk and spares the head and legs]); 10) any previous treatments and the responses to such (ie, antibiotic-responsive skin diseases suggest a bacterial cause; pruritus that responds to small doses of glucocorticoids, antihistamines, or essential fatty acids suggests allergic dermatitis); 11) frequency of bathing and when the last bath was given (recent bathing may obscure or change important clinical lesions, excessive bathing and wetting of the skin can predispose to skin disease); 12) presence of fleas, ticks, or mites; 13) other contact animals (ie, evidence of contagion, which suggests fleas, scabies, cheyletiellosis, or dermatophytosis); 14) the environment of the animal (housing changes can influence the development of certain skin diseases, eg, contact dermatitis, contagious diseases); and 15) signs or reports of systemic illness (endocrine [eg, hypothyroidism and hyperadrenocorticism] disorders and metabolic diseases [eg, diabetes mellitus, renal disease, liver disease] should be noted, because the skin can be the first place signs of systemic illness are noted).

PHYSICAL EXAMINATION

A complete physical examination should always be performed. Many skin diseases are manifestations of systemic diseases, eg, hypothyroidism, hyperadrenocorticism, hepatocutaneous syndrome, systemic lupus erythematosus.

A good dermatologic examination requires very close inspection of the entire hair coat and skin under strong lighting; flashlights may be necessary to examine the skin of large animals. It is important to examine the ventrum of the animal, where many primary lesions and cutaneous parasites are found.

Clinical lesions are described in a variety of ways. Gross lesions can be described as focal, multifocal, or diffuse in distribution, followed by a description of the affected region (eg, mucocutaneous, truncal). On closer inspection, lesions may be further described as primary or secondary.

Primary lesions include macules or patches (non-elevated areas of discoloration); papules or plaques (elevated lesions, the latter coalescing); pustules, vesicles, or bullae (fluid-filled lesions); wheals (flat-topped, steep-walled, solid elevations of the skin arising from histamine release); or nodules or tumors (large solid elevations of the skin). Secondary lesions include epidermal collarettes (late stage of a pustule), scars, excoriation (areas of self-trauma), erosions or ulcers (loss of the epidermis), fissures, lichenification (increased thickening and hyperpigmentation of the skin), and calluses. Some lesions may be either primary or secondary, depending on the cause of the disease. These include alopecia, scale, crusts, follicular casts (plugging of hair follicles with visible keratin), comedones (blackheads), and pigmentary changes.

ANIMAL DISEASE

The control of animal diseases and the promotion and protection of animal health are essential components of any effective animal breeding and production programme. Despite remarkable technical advances in the diagnosis, prevention and control of animal diseases, the condition of animal health throughout the developing world remains generally poor, causing substantial economic losses and hindering any improvement in livestock productivity.

In developing countries, animal health services were established with the main objective of controlling major contagious and infectious diseases, such as foot-and-mouth disease, rinderpest and contagious pleuropneumonia, as well as parasitic diseases, such as trypanosomiasis and tick-borne diseases. This was obviously the first priority, since the control of these diseases is a prerequisite to any successful livestock development programme.

With the present concern for sustainable economic development, more attention is now being given to other diseases that affect livestock productivity, such as helminthiasis, nutritional diseases, reproductive disorders, etc.

The successful control of disease depends initially on its timely and accurate recognition and on the presence of sound diagnostic capabilities based on effective working links between laboratories and field services. Emergencies created by outbreaks of major infectious diseases demonstrate the need for establishing, strengthening and improving such diagnostic services. As well, particular attention should be given to the development of an efficient animal disease information system.

Beyond the national level, a general increase in the movement of animals and animal products underlines the importance of international cooperation in the prevention and control of animal diseases. Most animal health services in developing countries do not have at present adequate technical and administrative infrastructures to carry out the tasks and duties necessary for the efficient control of animal diseases and for consumer protection.

In many developing countries, there is either a shortage of skilled veterinary personnel or their services are not correctly utilized. The problem is exacerbated by deficient veterinary infrastructures and inadequate disease control programmes, veterinary legislation and information services, as well as a lack of transport, communications, veterinary products and equipment. The most common problem is the shortage of funds to sustain the activities of veterinary staff. In some developing countries, the animal health services are not given the appropriate legal power in the administrative system.

These shortages significantly reduce the effectiveness of animal health services control measures against major animal diseases. By exploiting existing conditions, local resources and international help, possibilities for improving of animal health service programmes are increased. Veterinary education and training should receive the highest priority; however, more emphasis must be placed on the qualitative and practical aspects. Effective personnel development requires adequate planning of staff requirements, improved curriculums for undergraduate and postgraduate studies, training of auxiliary personnel and greater interregional cooperation to exploit existing training facilities fully, among other things. Animal health services should be further developed by improving their efficiency. While the control and prevention of major infectious diseases clearly remains a government responsibility, some veterinary tasks such as the treatment of individual animals could be undertaken in other ways. Privatization is one way of improving some sectors of animal health and of responding suitably to the needs of animal owners. Other ways include contracting out certain services, creating farmer cooperatives and producer associations, recovering government costs more efficiently and using the revenue thus generated for selective subsidies. Several countries have already taken steps to reorganize their veterinary services in this way.

Developing countries must address this problem. This publication aims to assist them in improving livestock production through better control of major animal diseases. It is not intended to be a comprehensive text describing in-depth all aspects of a complex subject with worldwide variations. Instead, it is meant to serve as a guideline, providing general background information on basic topics. Its main objective is to assist animal health authorities in their organization, planning and management activities.

The contents cover major problems facing official animal health services in developing countries in contributing to the production of food of animal origin and livestock development as integral components of general social, economic and agricultural development. Other priorities of animal health services include the protection of humans against diseases that may be transmitted by animals and the production of safe food.

Biological and pharmaceutical production may be the responsibility of some services, however, only aspects of the control and management of veterinary biologicals and drugs are included in this publication. The major issues dealt with in this publication are the objectives, functions, organization and management of animal health services. Without going into detail, relevant information, statements and recommendations make up the basic text. This general approach does not permit specific disease control or specific social, economic and ecological conditions to be dealt with.

ANIMAL MODELS OF DISEASE

A common justification for the creation of GA animals is that they will provide, or contribute to, 'improved', more predictive models of disease. This is an oversimplification because a) this is not necessarily always true, and b) even where a new GA model is more appropriate, it may be used alongside other, older models by different researchers. There is no mechanism for ensuring only the most relevant are used and that newer models are available to all researchers. In such cases the GA animal is not the new *definitive* model but just an *additional* one. The motivation for the research may merely be an interest in the model for its own sake, but a medical application may be used to justify the work since this is likely to be more acceptable publicly and politically. Basic, fundamental research carried out within academic research establishments is not regulated under Directive 86/609, so it may not undergo an ethical review with appropriate assessment and weighing of harms and benefits. This directive is under review and is expected to be adopted end 2010. The revised directive may incorporate basic, fundamental research with proper review, however only if implemented and enforced properly.

There is also currently no requirement for GA animals to be cryopreserved and stored within central archive facilities or depositories. Such methods can reduce repetition and duplication of work by providing a central resource for use by the wider scientific community and protect against adverse events such as environmental disasters or genetic drift. They also reduce the need for live transportation of GA animals, with associated welfare problems, because frozen gametes or embryos could be sent instead.

GA ANIMALS IN TOXICITY TESTING

GA mice and rats are increasingly used in genotoxicity and carcinogenicity testing, within studies that are done to fulfil regulatory requirements for the marketing of chemicals and pharmaceuticals. Such animals are likely to suffer equivalent (or even more severe) levels of pain and distress to those experienced by animals in traditional tests, but it has been claimed that fewer animals will be needed.

Eurogroup believes that reducing the numbers of animals used in research and testing is an important goal, provided that this can be done without increasing the level of suffering experienced by individual animals.

However, relatively severe adverse effects have been reported in some GA strains used in toxicity testing. For example, mortality rates are higher in *c-neu* and *c-myc* mice used in carcinogenicity testing than in conventional mice used in the same type of test. Many GA mice used in carcinogenicity tests are more susceptible to developing cancer and so will develop tumours more rapidly, which could make it more difficult to implement humane endpoints. Reducing numbers is thus not automatically a positive outcome for animals - the impact on individuals must be taken into account and it may be justifiable to use more animals who will suffer less. In any case, the contribution that biotechnologies can make to reducing animal numbers in carcinogenicity and genotoxicity is not consistent, largely due to actual or potential regulatory requirements. In carcinogenicity testing, GA mice were introduced to try to reduce animal numbers and the time taken to obtain test results.

However, there are proposals to add additional control groups (a positive control and treated and untreated controls using non-GA mice) that would decrease the magnitude of the reduction if they are adopted. It is also uncertain whether testing on one GA strain will be regarded as sufficient by regulators, in which case the reductions will be further diminished by requirements for results obtained using other strains.

For genotoxicity testing, GA models have distinct scientific advantages over existing *in vivo* assays when used as second tier tests for *in vitro* genotoxins. The reduction in numbers of animals used would be fairly substantial, perhaps from 50 to 20 per substance tested, but again it is not certain that a test on one GA model would be regarded as sufficient. There are potentially much greater savings in animals if GA tests can be used in place of very large tests of heritable mutation which are currently used, albeit rarely, for chemicals of high concern.

Conversely, using GA animal models in toxicity testing could increase the use of animals by making some tests more practical, or by increasing the amount of information they produce. For example, the use of GA animals could make investigations feasible that would otherwise require very large and impractical numbers of non-GA animals. Regulators might be inclined to ask for the GA test in cases where the conventional test would not have been requested (and could therefore presumably have been done without) because it was regarded as too cumbersome and possibly uninformative.

Eurogroup believes that, in toxicity testing as in the other research fields discussed in this document, the focus should be on developing *in vitro* alternatives to replace animals and not on developing different animal models.

ANIMALS AS 'BIOREACTORS'

This category of GA animal use includes:

- "Pharmed" animals who produce therapeutic substances *e.g.* pigs who express the blood protein Factor IX in milk, and goats that express the anti-clotting agent Atryn in their milk;
- Animals producing specialist materials *e.g.* goats who produce spiders' silk proteins in their milk for use to make 'biosteel'. This has both medical and non-medical applications (*e.g.* in sutures and bullet-proof vests respectively) (Nexia Biotechnologies, Quebec);

The substance produced may have an adverse effect on the animal, either at the point of expression, or if it can enter the animal's bloodstream. For example, a strain of rabbits genetically engineered to express human erythropoietin (EPO) in the mammary glands also expresses the protein at low levels in other organs, resulting in greatly elevated numbers of red blood cells, infertility and premature death.

Using animals in this way, and referring to them as 'bioreactors', reinforces the perception of animals as units of production and/or biological tools, rather than as sentient beings with the ability to experience pain, suffering and distress.

XENOTRANSPLANTATION

The use of GA animals to supply organs, tissues or cells for transplantation into humans is a highly controversial issue which has been the subject of a great deal of debate. There are many legal, scientific, human health, animal welfare and ethical concerns, which have been described in a number of documents. Only the ethical and welfare issues relating to animals are addressed here.

These include:

- The ethics of genetically modifying animals of any species as a source of cells, tissues and organs for human transplantation;
- The harms associated with the initial creation of GA animals as source animals;
- The suffering and/or distress associated with production and maintenance systems for high health status source herds. This includes hysterotomy-derivation, early weaning practices, and barren husbandry environments, which have a serious negative impact on animal welfare because they prevent animals from satisfying their physical, social and behavioural needs.

Furthermore, development of xeno technology to a point where it can be used still requires a great deal of pre-clinical research. To date, such research has included studies of efficacy, physiology, immunology, and infection risks in a range of species including primates, goats and dogs. This research, by its very nature, causes considerable suffering. Experiments involving organ transplantation require major surgery, which in itself causes suffering that is exacerbated by tissue rejection and immunosuppressive treatment.

Xenotransplantation is also an example of a biotechnology where over-optimistic claims are made to justify the approach, the funding and the use of animals. For example, in September 1995, the UK company Imutran *"envisaged the first xenotransplants of transgenic pig hearts into human patients taking place in 1996"*. Yet despite some progress, particularly with cell transplants, the transplant of whole organs is no closer and xenografts still rarely survive for more than a few months.

CLONING COMPANION ANIMALS

Eurogroup believes that, without doubt, some applications of modern biotechnology are trivial, scientifically unnecessary and ethically unjustifiable.

Examples include;

- The cloning of champion racing and show jumping horses for sport;
- The generation of a green fluorescent rabbit 'GFP Bunny' as transgenic "art";
- The cloning of companion animals for example cats, purely to satisfy humans' emotional requirements.

CONCERNS RELATING TO AGRICULTURAL PRODUCTION

Gene mapping was/is the most widely used technique in agriculture to enhance selective breeding schemes, however as more and more 'super' animals exist this is being overtaken by the import/export of embryos and/or sperm from cloned 'super' animals. Examples of agricultural applications of gene mapping and other genetic altering techniques that have given rise to ethical and animal welfare concerns include:

INCREASING PRODUCTIVITY OR CHANGING BODY COMPOSITION

Gene mapping has been used primarily to select individuals for breeding with the aim of increasing productivity *i.e.* growth rates, litter sizes and production traits such as egg laying, milk volume and meat quantity and quality (including the proportion of lean meat to fat). Whilst still being practiced to create 'super' individuals for subsequent breeding, gene mapping is being/has been replaced by the import/export of embryos and/or sperm from cloned 'super' livestock (primarily from the US).

Farmed species have also been genetically manipulated to alter the composition of meat and milk. For example, pigs and cows respectively have been genetically altered to have higher levels of Omega 3 in their muscle, and to express higher levels of casein in their milk.

INCREASING DISEASE RESISTANCE

Animals are genetically manipulated to be resistant to disease, for example, cattle have been engineered to express the antibiotic lysostaphin in their milk, which results in increased resistance to mastitis. Animals (including pigs, sheep, mice and rabbits) have also been modified to express antibodies providing immunity to specific diseases, for example mice have been generated with protection against prion disease.

MAKING ANIMALS MORE 'ENVIRONMENTALLY FRIENDLY'

An example of this application is the 'Enviropig', which has been engineered to contain the enzyme phytase in the pigs' saliva so that they can digest sources of dietary phosphorus.

This results in faeces with a lower phosphorus content, which in turn reduces the pollution of surface and ground water with phosphorus.

ETHICAL AND ANIMAL WELFARE CONCERNS

The selective breeding of farm animals has been conducted for thousands of years, and has given rise to a number of welfare concerns. However, Eurogroup believes that the use of cloning or other GA technologies to speed this process, or to introduce genes that could never be incorporated into the genomes of farm animals by any natural process, is a serious ethical and welfare issue. Directly altering an animal's genome is viewed by many as an unacceptable assault on the integrity of the animal that is incompatible with the concept of respecting farmed animals, and minimising the harms that are caused to them for human benefit. These views are important and should be respected as a legitimate part of the debate on biotechnology and farmed animal welfare.

Eurogroup also questions the necessity of further increasing production in farm animals. In many cases, productivity is already pushing animals to their physical and metabolic limits, so with any further increase there is an enhanced likelihood of animal welfare problems.

Enhancing selective breeding, by gene mapping or genetic modification, can also cause suffering if the trait that is selected for has a negative impact on the rest of the animals' physiology. For example, hens who produce high numbers of eggs suffer from osteoporosis because the majority of the calcium they ingest is used in eggshell production.

There can also be less direct effects on welfare, in that some GA animals may receive lower standards of husbandry than conventional animals. For example, clinical mastitis is a major welfare problem in dairy systems with sub-optimal standards of hygiene, and early detection is reliant on routine inspections by parlour staff at milking. The creation of cattle resistant to mastitis may encourage the perception that mastitis is no longer a problem. This could not only compromise standards of parlour hygiene, but may reduce the level of attention paid to each animal at milking. This would increase the potential for other clinical or welfare problems to go undetected. "High productivity" animals may also be at risk if their husbandry is not appropriate. It may be possible for them to be properly managed and cared for in the controlled environment of a breeding company or experimental farm, but there are serious concerns regarding the welfare of such animals once they are released into commercial agriculture.

CONCLUDING REMARKS

Modern biotechnologies have had, and will continue to have, a serious adverse impact on animals, particularly with regard to their use in scientific research and agriculture. This adverse impact relates to the numbers of animals used and the nature of the harms caused to them. In addition, directly altering an animal's genome, as occurs in many applications of biotechnology, is viewed by many as altering the integrity of the animal in a way that is incompatible with the concept of respecting animals, and minimising the harms that are caused to them for human benefit. Lastly, the technology is progressing at a rate that is outstripping public understanding and ethical and public debate.

The development and application of novel biotechnologies therefore poses new challenges for existing regulatory regimes in a number of fields of science, medicine, agriculture and the environment. Eurogroup believes that the broader issues surrounding the ethical and social acceptability of such uses of animals, as set out in this submission, cannot be effectively addressed within the current regulatory systems. The following principles are fundamental to ensuring that the lives and welfare of animals involved in all modern and future biotechnologies are awarded due priority.

- It is critically important that all relevant regulatory systems are updated to take into account the animal welfare, ethical and social implications and societal concerns of the development and intended use of all modern biotechnologies.
- Biotechnology is applied in many different fields so there needs to be effective liaison, co-ordination and definition of responsibilities within and between all the relevant legislative and regulatory bodies concerned with a particular issue. This includes, for example, the different bodies regulating use of animals in experiments and those setting requirements for product regulation.
- The regulatory framework for each technology must encompass a process which enables a critical scrutiny of the potential harms to animals and the intended benefits, and a careful and fair weighing of these. This applies to broad research directions as well as individual projects and the further application of new technologies that result from these. Critical assessment of justification needs to be done prior to the development and/or application of a technology and must then be reviewed regularly to check whether the harms and benefits are as expected so that appropriate action can be taken if necessary.
- A mechanism should be set in place to ensure that the justification and clinical relevance of all research involving the production and use of GA animals is critically scrutinised, such that animals are not used simply because the technology is available. This also needs to ensure that animal models of disease are regularly reviewed, so that redundant models are no longer routinely used for research purposes.
- There needs to be greater transparency with regard to the use of animals in biotechnology throughout Europe. Clearer information on the numbers of animals, and nature and level of any suffering that they experience, is essential in order to be able to identify issues of concern and assess trends. It is also vital that the public is well

informed and therefore able to engage in constructive debate on the associated ethical issues.

- Restrictions should be placed on the species of animal that it is permissible to genetically modify. Non-human primates should not be genetically modified or cloned for any purpose, nor used as source animals for cells, tissues or organs.
- The production of GA livestock where the intention is to modify traits such as increased lean to fat ratio, growth rate, or litter size should not be allowed, as levels of productivity are already causing serious welfare problems.
- There should be far greater effort devoted to developing and validating alternatives to animal use in all fields. There should be greater commitment to, and endorsement of, the principles of the Three Rs of reduction, refinement and replacement in animal experiments.
  Examples especially relevant to modern biotechnology are:
  - The development of GA germ cells for *in vitro* testing;
  - The production of drugs, proteins, or material by bacteria rather than 'bioreactor' animals;
  - Generating cells, tissues and organs for treatment or transplantation using a patients own cells, eg human bladders.

THE THREAT OF INFECTIOUS DISEASE

One of the most significant, though much overlooked, repercussions of animal domestication—and certainly the most relevant for this book—was the advent of infectious disease on an epidemic scale. Like violence, infectious disease was a scourge on early agricultural societies, resulting in great mortality—amongst both animal and human populations—and the disruption of food production. The growing intimacy between humans and other animals and increasing exploitation of animal resources, which ensued as a consequence of domestication, created a set of circumstances under which disease-causing microorganisms could flourish and transfer to, and between, human populations on a scale never before possible.

As the historian William H. McNeill explains, the increasing human manipulation and control of the natural world resulted in the disturbance of ecological balances; much in the same fashion as disease organisms upset the natural biological balance within a host's body. To a large extent, our hominid and early human ancestors would have been integrated into the natural ecosystem in which they lived, much the same as any other mammalian species. As our ancestors evolved, they developed into accomplished hunters and, by doing so, achieved a more or less supreme and unchallenged position in the animal kingdom. Within the African heartland, these formidable early human hunters probably maintained a relatively stable relationship to the natural environment. However, once they began to intrude into ecosystems within which they had not evolved, humans began to play real havoc with the delicate balances of nature. Early humans became very successful in exploiting the environment, creating multitudinous new niches for themselves in places and climates that had hitherto been unsuitable for human habitation. Both the domestication of fire and the use of animal skins and fur as clothing allowed humans to survive in colder climates and hunt animal populations previously untouched by human predation.

Once established in these areas, humans successfully used the natural resources and species found there to their advantage. Human expansionism and the ever-increasing exploitation of natural resources inevitably resulted in the alteration of pre-existing patterns of plant and animal distribution. As human groups began to adopt a sedentary lifestyle and produce their food through agriculture and livestock husbandry, the ecosystems where humans settled were to be changed irrevocably.

In the long run, the human manipulation of plants and animals meant that there were larger numbers of fewer species in areas where human settlements were located. This, in turn, created a happy hunting ground for disease-producing parasites, which took great advantage of the new ecological niches created by people.

The increasing densities of human populations offered a new food supply to disease organisms. Furthermore, the livestock kept by human communities and the wild scavengers that settlements attracted acted as ideal reservoirs for the microorganisms that would go on to blight human populations.

Hence, although they had achieved a supreme and more or less unchallenged position in the food chain by becoming highly skilled hunters and later agriculturalists, humans remained at peril from predators of a quite different kind: disease-producing microorganisms.

These predators would in fact turn out to be potentially more devastating than any of the ferocious beasts that had already been faced in the gradual ascent of the food chain. It is rather ironic that it was humankind's very evolutionary success and mastery of the natural environment which laid them bare to their new microscopic enemies.

This of course is not to say that prior to sedentism disease never afflicted human beings. As discussed earlier in this chapter, a wide variety of food-borne parasites and pathogens would have caused sickness and death in our pre-agrarian ancestors, in addition to rendering them easier prey for other predators. Further to this, bacterial and viral infections would have almost certainly struck the hunter-gatherers of earlier times.

Unsanitary living conditions would undoubtedly have been most favourable for the spread of enteric diseases; numerous individuals sharing cramped living quarters, particularly during winter time, would also have provided the ideal conditions for the spread of respiratory infection. Nevertheless, before the inception of agriculture, the microorganisms that caused epidemic disease would have had little opportunity to flourish for long within human communities or to decimate large populations since there were insufficient human or animal reservoirs to harbour and perpetuate disease. Humans, and our hominid ancestors, lived in relatively small groups, moving around nomadically in search of food. Consequently, many infections, particularly those that are transmitted by droplets, could not spread between human groups easily.

Likewise, given this lifestyle, infection would not have been readily acquired from contact with faeces or other waste. Faeces and other refuse would have been dispersed over a wide area, rather than concentrated in one particular or fixed area. If humans were afflicted by infection, the whole group probably suffered and, in the worst scenario, might even have been wiped out entirely. Nonetheless, only a limited number of individuals would have been affected. Given the small group size and restricted external contacts, disease would simply have died out before it could become virulent or affect large numbers of people. As Cockburn suggests, 'for each infection and set of circumstances, there is a minimum threshold of host population; if the population falls below this threshold, the infection will die out.

As a result, the acuteness of an infection is related to the size of the "herd"; small, isolated populations have chronic infections and large ones have more acute infections'. As humans began to adopt a sedentary lifestyle, the numbers of people living together in single locations increased, culminating in a greater concentration of and proximity to the middens and excreta which might harbour infection. Likewise, as the density of settlements increased, harmful pathogens could spread more easily. For example, droplet infections which originated in a single individual could more easily attack a larger number of people who had come into contact with that person—and subsequently those who came into contact with newly infected individuals—leading to a high rate of death and infirmity.

As the above discussion illustrates, the relationship between humans and disease is one of socio-ecological dynamics. The changing configurations of humans, animals and microorganisms that resulted from increasing human mastery over the natural world opened a new chapter in disease history. The processes of domestication and agrarianisation, therefore, led not only to fundamental and irrevocable transformations in the relationship between humans and other animals, but also altered the symbiosis between parasites and their hosts radically. As McNeill has argued, from the dawn of agrarianism onwards, disease and civilisation were to become inseparable. The establishment and advance (or fall) of human civilisations, he contends, inescapably went hand in hand with the advance of disease. While humankind flourished and multiplied so did disease-causing organisms. In short, epidemic infectious disease can only exist in what we commonly call 'civilised' communities; in large, complexly organised and densely populated areas where infection passes freely and unceasingly from individual to individual without necessarily even requiring an intermediate host.

Thus, while the enfoldment of other species into human society through domestication created—in the long term—a more stable future for humankind, the new-found intimacy between human and beast also created the ideal conditions for the spread of infectious disease on an epidemic scale. Furthermore, it is most likely that the animals that were domesticated were already the carriers of chronic infection. Again, the problem spawned by domestication was one of socio-ecological dynamics. With disease organisms only being able to survive at high population densities, the vast and gregarious herds in which wild cattle, sheep and horses lived prior to domestication had provided the suitable conditions for chains of infection to persist, transferring from animal to animal and between generations. In this way the biological balances between animals and disease-causing parasites had, over the course of time, become more or less stable. The genetic immunity against the effects of contamination that had been acquired by these animals over many generations meant that infections within wild herds probably only appeared in mild or relatively harmless forms.

The symptoms which the wild animals exhibited were likely akin to 'childhood diseases' which, while potentially debilitating, are generally not lethal to the afflicted. However, once these contaminated animals were brought to live within the realms of human social organisation, the relatively innocuous microorganisms that the animals bore acquired a far more deadly and virulent character for there, within human settlements, were large, vulnerable human populations off which they could feed? With little or no immunity against them, initial contact with new disease organisms would probably have been near-catastrophic for the early domesticators.

An ongoing relationship between parasite and host would need to be established over a period of centuries before sufficient immunities were built up. Only then would infection become as endemic to humans as it had been to the original animal carriers of the disease.

McNeill argues that it is likely that 'most and probably all of the distinctive infectious diseases of civilisation transferred to human populations from animal herds'. The most common infectious diseases, such as measles, influenza and smallpox, which have afflicted humans throughout the ages, closely resemble diseases which affect domesticated animals. Such human diseases can share a common ancestry with animal ones. Measles, rinderpest and distemper, for example, are all caused by pseudo-myxoviruses; these three viruses are very closely related and even share common antigens. As Fiennes explains, people who have suffered from measles tend to have antibodies in their sera which neutralise distemper. Likewise, dogs recovering from distemper display antibodies to measles. Although, if exposed to the measles virus, dogs will only produce a minute quantity of antibody to distemper they will, nonetheless, resist the distemper if exposed to it.

Similarly, sera taken from cattle immune to rinderpest can neutralise both measles and distemper. Moreover, humans suffering from measles can develop antibodies against rinderpest, and the rinderpest virus has immunising properties against canine distemper. Fiennes suggests that, due to its great virulence in cattle and the lack of apparent wildlife reservoirs for the disease, rinderpest is a relatively recent disease. Measles and rinderpest, he argues, have evolved in humans and cattle respectively as mutations of the distemper virus originally acquired from dogs, which themselves inherited the disease from their lupine ancestors. Similarly, there are clear connections between smallpox in humans and cowpox in cattle, and influenza in both humans and swine. Besides these diseases, there exists a large and important group of diseases, known as the zoonoses, which affect humans and the domesticated animals with which they share their lives.

A zoonosis is a disease or infection that can naturally be transmitted between vertebrate animals and humans. Tuberculosis, as discussed earlier, is one such disease. Humans first probably acquired the tuberculosis parasite through a close association with cattle. While closely related, the bovine and human tuberculosis bacilli are distinct and cause different clinical manifestations in each species. The bovine variant is, however, also capable of producing the disease in humans. Moreover, humans can act as a reservoir for *Mycobacteriumtuberculosis bovis* and reintroduce it into livestock populations that are tuberculosis-free. Other zoonoses of known ancient origin are, for example, rabies and anthrax.

Humankind's close association with dogs and meat-eating habits has provided the respective conditions under which these diseases can be transferred to human subjects. The increasing exploitation of animal domesticates also created new opportunities for the transmission of infection from animals to humans. Once humans began to exploit ruminants for their milk, a new and effective path for the transfer of zoonotic disease to humans was established through the consumption of dairy produce. With regard to the relationship between animal and human disease, McNeill proposes the maxim that 'the sharing of infection increases with the degree of intimacy that prevails between man and beast'. The greater the interdependence and residential proximity of humans and other animals, the greater the potential for disease to affect human-herd health. The relationship between the human-animal interdependence and vulnerability to disease is a theme that will be constantly returned to, both explicitly and implicitly, throughout this book. In the chapters that follow, I shall continue to explore the nature of humankind's increasing dependency on other animals and the consequences thereof in terms of health and disease. It will be argued that once infectious disease took hold of human communities, became part of everyday life and became associated with the conditions of, particularly food, animals; there arose a clear need to deal effectively with the manifestations of it. Sick animals threatened human food supplies. Conversely, sick humans were unable to harvest and maintain them adequately. In this way, both veterinary and human medicine gained their *raison d'etre*. The domestication of animals thus gave rise to the emergence of a veterinary regime. In the following chapter, I will look more closely at the very first phase of this process, examining how the veterinary regime was improved and increasingly intensified as human dependency on other animals continued to grow and grow.

VIRAL INFECTIONS

INFECTIOUS LARYNGOTRACHEITIS (ILT) CAUSATIVE AGENT: HERPES VIRUS

This viral infection of poultry typically affects chickens only, although occasional reports suggest pheasants also may be susceptible.

Method of Spread

The virus usually is spread through bird-to-bird contact, or contact with contaminated droppings or respiratory tract secretions. Recovered birds may be carriers and shedders of the virus, and may spread ILT to other poultry for many months.

Signs

Sudden death of an individual bird is often the first sign. Blood-stained feathers around the head and neck may be observed. The disease spreads slowly through a flock, and mortality is high.

Treatment and Prevention

Once the disease is diagnosed, there is no treatment for affected birds. Fortunately, an effective vaccine can be administered. Vaccination can prevent infection in uninfected birds during an outbreak, and can be given to prevent the disease in new stock. Diagnosis usually is made by microscopic examination of the trachea by a veterinary pathologist.

NEWCASTLE DISEASE VIRUS (NDV)

Newcastle virus is a virus that can infect most species of birds.

Method of Spread

Sick birds shed the virus in respiratory secretions and fecal matter.

Signs

In most instances the respiratory infection is quite mild in all but very young birds. However, egg layers usually show a moderate to severe egg production drop. It may take two to four weeks for egg production to come back to near normal levels.

Treatment and Prevention

The commercial poultry industry practices widespread vaccination for this disease as a preventative tool. There is no effective treatment for this viral infection.

INFECTIOUS BRONCHITIS (IB) CAUSATIVE AGENT: CORONA VIRUS

Method of Spread

Infected birds shed the virus through respiratory secretions and feces. (This viral disease affects chickens only.)

Signs

As with Newcastle disease, little or no death loss is common, except in very young chicks. However, if sexually immature birds become infected, they may experience permanent damage to their reproductive tract and never lay eggs. Mature layers infected with Infectious Bronchitis will lay eggs with misshapen, soft, wrinkled shells for several weeks. Broiler chickens will show poor weight gain and may develop secondary bacterial infections. Infected birds usually cough, because of excessive mucus in their trachea. This disease spreads rapidly through the entire flock. In uncomplicated cases, the flock recovers quickly.

Treatment and Prevention

There is no effective treatment. Prevention is by vaccination.

General Recommendations Concerning Poultry Respiratory Diseases

In any case of respiratory illness, it is important to know if you're dealing with a viral, bacterial, fungal or parasitic disease. The treatment for one disease may be ineffective or even harmful for others. To make a diagnosis, your veterinarian will perform several tests including bacterial cultures of the airways, blood tests, and necropsies (post-mortem examinations) of dead birds if they are available. Microscopic evaluation of affected tissues is helpful and can be performed at a diagnostic laboratory. A fecal test for parasites also should be done. Attempts to isolate virus may be required. Several general measures can be taken to reduce the incidence of respiratory illness in small flocks.

- Always purchase replacement stock from a reputable dealer, preferably one who is a member of the National Poultry Improvement Plan.
- Keep all new birds isolated from the rest of the flock for at least three weeks. During this time the birds should have their blood tested for antibodies, and a fecal parasite check performed.
- Keep birds isolated for two to three weeks after returning from a show. Respiratory outbreaks commonly occur after large groups of birds are mingled in these situations
- Screen all visitors to your farm. People can carry infectious agents from one farm to another on their shoes, hands, clothing, even on their hair. If a visitor requests to see your birds, ask that they not go near other birds the day of their visit. Request that they wear freshly laundered clothes and clean footwear.
- Try to keep age groups separate. Young poultry need time to develop immunity to diseases. Isolate any suspicious sick looking birds from the rest of the flock. Get a diagnosis as soon as possible. Dead birds should be immediately refrigerated (not frozen) until a necropsy can be performed by your veterinarian. The necropsy ideally should be done within several hours after death.
- Do not rely on 'home remedies' which often do not work, but tend to mask disease and make diagnosis more difficult.
- Your veterinarian may suggest a vaccination programme if appropriate for your needs.

VIRAL DISEASES (NON-RESPIRATORY)

MAREK'S DISEASE

Synonyms: acute leukosis, neural leukosis, range paralysis, gray eye (when eye affected)

Species affected: Chickens between 12 to 25 weeks of age are most commonly clinically affected. Occasionally pheasants, quail, game fowl and turkeys can be infected.

Clinical signs: Marek's disease is a type of avian cancer. Tumors in nerves cause lameness and paralysis. Tumors can occur in the eyes and cause irregularly shaped pupils and blindness. Tumors of the liver, kidney, spleen, gonads, pancreas, proventriculus, lungs, muscles, and skin can cause incoordination, unthriftiness, paleness, weak laboured breathing, and enlarged feather follicles. In terminal stages, the birds are emaciated with pale, scaly combs and greenish diarrhea.

Marek's disease is very similar to Lymphoid Leukosis, but Marek's usually occurs in chickens 12 to 25 weeks of age and Lymphoid Leukosis usually starts at 16 weeks of age.

Transmission: The Marek's virus is transmitted by air within the poultry house. It is in the feather dander, chicken house dust, feces and saliva. Infected birds carry the virus in their blood for life and are a source of infection for susceptible birds.

Treatment: none

Prevention: Chicks can be vaccinated at the hatchery. While the vaccination prevents tumor formation, it does not prevent infection by the virus.

INFECTIOUS BURSAL DISEASE

Synonyms: Gumboro, IBD, infectious bursitis, infectious avian nephrosis

Species affected: chickens

Clinical signs: In affected chickens greater than 3 weeks of age, there is usually a rapid onset of the disease with a sudden drop in feed and water consumption, watery droppings leading to soiling of feathers around the vent, and vent pecking. Feathers appear ruffled. Chicks are listless and sit in a hunched position. Chickens infected when less than 3 weeks of age do not develop clinical disease, but become severely and permanently immunosuppressed.

Transmission: The virus is spread by bird-to-bird contact, as well as by contact with contaminated people and equipment. The virus is shed in the bird droppings and can be spread by air on dust particles. Dead birds are a source of the virus and should be incinerated.

Treatment: There is no specific treatment. Antibiotics, sulfonamides, and nitrofurans have little or no effect. Vitamin-electrolyte therapy is helpful. High levels of tetracyclines are contraindicated because they tie up calcium, thereby producing rickets. Surviving chicks remain unthrifty and more susceptible to secondary infections because of immuno-suppression.

Prevention: A vaccine is commercially available.

EQUINE ENCEPHALITIS

Synonyms: EE, EEE, WEE

Note: This disease should not be confused with St. Louis Encephalits (SLE). Chickens are used as sentinels (test animals) in SLE suspect areas, such as southern Florida. While SLE is also carried by mosquitos, that is where the similarities between the two encephalitis diseases end. Chickens do not get SLE. *Species affected:* Equine encephalitis is a contagious disease of birds (especially pheasants), mammals (especially horses), and people. Birds are the major source of the virus.

Clinical signs: Two forms affect birds: eastern equine encephalitis (EEE) and western equine encephalitis (WEE). The clinical signs are identical and include reduced feed consumption, staggering, and paralysis. Surviving birds may be blind, have muscle paralysis, and have difficulty holding their head up. Damage to the bird's nervous system varies with species. In pheasants, there is pronounced leg paralysis, twisting of the neck, and tremors. Mortality is high. Chukar partridges and turkeys show drowsiness, paralysis, weakness, and death.

Transmission: Infected mosquitoes are the primary source of the virus. The *Culiseta melanuria* mosquito is the primary transmitter of the virus to poultry. Other mosquito species transmit the disease too, but feed mostly on other animals. Cannibalism of sick or dead birds by penmates is a major source of transmission within pens.

Treatment: none

Prevention: Remove the source of infection by establishing mosquito control: keep weeds mowed in a 50-foot strip around bird pens. This removes cover and resting areas for mosquitos. Eliminate mosquito breeding areas. Fog areas with malathion. It is possible to immunize birds, especially pheasants, with the vaccine prepared for horses. The recommended dose is one-tenth of a horse dose per bird.

BACTERIAL DISEASES

FOWL CHOLERA (PASTEURELLOSIS) CAUSATIVE AGENT: PASTEURELLA MULTOCIDA

Thousands of migrating waterfowl succumb to this disease annually, perhaps because of overcrowding in shrinking wetland habitats, coupled with the stress of the long migration. In addition to wild birds, chickens and domestic turkeys, ducks, geese and gamebirds also are susceptible.

Method of Spread

Recovered birds may carry the organism for a long time and serve as a source of infection.

Signs

Sudden death, without signs of illness, is often seen in turkeys and waterfowl. In addition to unexpected deaths, chickens also may develop swollen sinuses and wattles. Fowl cholera, if untreated, can kill a substantial portion of the flock.

Treatment and Prevention

This disease is treated with appropriate antibiotics following isolation and identification of the organism. Prevention may include vaccination on farms where repeated outbreaks are common. Isolation of domestic poultry from wild flocks is important.

CHICKEN AND TURKEY CORYZA CAUSATIVE AGENTS

Although the names of these diseases are similar, the organism that causes the disease in chickens (*Haemophilus paragallinarum*) is different from the organism that affects turkeys (*Bordetella avium*).

Method of Spread

These are common organisms in poultry flocks. The diseases are passed from age group to age group as replacement stock is introduced to the farm. A percentage of birds become asymptomatic carriers.

Signs

Both these bacterial infections produce foamy, watery eyes, discharge from the nostrils, and sometimes swollen sinuses. Unlike fowl cholera, deaths rarely occur. Affected chicks and poults do not grow well, and the flock appears uneven in size.

Treatment and Prevention

Appropriately administered antibiotics may be effective in alleviating signs of disease, but do not affect carrier status. Vaccines are available.

PATHOGENS TO ANIMALS

WAYS PATHOGENS SPREAD

In order to prevent the introduction of pathogens, one must understand how pathogens find their way onto backyard, hobby, and large corporate poultry or livestock operations. The spread of pathogens is primarily caused by the movement of animals, people, and contaminated equipment. Therefore, you can help prevent the spread of pathogens by controlling the movement of people and animals and avoiding contact with any potentially-contaminated equipment or objects.

Controlling Animal Movement and Contact

The easiest and most frequent way to transmit a pathogen is for an infected animal to come into contact with a healthy animal. Most disease is transmitted nose-to-nose or by other direct contact with sick animals. New additions to flocks or herds are a very common way to introduce pathogens. Stray pets that wander onto your farm or land can be another source of pathogen transmission.

If a sick animal is allowed into a show or fair, it may infect other nearby animals. In addition to stray pets; wild animals, free-flying birds, and insects can be responsible for the introduction of a pathogen.

People Movement People, vehicles, equipment, and clothing that are in contact with an infected animal may be contaminated with pathogens. These contaminated articles include equipment, machinery, and other objects used for the transportation, care, and management of livestock and poultry. If pathogens can be spread from animal to animal at shows and fairs, does that mean that we cannot take an animal to the show? We can purchase animals and go to the fair, but you should isolate those animals when you return. The wisest decision is to choose shows and make livestock and poultry purchases from places where disease prevention is always given high priority.

Practical Steps that Improve Isolation

Isolation (a form of quarantine) prevents contact between animals within a controlled environment. The idea behind isolation is to prevent contact between healthy animals and an animal that is or could be infected with a pathogen. Animals new to the herd or flock should be isolated away from the rest of the herd or flock for at least four weeks. Always isolate sick animals and only return them to their original group when they've fully recovered. Livestock returning from fairs or shows should also be isolated, since they could have picked up a new pathogen at the show.

After returning to the farm, you should isolate your show animals to avoid the possibility of infecting other animals on your farm. Ideally, this should be in a completely separate place to avoid close contact. At minimum it could be a separate pen in a different building or at least a separate corner of the barn. This may represent some extra work, but it can be very important. Isolate all purchased animals for four weeks. If they are incubating a serious disease, the signs (i.e., diarrhea, hard breathing, etc.) of that disease will likely be observed in that 4 week isolation period.

This gives you some time to do follow-up testing or give booster vaccinations if needed. Always purchase good, healthy animals. Do not buy sickly animals, even if they are being sold for a "cheap" price. Livestock or poultry at bargain prices can be expensive!

Since people can carry pathogens on their body or clothing, it is necessary to control the visitors that may come in contact with your livestock or poultry. Always make sure visitors wear clean boots and clothing. It is best if visitors come only when you are there to escort them around your farm. Locked gates and doors will keep people out when you're not around. Signs and notices help to alert visitors of the potential risk that they may pose. Perimeter fences will keep people from accidentally wandering onto your property. Question visitors about the farms or animals they have visited or have been near recently, and ask if they have visited a foreign country within the past 5 days.

There are ways to help keep out wild animals, free-flying birds, and insects. Although it is impossible to totally prevent all contact between wildlife and our livestock, we can make barnyards and surroundings unattractive to many of these species. Cutting the grass and weeds around the outside of buildings will help prevent rodents from entering. Keep grain spills or other potential sources of food cleaned up and unavailable to wildlife.

Clean up old board piles or woodpiles and inspect buildings for possible hiding or denning areas. Inspect the haymow or other protected areas for evidence that cats, raccoons, or other animals that are likely using the hay or the straw for nesting areas. Store feed where wild animals, including rodents and birds, cannot make contact with it. Dispose of all waste feed in a way that will not attract pests. Maintain barns and buildings in good repair making it more difficult for animals or birds to gain access. Keep doors and windows shut when not needed for ventilation. Place screens or netting on the windows.

Location and Construction of Buildings

When planning the location of a barn or building used to house your livestock and/or poultry, isolation is key. The buildings or pens should be constructed to promote isolation from outside sources of disease. The facility should be a substantial distance from road traffic. It is important to consider possible exposure and the distance from other flocks, herds, or populations of domestic or wild animals. It is especially crucial that there is no nose-to-nose or beak-to-beak contact with other animals. There should not be any contact with drainage water or waste runoff from other animals. When planning the organization of either a large- or small-scale animal operation, the risk of disease can be greatly reduced whenever you keep different species and ages of the same species well separated. This is because pathogens producing little or no disease in one species can produce significant disease in another species. Mild infections in older animals can produce severe disease in young animals.Disease susceptibility within the same species varies with age.

Because they have acquired resistance, older animals may shed pathogens without getting sick themselves. These same pathogens can be serious to younger animals. Salmonella and E. coli are good examples of pathogens that can spread and produce extra trouble in young or newborn animals when they are not well separated from older stock.

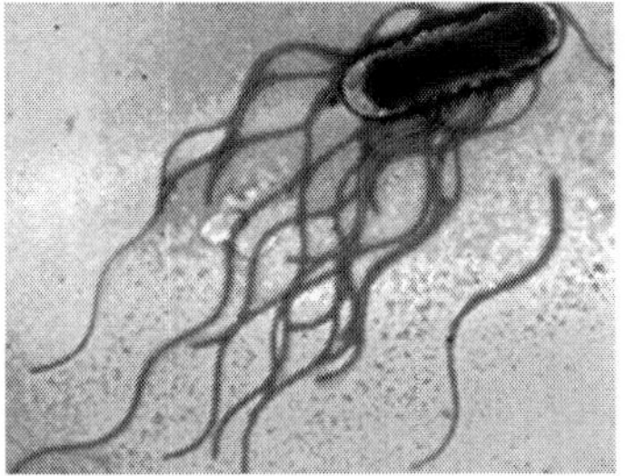

Fig. Salmonella magnified 3000 X

Various ways may be available to achieve species/age separation. They will be different depending on many factors such as the value of the animals, the economic and labour resources available to the herd/flock owner, and such other factors as farm size and marketing opportunities. They may include separate buildings, well-separated pens, different caretakers, or, ideally separate premises for different species and ages. Certain types of farm operations are able to ensure separation of ages by using the "all-in/all-out" management practice. All-in/all-out management allows only one age at a time on a premise. No new or younger animals are brought in until all of the older animals are removed and the barn has been cleaned. This allows for cleaning and disinfecting before a new group of animals is brought onto the premises. The farm environment can be a very comfortable place where pathogens can survive and multiply. Animal buildings, barns and pastures, as well as litter and manure surfaces, are often damp environments favourable for a dangerous increase in pathogen populations. Depending on the number of animals, very large accumulations of manure and litter may develop and become areas where pathogens can survive and multiply for many weeks or months.

SANITATION

How can you avoid bringing your animals to pathogens? The best way is to maintain a clean, dry, and sanitary environment. Cleaning is very important in reducing pathogen levels. Cleanliness means freedom from dirt, filth, and debris. Although buildings and equipment can appear clean when they are not visibly dirty, many microscopic contaminating pathogens can continue to be present. They remain and survive by clinging to surfaces, and by hiding in tiny cracks and crevices. The use of a disinfectant kills these remaining pathogens

Proper disinfection results in reduction of pathogens. Reducing the amount of pathogens around your animals will decrease the risk of disease. Disinfectants are chemical agents that kill pathogens on contact. However, it is important to clean before disinfecting so that the pathogens become fully exposed to the disinfectant. Pre-cleaning is doubly important because a disinfectant can be used up or inactivated by dirt. Disinfection and thorough, prompt drying are the last steps in the sanitation process. Without quick, thorough drying, any pathogens surviving the effects of the disinfectant can re-multiply to high numbers.

Hygienic Manure

Animal body wastes (feces, urine, etc.) ordinarily accumulate right in the environment (surroundings) where the animals spend most of their lives. In humans, of course, this does not occur because of toilets, plumbing and sewage treatment/disposal systems. Since flush toilets are not practical for animals, this ordinarily unavoidable problem for animals is partially reduced when manure or litter is managed in a way that, at least lowers the level of exposure to potential pathogens. Accumulated manure must be managed to reduce its volume, its odor, and to kill pathogens and weed seeds. The essential parts of manure management include collection, transfer, and storage. Spreading manure onto fields is the most common method of disposal. The sun will dry manure after it is spread onto fields which will kill many pathogens. A proper level of airflow over manure surfaces promotes drying and the decrease of many pathogen populations. In contrast, stagnant air contributes to the build- up of moisture, and an increase in pathogen populations. Chemical treatments can be beneficial in manure management. Raising the pH to at least 12 for 30 minutes will kill most of the microorganisms present. Lime is usually used to raise the pH. Treatments that produce anaerobic conditions (very low oxygen) are also used. Anaerobic lagoons take advantage of a natural process where manure is digested by beneficial anaerobic bacteria. In contrast, aerobic lagoons add oxygen to the manure.

The addition of oxygen allows more common bacteria to survive and multiply and for the bacteria to break down the waste material. These bacteria convert the manure into carbon dioxide, water, and more beneficial lagoon bacteria. In animal pens or holding areas, we want the bedding and floor dry. Management of areas where water spillage or water accumulation is highest is very important. Good drainage and proper ventilation of buildings will help reduce the dangers of dampness. The frequent removal of wet litter and/or bedding and a continuous, modest flow of air over manure/litter surfaces will help to produce the drying needed to suppress bacteria.

THREATS TO ANIMAL HEALTH FROM THE VISIBLE TO THE INVISIBLE

Animals may be injured or die from the attacks by something as large and dangerous as a coyote or wolf to something just as dangerous, but only as small, as a molecule. This section takes you on a voyage into a world of animal health dangers. This fascinating voyage ranges from dangers that are visible to the naked eye (predators), to some that are more easily seen with a hand lens (internal and external parasites), to some that can only be seen with a microscope (bacteria and viruses).

The voyage continues all the way on down to the sub-microscopic world of disease-producing molecules! More about these visible and invisible hazards to animal health and a short discussion about their prevention is presented below. The discussion is very basic and introductory.

We know that disease-causing pathogens that we cannot see threaten our livestock. In addition, there are also other threats that can be easily seen. Predators may easily be detected; however, many often appear at night or when people are not around. There are ways to help keep out predators that could potentially physically attack and harm your animals.

First, remove all easily accessible food supplies. This may be very difficult depending on the size of the farm and the amount of livestock feed on-hand. Keeping feed bins in good repair and sealed off will help prevent predators from entering areas where feed is stored. Keeping feed bins and feeding areas clean is very important.

An accumulation of waste feed in and around feed bunks attracts animals. A second suggestion is to remove water supplies. This is even more difficult on most farms. Stock tanks often provide a constant water supply and are attractive to predators such as raccoons.

Preventing any unnecessary pools of water will help. A third suggestion is to modify habitat and reduce access. Clearing brush and keeping weeds away from barns and buildings will help deter animals just like it will help deter rodents. Finally, you can trap or control predators. There are a variety of traps available to catch animals. Barns and buildings should be kept in good repair. Predators often enter barns though open doors, or cracks and holes that may exist. Closing doors and patching cracks and holes helps to reduce the problem. Wire mesh or screening on windows can also help.

EXTERNAL PARASITES

Small yet visible threats to livestock include external parasites such as ticks, flies, fleas, lice, mosquitoes, mites, grubs, etc. Parasites are a threat to livestock health just as microbial (invisible) pathogens are a threat. Parasites can transmit and spread microbial pathogens in addition to the harm and damage that they naturally cause by irritating animals and sapping their energy. The most common way to control external parasites is through the use of pesticides or insecticides. Pesticides kill and help control the parasite populations. Pesticides are applied as sprays, dips, pour-ons, dusts, injectables, pastes, boluses, etc. Ear tags impregnated with insecticide are commonly used in cattle.

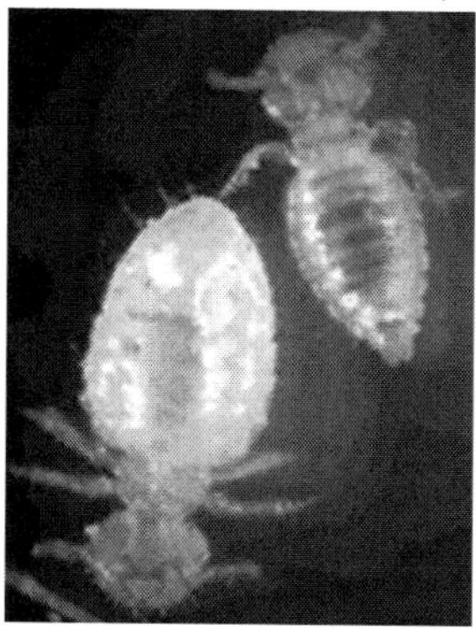

Fig. Lice

Pesticides are very effective however, pesticides alone will not control a threat such as flies. Keeping the environment clean and sanitary helps eliminate fly breeding areas. Manure management will help reduce fly breeding areas. Fly eggs and larvae in thinly spread manure are killed by drying and heat.

INTERNAL PARASITES

Livestock and poultry can be attacked by a variety of large and small worm-like parasites such as roundworms and tapeworms. These internal parasites mainly invade the digestive passages while some also infest an animal's breathing passages. Other parasites can go even deeper into the "donut" or animal body reaching various vital organs and body tissues. Most parasites enter an animal's body when the animal eats the egg (ova) or an early life stage of the parasite. These ova or intermediate life stages come from the adult parasite reproducing and living inside an animal. They are typically passed by way of animal droppings onto the ground, or into the bedding or litter. As a result, an effective preventive strategy for many internal parasites rests on keeping animals from eating feed or licking surfaces contaminated by animal waste. It is a wise practice to keep animal yards, pens and buildings or other concentration points as clean from urine and accumulated fecal material as is practicable.

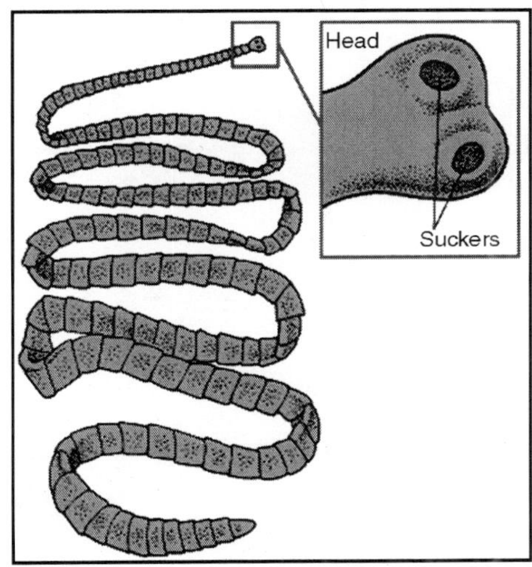

Fig. Tapeworm

Various powerful chemicals are sometimes used to treat different types of infestation. Their improper or inappropriate use may produce more damage to your animals than would be done by the parasites alone. Consequently, it is best to seek guidance from your local veterinarian before you treat for worms. In the final analysis, prevention is often less expensive than treatment.

Bacteria and Viruses

Bacteria and viruses are visible only when they are magnified hundreds to many thousands of times. They are not only able to attack the skin and digestive tract or respiratory linings of an animal's body, but, are often able to devastate the entire body including such organs as the brain, heart, liver and spleen. Their extremely small size makes it possible for these pathogens to survive long periods of times outside an animal's body. They can survive in fur, hair and feathers, in nasal and other discharges from a sick animal, and in animal urine and fecal droppings.

Viruses survive, and bacteria can actually multiply, in animal bedding, litter, and manure. Many survive long periods of time in the tiny particles of dust or soil present in the farm environment. With many tiny, scattered hiding places they can easily be carried to a new farm or group of animals riding on a person's clothing, on the surfaces of boxes, crates or equipment, and on the wheels of cars and trucks. Bacteria are single-celled microorganisms. They may live free in the environment or within a living cell. E. coli (Escherichia coli), Streptococcus, Staphylococcus, and Salmonella are a few examples of bacteria that can cause disease.

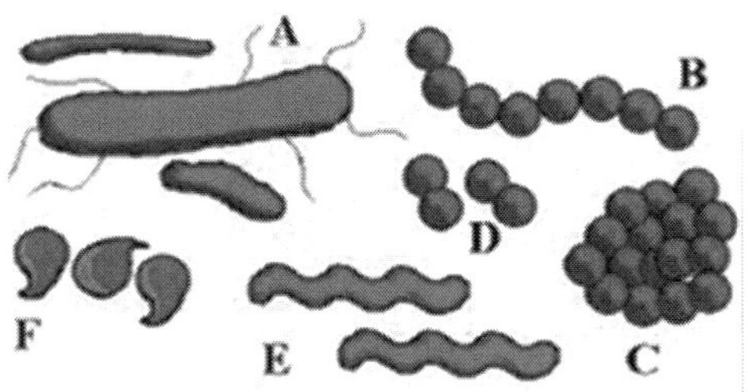

Fig. Bacteria come in a wide variety of shapes: A: Rods; B: Pour ir chains; C: Round in clusters; D: Round in twos; E: Spira; F: Cormma

Viruses are tiny organisms that only grow inside the cells composing the animal's body. All viruses rely on a live animal host to reproduce. Examples of viruses that affect humans include the common cold (rhinovirus) or the flu (influenza) virus. Viruses can infect animals and cause respiratory symptoms (influenza viruses), diarrhea (rotavirus and coronaviruses), and numerous other disorders. Although common viral or bacterial pathogens are unwelcome visitors or residents, certain ones can be especially troublesome. These special pathogens produce unusually high losses and/or unusual behaviour such as extensive tenderfootedness, incoordination, or slobbering. Milk or egg production may cease or drop sharply. Your daily activities in caring for and feeding your animals put you in an excellent position where you could be among the first to spot the possible emergence of an especially unwelcome pathogen.

As previously emphasized, isolation, traffic control, hygiene, and sanitation are the main ways to keep these essentially invisible pathogens from spreading to, and from reaching levels that can infect your animals! Medications, antibiotics, and vaccines are additional measures available to minimize the effects of bacterial or viral infections. Although powerful allies in an animal's battle with one or more pathogens, they are really the second line of defence. The first line consists of all the steps you take to keep these microbes out or their numbers down to begin with. Again, those primary steps are herd/flock isolation, traffic control, hygiene, and sanitation.

Dangerous Molecules Prion

A prion is a very unusual infectious agent that is capable of causing an infection or disease. It is believed to be a self-reproducing protein structure that is similar to a virus. Prions cause prion diseases such as transmissible spongiform encephalopathies (TSE's). Unlike other infectious agents, prions produce no body-defending immune response. Mold Toxins. Mold growth takes place in feeds when they are damp. Mold does not always mean that you cannot use the feed. Most molds are not toxic when fed to livestock; however, some are very toxic. The toxic by-products produced by molds (fungi) are known as mycotoxins (mold toxins). Mold toxins are very diverse because they are produced by many different molds.

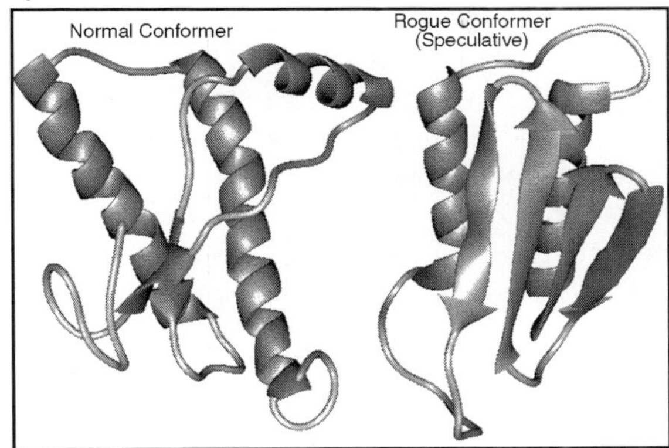

Fig. Prion

Fungi that have the ability to produce mycotoxins are very common in grain and other livestock feeds and in the facilities and equipment used for transportation and storage of feed. They can be very dangerous causing reduced growth rates, lowered immunities, and increased susceptibility to various infectious diseases. Many feed companies are working on ways to sample and test feeds and grains for mold toxins before their sale.

Animals feeds must be kept dry. We must realise that feeding any moldy feedstuffs is a risk to the health of our animal. There is less risk in feeding moldy feeds to fattening animals than for lactating or pregnant animals. The risk is also different among different species of animals. Dryness is the simplest way to control the growth of mold. Take the following steps when evidence of mold growth (musty odor, visible mold) is suspected.

- Stop the moisture source (fix the leak) correct condensation problems in outside storage bins.
- Thoroughly dry or discard all porous items.
- Scrub mold off hard surfaces with detergent and water, and thoroughly dry. Chlorine-containing products are of help in killing mold spores.

Bacterial Toxins

Many bacterialpathogens have the ability to produce toxins which add to the disease they produce, thus making them a double threat to your animals. Some toxin-producing bacteria form their poisons outside the body (botulism), while others do so inside the body (tetanus, black leg, and gangrene). These toxic bacteria can present a much greater risk than many ordinary bacteria.

Vaccines are used to aid in their prevention, particularly where risks of exposure or infection are high.

Safeguarding Animal Health

The position of a flock or herd is not unlike that of a populous city of which the public health largely depends on the functions of an intelligent "health officer." The owner, above all, should function as a health officer to his/her flock or herd. This element of animal management completes the picture of what it takes to keep animals safe and healthy. The health officer idea is especially important to many young people. After all, in the next few years, they may become the owners or managers of even larger populations of animals. They need to be alert to threats to the health of their own animals, and to those belonging to others. They should be quick to recognize and properly respond to unusual diseases and to oversee and manage their own operations to prevent or minimize the effects of common diseases. The search for and application of disease prevention knowledge can be an enjoyable, enriching lifelong experience. An alert, active disease prevention "mind set" provides many dividends! By protecting your own animals from pathogens you are also helping to protect the animals of others.

LABORATORY PROCEDURES FOR SKIN DISEASES

SKIN SCRAPINGS

Skin scrapings are part of the basic database for all skin diseases. There are two types of skin scrapings, superficial and deep. Superficial scrapings do not cause capillary bleeding and provide information from the surface of the epidermis. Deep skin scrapings collect material from within the hair follicle; capillary bleeding indicates that the sampling was deep enough. Skin scrapings are used primarily to determine the presence or absence of mites. Skin scrapings are best performed using a skin-scraping spatula, which is a thin metal weighing spatula commonly found in pharmacy or chemical supply catalogues. These spatulas are reusable and will not injure patients.

Examination of Hairs

Microscopic examination of hair shafts can be used to look for evidence of self-trauma, dermatophyte infections (requires clearing agents and special staining), dysplastic hairs, and, sometimes, genetic diseases of the hair coat.

Combing of the Hair Coat

This technique, commonly referred to as "flea combing," is useful to collect large amounts of skin debris and trap cutaneous parasites. Combings are particularly useful to find fleas, ticks, lice, and some mites. A clean scrub brush or curry comb can be used to collect material into a flat container (eg, pie plate) in large animals.

Cytology

Cutaneous and auricular cytology is helpful to identify bacterial, fungal, and, possibly, neo-plastic skin diseases. At least 4-6 impression smears should be made; several slides should be saved for examination at a reference laboratory if necessary.

When performing impression smears of the skin, the glass slide should be placed directly over the site to be sampled. An index finger or thumb should be placed directly over the slide and very firm pressure exerted. Alternatively, clear acetate tape can be used to sample the skin. Adequate sampling will produce a "thumb print" from the surface. At least one slide should be heat fixed with a match or lighter before staining. In most cases, a Romanowsky-type stain is adequate. In pruritic patients, material should be scraped from beneath nail beds and smeared onto glass slides for heat fixing, staining, and cytologic examination. Specimens should be examined under 4×, 10×, and oil immersion magnification.

Fungal Cultures

Dermatophyte infections are best identified with a fungal culture on either dermatophyte test medium or on plain Sabouraud agar. Plates that are easily inoculated are preferred; glass, screw-topped jars are difficult to inoculate and obtain samples from and are best avoided. Cats are best sampled using a new toothbrush aggressively combed over the affected lesions. Dogs can be sampled with either a toothbrush or via a hair plucking technique. In large animals, hairs should be gently wiped with alcohol before collecting to minimize contaminant growth. Intermediate and deep fungal organisms are best cultured at a reference laboratory using a skin biopsy specimen (6-8 mm in size).

Bacterial Cultures

Intact pustules can be cultured by rupturing the pustule with a sterile needle and swabbing the lesion with a sterile culture swab. Lesions should not be scrubbed before sampling. Deep pyodermas are best cultured from a skin biopsy (6-8 mm). The reference laboratory should be informed as to what pathogens are suspected, because this may affect how the exudate is cultured. Systemic and topical agents should be withheld for at least 72 hr before sampling.

Biopsy

Skin biopsies are indicated in any case that appears severe, unusual, or does not respond to appropriate therapy. Lesions should not be scrubbed before biopsy, because surface pathology is important in the diagnosis of many skin diseases. Several samples from a variety of lesions should be submitted for examination. Primary lesions should be sampled whenever possible; otherwise, the report is often not very helpful in making a diagnosis or narrowing a list of differential diagnoses. Biopsy specimens require examination by a pathologist familiar with skin diseases of animals. Direct immunofluorescence is not necessary to diagnose autoimmune skin diseases; routine histopathology is the test of choice.

Routine Blood and Urine Tests

In most dermatologic cases, these tests do not help to make a definitive diagnosis. If systemic signs of an illness are present, then a CBC, serum chemistry panel, and urinalysis may be helpful to identify the cause. In dogs with recurrent infections, these tests may identify an underlying subclinical disease.

Intradermal Skin Testing

This test is not necessarily required to make a diagnosis of atopic dermatitis. A positive intradermal skin test reaction indicates past exposure to a particular allergen. Inhalant allergies are best diagnosed based on a compatible history, physical examination findings, and judicious use of intradermal skin testing or in vitro testing for allergies. Intradermal skin testing is recommended for animals in which immunotherapy is indicated because of the severity or duration of allergic signs. Potential drug interactions that can interfere with testing should be considered before intradermal skin testing is performed.

In Vitro Diagnostic Tests

In vitro diagnostic tests (ELISA or RAST tests) are an alternative to intradermal skin testing. Although in vitro tests are considered less reliable because of the large number of false-positive reactions, most complications in interpretation are the result of poor patient selection. Like intradermal skin tests, in vitro tests reflect exposure and must be interpreted in light of the patient's clinical signs and history.

SKIN PROBLEMS IN DOGS

Understanding that there are over 160 different skin disorders of dogs, some of which create chronic difficulties, is key in helping your veterinarian solve the issue at hand. As a team, you and the veterinarian should be proactive in defining the problem accurately and in a timely manner. In order to achieve satisfactory results, it will require the doctor's expertise and perseverance coupled with your permission and financial commitment.

There are few challenges in veterinary medicine more daunting than treating a patient for a long-term skin disorder. Chronic dermatitis cases take up about 10 per cent of animal hospital file folders; and these patient folders tend to be the thickest due to the multiple pages of patient history, lab test results, biopsy reports, medications and supplements dispensed, and even dermatology specialist referral summaries. Reading through all that data you would find an oft-repeated theme ... "Control is the goal since for sure there's no cure."

CURABLE VS. INCURABLE

To simplify a bit, there are just two kinds of skin disorders in dogs: curable and incurable. Veterinarians need to understand what is really happening to and within the skin before appropriate therapeutic strategies can be employed. Since it takes a new, healthy skin cell about four weeks to mature and be present near the skin surface even curable skin diseases may take weeks to resolve. For the incurable cases, controlling an ongoing skin disorder through selected diets, medications, shampoos, sprays, fatty acids and vitamin supplements is the best we can do.

Managing a chronic skin disorder presupposes that an exact diagnosis has been established. Making that diagnosis requires certain diagnostic protocols be done so that the doctor has a clear understanding of the pathological processes impacting the patient. A multitude of different causes may very well manifest themselves in very similar appearing visual signs.

For example "itchy skin" (pruritus) is not a diagnosis, nor is "allergy." The veterinarian needs to establish what is causing the pruritus and to what the dog is allergic. Diligent detective work has to be done and it's no small task, as evidenced by a recently published veterinary dermatology textbook that lists over 160 skin disorders of dogs!

If you ever find yourself in a situation where you leave the veterinary clinic with yet another assortment of medications or skin care products, and the plan of action is "let's try these for a while and we'll see if they help," you need to insist on a more proactive approach to actually obtain a definitive diagnosis. It's time to get busy with whatever testing is needed to find the cause of the dog's skin troubles. Only then can we recognize the curable from the controllable.

CURABLE CHRONIC SKIN DISORDERS

Of the curable skin disorders the most commonly seen is reoccurring bacterial dermatitis where the dog displays circular patches alopecia (hair loss), scales and crusts, and tiny inflamed eruptions that evolve into additional crusty patches. At every dermatology seminar we are reminded that most chronic bacterial dermatitis cases need to have cultures and antibiotic sensitivity tests run. And then, the appropriate antibiotic must be used for 8 to 12 weeks and sometimes much longer. Healthy dogs seldom develop bacterial dermatitis, therefore underlying predisposing factors should be considered.

Other causes of curable but chronic skin disorders are Malassezia (yeast) infections, seen very commonly in Cocker Spaniels and West Highland White Terriers. Malassezia will cause a greasy and odorous skin. Fungal (ringworm) infections,seborrhea (oily and flaky skin) due to low fatty acid and protein in the diet, and dermatitis/alopecia due to parasites such as fleas and mites.

These curable disorders, if not properly treated, can be present throughout the dog's life and can be mistakenly assumed to be incurable!

INCURABLE SKIN DISORDERS

The incurable, chronic skin disorders can be a nightmare for the unfortunate dog and frustrating to the veterinarian and dog owner. Hormonal imbalances such ashypothyroidism in Golden Retrievers and Cushings disease (adrenal gland disorder) often seen in small breeds, generally are not curable but be managed and will display remarkable improvement once proper therapy is instituted. Chronic dermatitis due to flea saliva, food allergy, and contact or inhalant allergy will miraculously vanish once we discover the offending antigen and then prevent dog-antigen contact.

DERMATOLOGICAL (SKIN) DISEASE

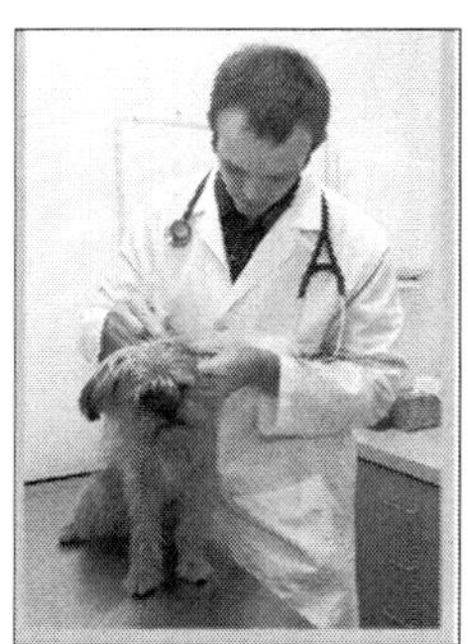

Skin disorders are one of the most common reasons pets visit their veterinarians. Problems can develop wherever there is skin, including the ears, around the lips, the bottom of paws, and around the anus. Whatever the symptoms, problems with your pet's skin are hard to ignore. Although the causes are varied, most skin problems make themselves known with one or more of the following signs: itchiness (scratching, licking, chewing, rubbing, scooting-dragging the bottom across the floor, shaking the head), sores, rashes, hair loss or a thinning coat, bumps, seeing fleas or ticks, or noticing a bad smell, even after bathing.

COMMON DISORDERS

Common causes of skin problems include parasites (fleas, ticks, mites and lice), atopy (an allergy to things breathed in or absorbed through the skin), food allergy, anal gland disorders (infection, impaction), infection/inflammation (abscesses, hotspots, scabs, ear hematomas, lick granulomas), and tumors (papillomas or warts). Underlying illnesses can also manifest as problems in the skin (*i.e.* endocrine diseases, cancer).

Parasites

Parasites such as fleas and ticks can be seen directly on the skin. Fleas are tiny (about 1mm) and dark, and usually seen moving quickly on the skin when you part the fur. There is usually flea "dirt" (which is digested pet blood, the flea's source of nutrition) seen on the skin and throughout the fur. Anytime flea dirt is found, there are fleas on your pet. Anytime there are fleas on your pet, there are or will soon be 1000's of fleas in your house! Both fleas and flea dirt can be found easily by combing your pet with a flea comb (a comb with lots of closely spaced teeth). Ticks are variable in size, ranging from less than a millimeter to over a centimeter just after feeding. Mites (Demodex, Sarcoptes) and most lice are too small to see and are diagnosed by your veterinarian using a microscope. Fleas, ticks and mites can transmit other diseases that can be zoonotic (diseases that affect people as well as animals) such as Plague, Lymes Disease, and Scabies. Most lice are species specific and usually do not transmit zoonotic diseases. They are gross, but do not usually cause medical problems for humans.

Ringworm

Another skin condition that can be seen in dogs, but is more often found on cats is ringworm, or dermatophytosis. Ringworm is not a "worm"at all, but a fungal infection. This is a highly contagious infection of the skin that is zoonotic (can be transmitted to people from animals) and causes a very itchy, scabby rash and hair loss, or sometimes no symptoms at all. One of the biggest problems with ringworm is that carrier animals (animals that have the fungal organisms in their fur but not the disease so there are no clinical signs) can transmit the infection.

Atopy

Allergies to pollens, molds, organic fibres (wool) and other tiny particles found in our environment are extremely common in our pets. Dogs and cats can develop allergies to the same things which we are allergic. Instead of responding as we do with red, runny, itchy eyes, sneezing and sinus problems, our pets usually get itchy skin. They often lick their paws, chew at their skin or start to have problems with their ears (waxy buildup, redness, odour or just shaking their head a lot). Sometimes the only sign you may notice is the fur starts to turn colours, usually a rusty brown. This is due to your pet licking and chewing their fur or increased tearing from the eyes, both of which can indicate that your pet has developed an allergy.

Food Allergy

Food allergies can manifest similar to atopy, but often have added gastrointestinal signs such as vomiting, diarrhea or excessive gas. These pets may have chronic (long term, recurrent) ear infections and waxy buildup as the only sign.

Ear Problems

Because the ears are an extension of the skin, disorders commonly seen in the skin (allergies, infections) often affect the ears as well. Infections with bacteria and yeast can lead to odour, redness, discharge, pain and inflammation. Excessive shaking of the head and scratching at the ears can lead to an aural hematoma, a swollen external ear flap (pinna). Certain breeds (Cocker Spaniels) are prone to chronic ear problems due to excessive wax production and an exaggerated response to inflammation.

Anal Glands

Anal glands are normal scent glands located in the tissue around the anus. They contain a foul smelling material used by animals to mark their territory. Normally, the material is released when pets have a bowel movement. If stools are too soft, or your pet has been constipated, the anal gland material does not empty properly and can buildup inside the gland. This leads to itchiness, causing your pet to lick excessively, scoot across the floor (usually when you have company!), or sit down often with the tail tucked between the legs. Other problems seen when the anal glands do not empty regularly is that the material inside can become too thick. This can lead to a blockage and formation of an impaction or an infection. Signs that this has occurred include a bulge on either side of the anus at about 8:00 and 4:00 position, or you may actually see a small hole with bleeding or drainage, indicating that the gland has ruptured.

Infections/Inflammation

Skin infections can be secondary to many primary problems such as parasites, allergies, trauma (bites and scratches from fighting), and tumors. Signs include a rash that is moist and very red, and many small red bumps all over or in little patches. Sometimes you will notice multiple crusts and flakes with the loss of clumps of fur, or you may find a painful swelling or discharge. Usually, there is a bad odour associated with these lesions, a sign that there is an infection with either bacteria or yeast. Inflammation is the response of tissues to trauma, and inflammatory lesions can be caused by parasites, allergies, or anything that leads to excessive licking, scratching, and self-trauma. Acral Lick Granuloma, or "lick sore" is a common skin disorder in dogs. A large firm, hairless, lump will arise, often on the feet or legs, in pets that constantly lick at the area. Eventually, the spot will become darkened (hyperpigmentation), and the skin becomes rough and thickened (lichenification). Sometimes boredom and anxiety are the causes. In other dogs, the type of fur they have makes them at risk for developing inflammatory lesions between the toes or on the paws. Folliculitis (inflamed hair follicles), also called interdigital cysts by some, are seen commonly in Labrador Retrievers. They look like small red boils and are often quite painful, and can become infected due to excessive licking.

Tumors

A tumor is a mass of tissue that grows independently from the tissue around it. It can be benign (does not spread to other areas, is stable) or malignant (spreads to other areas). Tumors of the skin are seen more commonly in dogs than cats. Some of the more common tumors seen include papillomas and adenomas which are benign skin growths and mast cell tumors which tend to be malignant (although Boxers tend to get benign mast cell tumors). It is difficult to identify a dermal tumor and determine if it is benign or malignant just by looking at it, this is often why your veterinarian may recommend surgical biopsy to help identify a tumor.

Autoimmune Disease

The immune system, that part of the body responsible for fighting off infections and keeping your pet healthy, can sometimes turn against itself. Autoimmune diseases (diseases where the body attacks itself) specific to the skin include a group of disorders known as Pemphigus. This disorder is characterized by bullous (bubble or bladder like), blisters and crusty pustules on the skin of the nose, paw pads, ears and lips. Another disorder is called Lupus. This disease causes the formation of ulcers, loss of colour around the lips and eyes, and hyperkeratosis (over production of the top layers of the skin into a thick, horny growth) of the nose and paw pads.

DIAGNOSIS

Diagnosing the cause of skin diseases involves getting an accurate and thorough history. Your veterinarian must know your pet's diet, including all treats given, medications, especially those OTC (over the counter) medicines and supplements you give, grooming products used, and travel history. It is very important to let your doctor know if your pet has been ill recently, and you should be prepared to give as much detail about the symptoms you are seeing as possible. If necessary, bring in labels of medication, supplements and different food or treats so that, together, you will both have as much information as possible to figure out what is going on. If more information is needed beyond the history and physical examination, your veterinarian may recommend blood tests to get information about the overall health and internal condition of your pet, skin scrapes, needle aspirate cytology (looking at cells under the microscope), biopsies, or cultures (growing bacteria in the lab and testing for sensitivity to antibiotics). In some cases, biopsies, special food trials or even a referral to a dermatologist for allergy skin testing may be recommended.

TREATMENT AND PROGNOSIS

The treatment of skin disease will vary, but will depend on treating the underlying cause at the same time as treating the secondary symptoms. Some simple treatments may involve using bandages or Buster/Elizabethan collars to prevent self-trauma. Most treatments will be based on test results, but often include parasite control (monthly flea/heartworm preventatives), antibiotics, or medicated shampoos and conditioners. Other useful treatments include anti-inflammatory drugs (drugs to decrease the redness/heat/pain/swelling response), antihistamines, topical ear cleaners and medicated drops, immune suppressive drugs (for autoimmune diseases and atopy), hypoallergenic diets (usually prescription pet foods with a limited number of ingredients) or dietary supplements (omega-3,6 fatty acids), or possibly surgery (to drain abscesses, hematomas, or remove tumors). Some newer treatments involving phototherapy (light therapy) and acupuncture have also shown success in controlling some of the more chronic disorders. In most cases, the prognosis is excellent for providing your pet with relief and restoring comfort, however most skin disorders involve control rather than cure. Because the causes are often chronic in nature, diligence, commitment and constant open communication with your veterinarian are critical to long-term success.

ANIMAL RABIES PREVENTION AND CONTROL

Rabies is a fatal viral zoonosis and a serious public health problem. All mammals are believed to be susceptible to the disease. Rabies is an acute, progressive encephalitis caused by a lyssavirus. Worldwide, rabies virus is the most important lyssavirus. In the United States, multiple rabies virus variants are maintained in wild mammalian reservoir populations such as raccoons, skunks, foxes, and bats. Although the United States has been declared free of canine rabies virus variant transmission, reintroduction of this variant is always a risk. Rabies virus usually is transmitted from animal to animal through bites. The incubation period is highly variable. In domestic animals, the incubation period is generally 3–12 weeks but can range from several days to months, rarely exceeding 6 months. Rabies is communicable during the period of salivary shedding of rabies virus. Experimental and historic evidence indicates that dogs, cats, and ferrets shed virus a few days before clinical onset and during illness. Clinical signs of rabies and include inappetance, dysphagia, cranial nerve deficits, abnormal behaviour, ataxia, paralysis, altered vocalisation, and seizures. Progression to death is rapid. There are currently no known effective rabies antiviral drugs.

METHODS

NASPHV periodically updates the recommendations to prevent and control animal rabies. The revision includes reviewing recent literature, updating licensed vaccine product information as provided by the manufacturers, and soliciting input from NASPHV members and stakeholder groups. During July 15–16, 2010, NASPHV members and external expert consultants met in Atlanta, Georgia. A committee consensus was required to add or modify existing language or recommendations. After the meeting, the updated draft was circulated via e-mail for final review by all voting committee members. The 2011 guidelines include several updates. First, the national case definition for animal rabies was added to clarify how rabies cases are defined for public health surveillance purposes.

Second, the diagnostics section was expanded to:

- Clarify that the CDC rabies laboratory is available for confirmatory testing and on an emergency basis to expedite exposure management decisions,
- Include information on testing methodology appropriate for field testing of surveillance specimens, and
- Clarify that no reliable antemortem rabies tests are available for use in animals.

Third, the research section was expanded to include additional topics that warrant further study. Finally, the table of rabies vaccines licensed and marketed in the United States was updated, and additional references were included to provide scientific support for information provided in the recommendations.

Principles of Rabies Prevention and Control

- *Case Definition*. An animal is determined to be rabid after diagnosis by a qualified laboratory as specified in Part I.A.9. The national case definition for animal rabies requires laboratory confirmation by either
  - A positive direct fluorescent antibody (DFA) test (preferably performed on central nervous system tissue); or
  - Isolation of rabies virus (in cell culture or in a laboratory animal)
- *Rabies Virus Exposure*. Rabies virus is transmitted when the virus is introduced into bite wounds, into open cuts in skin, or onto mucous membranes from saliva or other potentially infectious material such as neural tissue. Questions regarding possible exposures should be directed promptly to state or local public health authorities.
- *Public Health Education*. Essential components of rabies prevention and control include ongoing public education, responsible pet ownership, routine veterinary care and vaccination, and professional continuing education. The majority of animal and human exposures to rabies virus can be prevented by raising awareness concerning rabies virus transmission routes, avoiding contact with wildlife, and following appropriate veterinary care. Prompt recognition of possible exposure and prompt reporting to medical professionals and local public health authorities is critical.
- *Human Rabies Prevention*. Rabies in humans can be prevented either by eliminating exposures to rabid animals or by providing persons who have been exposed with prompt local treatment of wounds combined with the appropriate administration of human rabies immune globulin and vaccine. Exposure assessment should occur before rabies

postexposure prophylaxis (PEP) is initiated and should include discussions between medical providers and public health officials. The rationale for recommending pre-exposure prophylaxis and details of both pre-exposure and post-exposure prophylaxis administration are available in the current recommendations of the Advisory Committee on Immunisation Practices (ACIP). These recommendations, in addition to information concerning the current local and regional epidemiology of animal rabies and the availability of human rabies biologics, are available from state health departments.

- *Domestic Animal Vaccination*. Multiple vaccines are licensed for use in domestic animal species. Vaccines available include inactivated or modified live-virus vectored products, products for intramuscular and subcutaneous administration, products with durations of immunity from 1 to 4 years, and products with varying minimum age of vaccination. The recommended vaccination procedures and the licensed animal vaccines are specified in Parts II and III of this compendium, respectively. Local governments should initiate and maintain effective programmes to ensure vaccination of all dogs, cats, and ferrets and to remove stray and unwanted animals. Such procedures in the United States have reduced laboratory-confirmed cases of rabies in dogs from 6,949 in 1947 to 93 in 2009 and are responsible for the elimination of the canine rabies virus variant. Because more rabies cases involving cats are reported annually than dogs, vaccination of cats should be required. Animal shelters and animal control authorities should establish policies to ensure that adopted animals are vaccinated against rabies.
- *Rabies in Vaccinated Animals*. Rabies is rare in vaccinated animals. If suspected, the case should be reported to public health officials, the vaccine manufacturer, and the USDA Animal and Plant Health Inspection Service, Center for Veterinary Biologics. The laboratory diagnosis should be confirmed and the virus variant characterised by the CDC rabies reference laboratory. A thorough epidemiologic investigation should be conducted, including documentation of the animal's vaccination history and a description of potential rabies exposures.
- *Rabies in Wildlife*. Controlling rabies in wildlife reservoirs is difficult. Vaccination of free-ranging wildlife or selective population reduction is useful in some situations; however, the success of these procedures depends on the circumstances surrounding each rabies outbreak. Because of the risk for rabies in wild animals (especially raccoons, skunks, coyotes, foxes, and bats), the American Veterinary Medical Association, the American Public Health Association, the Council of State and Territorial Epidemiologists, the National Animal Control Association, and the National Association of State Public

Health Veterinarians (NASPHV) strongly recommend the enactment and enforcement of state laws prohibiting the importation, distribution, translocation, and private ownership of these animals.

- *Rabies Surveillance.* Enhanced laboratory-based rabies surveillance and variant typing are essential components of rabies prevention and control programmes. Accurate and timely information and reporting is necessary to guide human PEP decisions, determine the management of potentially exposed animals, aid in discovery of emerging pathogens, describe the epidemiology of the disease, and assess the need for and effectiveness of vaccination programmes for domestic animals and wildlife. Every animal submitted for rabies testing should be reported to CDC to evaluate surveillance trends. Electronic laboratory reporting and notification of animal rabies surveillance data should be implemented. Optimal information on animals submitted for rabies testing should include species, point location, vaccination history, rabies virus variant (if rabid), and human or domestic animal exposures. A case of rabies in an animal with a history of importation into the United States within 60 days is immediately notifiable by state health departments to CDC; reporting of indigenous cases should follow standard notification protocols.
- *Rabies Diagnosis*
  - *DFA.* The DFA test is the gold standard for rabies diagnosis. The test should be performed in accordance with the established national standardised protocol by a qualified laboratory that has been designated by the local or state health department. Animals submitted for rabies testing should be euthanised in a way that maintains the integrity of the brain and allows the laboratory to recognise the anatomical parts. Except for very small animals, such as bats, only the head or brain (including the brain stem) should be submitted to the laboratory. To facilitate prompt laboratory testing, submitted specimens should be stored and shipped under refrigeration (rather than frozen) without delay. Thawing frozen specimens will delay testing. Chemical fixation of tissues should be avoided because it can cause substantial testing delays and might preclude reliable testing. Questions about testing fixed tissues should be directed to the local rabies laboratory or public health department.
  - *Emergency Rabies Testing.* Emergency rabies testing should be available to expedite exposure management decisions. When state health departments need confirmatory testing (*e.g.*, for inconclusive results, unusual species, or mass exposures), the CDC rabies laboratory can provide results within 24 hours of submission.

- *Direct Rapid Immunohistochemical Test (DRIT).* DRITs are being used by trained field personnel in surveillance programmes for specimens not involved in human or domestic animal exposures. All positive DRIT results need to be confirmed by DFA testing at a qualified laboratory.
- *Unlicensed Test Kits.* No USDA-licensed rapid test kits are commercially available for rabies diagnosis. Unlicensed tests should not be used for several reasons: the sensitivity and specificity are not known; the tests have not been validated against current standard methods; the excretion of virus in the saliva is intermittent and the amount varies over time; any test result would need to be confirmed by more reliable methods such as DFA testing on brain tissue; and the interpretation of results might place exposed animals and persons at risk.

- *Rabies Serology.* Certain jurisdictions require evidence of vaccination and rabies virus antibodies for animal importation. Rabies virus antibody titers are indicative of a response to vaccine or infection. Titers do not directly correlate with protection because other immunologic factors also play a role in preventing rabies, and the ability to measure and interpret those other factors is not well-developed. Therefore, evidence of circulating rabies virus antibodies in animals should not be used as a substitute for current vaccination in managing rabies exposures or determining the need for booster vaccinations.
- *Rabies Research.* Information derived from well-designed studies is essential for the development of science-based recommendations. Data are needed in several areas, including viral shedding periods for domestic livestock and lagomorphs, potential shedding of virus in milk, earliest age at which rabies vaccination is effective and the protective effects of maternal antibodies, duration of immunity, PEP protocols for domestic animals, models for treatment of clinical rabies, extra label vaccine use in domestic animals and wildlife rabies reservoirs, host-pathogen adaptations and dynamics, and the ecology of wildlife rabies reservoir species, especially in relation to the use of oral rabies vaccines.
- Prevention and Control Methods in Domestic and Confined Animals
- *Pre-exposure Vaccination and Management.* Parenteral animal rabies vaccines should be administered only by or under the direct supervision of a licensed veterinarian on the premises. Rabies vaccinations may also be administered under the supervision of a licensed veterinarian to animals being held in animal control shelters before release. The veterinarian who signs the rabies vaccination certificate must ensure that the person administering vaccine is identified on the certificate

and is appropriately trained in vaccine storage, handling, administration, and in the management of adverse events. This practice ensures that a qualified and responsible person is held accountable for properly vaccinating the animal. Within 28 days after initial vaccination, a peak rabies virus antibody titer is reached, and the animal can be considered immunised. An animal is currently vaccinated and is considered immunised if the initial vaccination was administered at least 28 days previously or booster vaccinations have been administered in accordance with this compendium.

- Regardless of the age of the animal at initial vaccination, a booster vaccination should be administered 1 year later. No laboratory or epidemiologic data exist to support the annual or biennial administration of 3- or 4-year vaccines after the initial series. Because a rapid anamnestic response is expected, an animal is considered currently vaccinated immediately after a booster vaccination.
  - *Dogs, Cats, and Ferrets.* All dogs, cats, and ferrets should be vaccinated against rabies and revaccinated in accordance with Part III of this compendium. If a previously vaccinated animal is overdue for a booster, the animal should be revaccinated. Immediately after the booster, the animal is considered currently vaccinated and should be placed on a booster schedule, depending on the labeled duration of the vaccine used.
  - *Livestock.* All horses should be vaccinated against rabies. Livestock, including species for which licensed vaccines are not available, that have frequent contact with humans (*e.g.*, in petting zoos, fairs, and other public exhibitions) should be vaccinated against rabies. Consideration also should be given to vaccinating particularly valuable livestock.
  - Captive Wild Animals and Hybrids
    i. Wild animals or hybrids (the offspring of wild animals crossbred to domestic animals) should not be kept as pets. No parenteral rabies vaccines are licensed for use in wild animals or hybrids.
    ii. Animals that live in exhibits and in zoological parks and are not completely excluded from all contact with rabies vectors can become infected. Moreover, wild animals might be incubating rabies when initially captured. Therefore, wild-caught animals susceptible to rabies should be quarantined for a minimum of 6 months. Employees who work with animals at such facilities should receive pre-exposure rabies vaccine. The use of pre-exposure or postexposure rabies vaccinations for handlers who work with animals at such facilities might reduce the need for euthanasia of captive animals that expose handlers. Carnivores and bats should be housed in a manner that precludes direct contact with the public.

- *Stray Animals.* Stray dogs, cats, and ferrets should be removed from the community. Local health departments and animal control officials can enforce the removal of strays more effectively if owned animals are required to have identification and are confined or kept on leash. Stray animals should be impounded for at least 3 business days to determine whether human exposure has occurred and to give owners sufficient time to reclaim animals.
- *Importation and Interstate Movement of Animals*
  - *International.* CDC regulates the importation of dogs and cats into the United States. Importers of dogs must comply with rabies vaccination requirements and complete CDC form 75.37. These regulations require dogs imported from rabies-endemic countries to be vaccinated for rabies and confined for varying periods depending on age and prior vaccination status. The appropriate health official of the state of destination should be notified within 72 hours of the arrival of any imported dog required to be placed in confinement under these regulations. Failure of the owner to comply with these confinement requirements should be reported promptly to the CDC Division of Global Migration and Quarantine.
  - Federal regulations alone will not prevent the introduction of rabid animals into the United States. All imported dogs and cats are subject to state and local laws governing rabies and should be currently vaccinated against rabies in accordance with this compendium. Failure of an owner to comply with state or local requirements should be referred to the appropriate state or local official.
  - *Areas with Dog-to-Dog Rabies Transmission.* Canine rabies virus variants have been eliminated in the United States. Rabid dogs have been introduced into the continental United States from areas with dog-to-dog rabies transmission. The movement of dogs for the purposes of adoption or sale from areas with dog-to-dog rabies transmission increases the risk for introducing canine-transmitted rabies to areas where the disease does not exist and should be prohibited.
- *Adjunct Procedures.* Methods or procedures that enhance rabies control include the following:
  - Identification. Dogs, cats, and ferrets should be identified (*e.g.*, metal or plastic tags or microchips) to allow for verification of rabies vaccination status.
  - *Licensure.* Registration or licensure of all dogs, cats, and ferrets is an integral component of an effective rabies control programme. A fee frequently is charged for such licensure, and revenues collected are used to maintain rabies or animal control activities.

Evidence of current vaccination should be an essential prerequisite to licensure.

- *Canvassing.* House-to-house canvassing by animal control officials facilitates enforcement of vaccination and licensure requirements.
- *Citations.* Citations are legal summonses issued to owners for violations, including the failure to vaccinate or license their animals. The authority for officers to issue citations should be an integral part of each animal control programme.
- *Animal Control.* All local jurisdictions should incorporate stray animal control, leash laws, animal-bite prevention, and training of personnel in their programmes.
- *Public Education.* All local jurisdictions should incorporate education covering responsible pet ownership, bite prevention, and appropriate veterinary care in their programmes.

Postexposure Management

This chapter refers to any animal exposed to a confirmed or suspected rabid animal. Wild mammalian carnivores or bats that are not available or suitable for testing should be considered rabid.

- *Dogs, Cats, and Ferrets.* Any illness in an animal that has been exposed to rabies should be reported immediately to the local health department.

  i. Dogs, cats, and ferrets that have never been vaccinated and are exposed to a rabid animal should be euthanised immediately. If the owner is unwilling to euthanise, the animal should be placed in strict isolation for 6 months. Isolation in this context refers to confinement in an enclosure that precludes direct contact with people and other animals. Rabies vaccine should be administered after entry into isolation or up to 28 days before release to comply with pre-exposure vaccination recommendations. No USDA-licensed biologics for postexposure prophylaxis of previously unvaccinated domestic animals exist, and evidence indicates that the use of vaccine alone does not reliably prevent the disease in these animals.

  ii. Animals overdue for a booster vaccination should be evaluated on a case-by-case basis based on severity of exposure, time elapsed since last vaccination, number of previous vaccinations, current health status, and local rabies epidemiologic factors to determine need for euthanasia or immediate revaccination and observation with isolation.

  iii. Dogs, cats, and ferrets that are currently vaccinated should be revaccinated immediately, kept under the owner's control, and observed for 45 days. The rationale for an observation period is based in part on the potential for overwhelming viral challenge, incomplete vaccine efficacy, improper vaccine administration, variable host immunocompetence, and immune-mediated fatality (*i.e.*, early death phenomenon).

- *Livestock.* All species of livestock are susceptible to rabies; cattle and horses are the most frequently reported infected species. Any illness in an animal exposed to rabies should be reported immediately to the local health and agriculture officials.
  i. Unvaccinated livestock should be euthanised immediately. For animals that are not euthanised, on a case-by-case basis, they should be observed and confined for 6 months.
  ii. Livestock exposed to a rabid animal and currently vaccinated with a vaccine approved by USDA for that species should be revaccinated immediately and observed for 45 days.
  iii. Multiple rabid animals in a herd or herbivore-to-herbivore transmission are uncommon; therefore, restricting the rest of the herd if a single animal has been exposed to or infected by rabies is usually not necessary.
  iv. Handling and consumption of tissues from animals exposed to rabies might carry a risk for rabies virus transmission. Risk factors depend in part on the sites of exposure, the amount of virus present, the severity of the wounds, and whether sufficient contaminated tissue has been excised. If an exposed animal is to be custom- or home-slaughtered for consumption, the slaughter should occur immediately after the exposure, and all tissues should be cooked thoroughly. Persons handling animals, carcasses, and tissues that have been exposed should use barrier precautions. Historically, federal guidelines for meat inspectors required that any animal known to have been exposed to rabies within 8 months be rejected for slaughter. The USDA Food and Inspection Service (FSIS) and state meat inspectors should be notified when such exposures occur in food animals before slaughter. Rabies virus is widely distributed in tissues of rabid animals. Tissues and products from a rabid animal should not be used for human or animal consumption or transplantation. Pasteurisation and cooking inactivate rabies virus; therefore, inadvertently drinking pasteurised milk or eating thoroughly cooked animal products does not constitute a rabies exposure.

- *Other Animals.* Other mammals exposed to a rabid animal should be euthanised immediately. Animals maintained in USDA-licensed research facilities or accredited zoological parks should be evaluated on a case-by-case basis in consultation with public health authorities.

Options might include isolation, observation, or administration of rabies biologics (*i.e.*, immune globulin or vaccine or both).

Management of Animals that Bite Humans

- *Dogs, Cats, and Ferrets.* Rabies virus is excreted in the saliva of infected dogs, cats, and ferrets during illness and/or for only a few days before illness or death. Regardless of rabies vaccination status, a healthy dog, cat, or ferret that potentially exposes a person through a bite should be confined and observed daily for 10 days from the time of the exposure; administration of rabies vaccine to the animal is not recommended during the observation period to prevent confusion between signs of rabies and rare adverse reactions. Any illness in the animal should be reported immediately to the local health department. Animals should be evaluated by a veterinarian at the first sign of illness during confinement. If signs suggestive of rabies develop, the animal should be euthanised and the head submitted for testing as described in Part I.A.9. Any stray or unwanted dog, cat, or ferret that potentially exposes a person to rabies may be euthanised immediately and the head submitted for rabies examination.
- Other Animals. Other animals that might have exposed a person to rabies should be reported immediately to the local health department. Management of animals other than dogs, cats, and ferrets depends on the species, the circumstances of the exposure, the epidemiology of rabies in the area, and the animals' history, current health status, and the potential for exposure to rabies. The shedding period for rabies virus is undetermined for most species. Previous vaccination of these animals might not preclude the necessity for euthanasia and testing.

Outbreak Prevention and Control.

The emergence of new rabies virus variants or the introduction of non-indigenous viruses poses a significant risk to humans, domestic animals, and wildlife.

A rapid and comprehensive response includes the following measures:

- Characterise Virus. Characterise the virus at the national reference laboratory.
- *Identify and Control Source.* Identify and control the source of the virus introduction.
- *Enhance Surveillance.* Enhance laboratory-based surveillance in wild and domestic animals.

- *Increase Vaccination.* Increase animal rabies vaccination rates.
- Restrict Animals. Restrict the movement of animals.
- *Evaluate Need to Reduce Vector Population.* Evaluate the need for vector population reduction.
- *Coordinate Response.* Coordinate a multiagency response.
- *Provide Outreach.* Provide public and professional outreach and education.

- *Disaster Response.* Animals might be displaced during and after man-made or natural disasters and need emergency sheltering. Animal rabies vaccination and exposure histories often are not available for displaced animals. Disaster response creates situations in which animal caretakers might lack appropriate training and pre-exposure vaccination. In such situations, implementing and coordinating rabies prevention and control measures is critical to reduce the risk for rabies transmission and the need for human PEP.

Such measures include the following:

- *Coordinate Relief.* Coordinate relief efforts of individuals and organisations with the local emergency operations center before deployment.
- *Examine Animals.* Examine each animal at a triage site for possible bite injuries or signs of rabies.
- *Isolate Animals.* Isolate animals exhibiting signs of rabies, pending evaluation by a veterinarian.
- *Check Animal Identifiers.* Ensure that all animals have a unique identifier.
- *Vaccinate.* Administer a rabies vaccination to all dogs, cats, and ferrets unless reliable proof of vaccination exists.
- *Adopt Caretaker Standards.* Adopt minimum standards for animal caretakers as feasible, including personal protective equipment, pre-exposure rabies vaccination, and appropriate training in animal handling.
- *Maintain Documentation.* Maintain documentation of animal disposition and location (*e.g.*, returned to owner, died or euthanised, adopted, relocated to another shelter, and address of new location).
- Provide Facilities for Animals that Have Been Exposed. Provide facilities to confine and observe animals involved in exposures.
- Report Human Exposures. Report human exposures to rabies to appropriate public health authorities.
- *Prevention and Control Methods Related to Wildlife.* The public should be warned not to handle or feed wild animals. Wild animals and hybrids that expose persons, pets, or livestock to rabies should be

considered for euthanasia and rabies diagnosis. A person exposed by any wild animal should immediately report the incident to a health-care provider who, in consultation with public health authorities, can evaluate the need for PEP.

Translocation of infected wildlife has contributed to the spread of rabies; therefore, the translocation of known terrestrial rabies reservoir species should be prohibited. Whereas state-regulated wildlife rehabilitators and nuisance wildlife control operators might play a role in a comprehensive rabies control programme, minimum standards for persons who handle wild animals should include rabies vaccination, appropriate training, and continuing education.

- *Carnivores.* The use of oral rabies vaccines (ORV) for the mass vaccination of free-ranging wildlife should be considered in selected situations with the approval of the appropriate state agencies. Success has been documented using ORV to control rabies in wildlife in North America. The currently licensed vaccinia-vectored ORV is labeled for use in raccoons and coyotes. The distribution of ORV should be based on scientific assessments of the target species and followed by timely and appropriate analysis of surveillance data; such results should be provided to all stakeholders. In addition, parenteral vaccination (trap—vaccinate—release) of wildlife rabies reservoirs may be integrated into coordinated ORV programmes to enhance their effectiveness. Continuous and persistent programmes for trapping or poisoning wildlife do not reduce wildlife rabies reservoirs statewide. However, limited population control in high-contact areas (*e.g.*, picnic grounds, camps, and suburban areas) might be indicated for the removal of selected species of wildlife at high risk for having rabies. State agriculture, public health, and wildlife agencies should be consulted for planning, coordination, and evaluation of vaccination or population reduction programmes.
- *Bats.* From the 1950s through 2011, indigenous rabid bats have been reported from every state except Hawaii and have caused rabies in at least 43 humans in the United States. Bats should be excluded appropriately from houses, public buildings, and adjacent structures to prevent direct association with humans. Such structures should then be made bat-proof by sealing entrances used by bats. Controlling rabies in bats through programmes designed to reduce bat populations is neither feasible nor desirable.

11

Preventive Medicine for Veterinary

The foundation of a medical programme for zoo animals is preventive medicine. Preventive medical programmes should be adaptive and include attention to individual specimens as well as the herd, troop, or flock. Components of the programme include quarantine of new arrivals, periodic fecal examinations and treatments for parasites, booster vaccinations, health screening procedures, nutrition evaluation, necropsy examination of deceased specimens, and a comprehensive pest control programme. Animals should be evaluated to ensure their health complies with local, state, and federal health requirements before shipment to other zoos or before release in managed reintroduction programmes. Preshipment evaluations can also be used as an opportunity to assess the overall health status of the group in which the animal has been living.

QUARANTINE

Animals entering a collection must undergo quarantine. Quarantine facilities should be designed to allow handling of animals and proper cleaning and sanitizing of enclosures. Shipping crates should be cleaned and disinfected before they leave the quarantine area, and the crates' contents disposed of appropriately. Quarantine facilities require barriers against ingress of potential vectors and vermin. Separate keepers who are skilled at recognizing signs of stress and disease and who will carefully monitor feed intake and fecal characteristics should care for quarantined animals.

Quarantine entry should be strictly controlled. Only essential personnel should be allowed into the quarantine facility. Individuals leaving the quarantine facility should not return to other animal areas without showering and changing clothing. The duration of quarantine should be appropriate to ensure that infectious diseases are not introduced into the permanent collection when the quarantined animals are released to exhibits. Quarantine facilities should follow the "all-in/all-out" principle, ie, if additional animals are added to an ongoing quarantine, the quarantine period should be restarted. During quarantine, animals should receive appropriate vaccinations and diagnostic testing (eg, tuberculosis, heartworm). They should be examined and treated for ecto- and endoparasites and screened for enteric bacterial pathogens. Before release, animals should receive physical and laboratory examinations, which may include radiographs, serology, hematology, and clinical chemistries. Serum should be frozen for future reference and possible epidemiologic studies. All procedures and results should be recorded in each individual animal's medical record, which is an essential component of the medical programme. Each animal should also be identified by some permanent method (eg, tattoo, tag, band, eartag, transponder) to ensure future identification.

When new animals are introduced to enclosures, caution and forethought are necessary to prevent self-induced trauma. Visual barriers, eg, suspending canvasses from fences or enclosure walls or obscuring glass with soap to provide a visual cue, are standard management steps to protect newly introduced specimens from accidents during acclimation to a new exhibit.

PARASITE CONTROL

Like domestic animals, zoo animals are vulnerable to a wide variety of ecto- and endoparasites, and similar drugs are used for treatment. Care must be exercised in the choice of medications due to species-specific sensitivities to some drugs. Young animals and those stressed by shipment, disease, or injury are the most likely to be adversely affected by parasites. At these times, commensal parasites (especially protozoa) can cause disease. Acute diarrhea can result from massive infections of Coccidia,Trichomonas, Giardia, or Balantidium spp. Amebiasis, which is fairly common in primates and reptiles, can be fatal in a compromised animal. Intestinal parasites may be a major, continuous problem in species kept in naturalistic exhibits or on dirt substrate or pasture, especially in young, newly introduced, or stressed individuals. Of most concern are parasites with direct life cycles. Incorporating anthelmintics directly into the feed is helpful. As in domestic species, anthelmintic resistance may develop and necessitate rotating medication. Parasites with indirect life cycles are less frequently a problem if the exhibit area is free of intermediate hosts.

VACCINATION

Vaccination programmes for carnivores, non-human primates, equids, artiodactylids, and birds should be developed. Vaccination of zoo carnivores is essential because of their susceptibility to various diseases such as feline panleukopenia, feline rhinotracheitis, feline calicivirus, rabies, canine distemper, and canine parvovirus. Previously, only killed virus vaccines were recommended, but recent studies have shown that some modified live vaccines are safe for use in select species. Further studies are required because some modified live vaccines (especially canine distemper) produce fatal disease in certain species. A canarypox-vectored recombinant canine distemper vaccine has proven safe for use in those species susceptible to modified live virus vaccine-induced disease. Appropriateness of rabies vaccination depends on the circumstances of each collection. If indicated in rabies-endemic areas for the protection of individual animals, only a killed rabies vaccine should be used. The decision to vaccinate zoo animals for less common diseases for which a vaccine is available should be made on an individual basis. Newer recombinant and subunit vaccines are being developed for a variety of infectious diseases for domestic animals and humans. These vaccines should be used with caution until safety and efficacy studies have been completed for zoologic species.

NECROPSY

All dead animals should be necropsied. This should include gross and histopathologic evaluation of tissue and viral, bacterial, or fungal cultures when appropriate. Tissues should also be saved for potential future examinations. A thorough pathology examination allows evaluation of medical, management, and nutritional programmes. It is also valuable in identifying problems requiring immediate action to safeguard the health of the collection. Variations in anatomy should be recorded because such observations may aid in future diagnostic procedures or therapy in the species.

PEST CONTROL

A successful control programme is continuous and requires a concerted effort by zoo staff to minimize harborage and food for pests, in addition to the use of mechanical and chemical control methods. Choice of agent, method of use, and storage may minimize zoo animals' access to pesticides and the risk of secondary poisoning. Common zoo pests may serve as important disease vectors. For example, cockroaches are intermediate hosts for GI parasites of primates and birds; rodents can harbour and spread Listeria, Salmonella, and Leptospira spp and Francisella tularensis. Wild and feral carnivores such as foxes, raccoons, and domestic dogs and cats can devastate animal collections through predatory attacks and may be important vectors for viral diseases such as rabies, parvovirus, and canine distemper. Raccoons may also transmit Baylisascaris parasites, which can cause larval migration resulting in fatal neuropathy in some species. Pigeons, geese, ducks, and starlings are potential reservoirs for avian diseases; they consume or contaminate animal food and deposit droppings everywhere. Arthropod vectors can transmit pathogens such as West Nile virus.

VETERINARY MEDICINE

Recent developments in both the facilities and curriculum have produced a modern, exciting veterinary course at Cambridge. The number of veterinary places at Cambridge is about 70 per year making it one of the smallest veterinary schools. This facilitates a strong cohesion between students, whilst enabling close contact with staff and expediting small group teaching - a particular strength at Cambridge. Veterinary students are spread over the whole university and Clare College typically admits about 4 veterinary undergraduates a year, though, as explained in the general notes, it imposes no upper limit on the numbers in any subject. We also take about 12 medical undergraduates. Much of the preclinical teaching is shared, in the Medical and Veterinary Sciences Tripos. The College is thus able to devote a considerable amount of resources to looking after this group of students.

The course, leading eventually to the degree of Bachelor of Veterinary Medicine (Vet MB) is a six year one. After admission to the degree of Vet MB at the end of the course, graduates are registered asMembers of the Royal College of Veterinary Surgeons and are thus entitled to practise as fully-qualified veterinary surgeons. Most students at Cambridge spend the first three years of the course reading for an honours BA degree. The first two of these years are spent studying the major pre-clinical sciences in the Medical and Veterinary Sciences Tripos to provide a sound scientific basis for the detailed study in the last three clinical years of animal health, veterinary pathology, public health, medicine, and surgery, etc. There is continual discussion, involving both the Royal College of Veterinary Surgeons and the General Medical Council as well as the relevant faculties of the University, about modernising and streamlining the curriculum for medical and veterinary students. A major overhaul of the course was carried out in October 2000, and the pre-clinical course is being reviewed again now (2012). The current course includes such subjects as Homeostasis, Molecules in Medical Science, Veterinary Anatomy and Physiology, Biology of Disease, Mechanisms of Drug Action, Neurobiology with Animal Behaviour, Comparative Vertebrate Biology, Veterinary Reproduction and will constitute a core of pre-clinical knowledge on which to base further study. There are also short courses on Principles of Animal Management and Preparing for the Veterinary Profession, aimed at a more practical appreciation of modern husbandry practices and to begin veterinary professional training which continues throughout the six years.

Under regulations set by the Royal College, students must attain a certain standard in each of these pre-clinical sciences before they are allowed to proceed to the clinical part of the course. There are, therefore, examinations - the '2nd Vet MB' - in each of these subjects to be passed, but most students obtain passes in these examinations as part of the Tripos examinations for the B.A degree. In the third pre-clinical year there is a very wide choice of options open to the veterinary student. He or she may opt to study one of the medical science subjects in depth. This usually involves either a written dissertation or a research project which can often lead to a published paper. Alternatively, there are more general courses within the medical and natural sciences on offer, or it may be possible to study another Cambridge Tripos for a year.

It is important to appreciate that there is a strong emphasis on science in the Cambridge preclinical course. Veterinary students obtain an honours BA of standing with a Natural Sciences degree. Many of the lectures and practicals are shared with medical students, and standards are high. Nevertheless, even though much of the teaching is shared with medical and science students at present, there is a strong sense of identity among the pre-clinical veterinary students. There are short courses in animal handling and informal contact with the clinical Veterinary School is encouraged, especially through the very active University Veterinary Society. It is widely agreed that veterinary graduates with such a strong scientific background, together with well developed critical skills, should make better and more informed practitioners, as well as being very well equipped for a range of other professions including research and academia. Intercalated science degrees are becoming much more common in the other veterinary schools, but not as such an integral part of the course as at Cambridge.Entry to the clinical Veterinary School for the second three years of the course is automatic, provided the student has passed all the necessary 2nd Vet MB exams and has been awarded their degree. During the pre-clinical years, students are also expected to have completed 12 weeks working on farms (pre-clinical extramural studies, EMS). This formal farm practice experience can only be undertaken after arrival at Cambridge and an induction course, and will include time spent working with sheep, dairy cattle, pigs and horses.

The sixth year of the course is now lecture-free, giving students more time to work with clinicians at the Veterinary School and to acquire skills. There is also the opportunity of an elective, specialising in some aspects of clinical veterinary medicine during the last year. During the three clinical years, students spend part of their vacations at veterinary practices experiencing the work of a veterinary surgeon at first hand and learning veterinary medicine and surgery 'in the field' (clinical EMS).

A typical formal workload for a first year veterinary student would consist of 9-12 lectures, 2 dissection sessions, 4 other practical classes, together with 3 supervisions per week. Typically two to four students are supervised together and for some supervisions an essay has to be prepared. Each week the supervisions provide an opportunity for each student to discuss each course with an academic who is a specialist in that field.

During the course, academic and professional work is overseen by the College's Directors of Studies in Pre-clinical and Clinical Veterinary Medicine. There is also close contact with a number of the college Teaching Fellows in many of the pre-clinical subjects. Before embarking on the veterinary course, every student must have been exempted from the First MB examination. Details of what this entails are given in the Cambridge Admissions Prospectus. It is only fair to point out that competition for places to read Veterinary Medicine at Cambridge is severe. On the other hand, our willingness to interview more applicants gives you every opportunity to demonstrate your worth.

ADMISSIONS

Most veterinary applicants to Clare are interviewed in December. Candidates are also required to sit the Biomedical Admissions Test (the BMAT) in their schools in the November before the interview. Usually two interviews are conducted, each with two interviewers and lasting for about 20min. Questions are aimed at testing the candidates' ability to extrapolate and think laterally, rather than a simple test of knowledge per se. A small number of applicants are not interviewed if their academic record to date makes it very unlikely that they would be given a place. Successful candidates are made a conditional offer; usually A*A*A at A2 level, including at least two science or maths subjects. Candidates offering only two science A2s will normally be expected to have an A-grade in a third science at AS level. Exceptional candidates offering just one science at A2-level will be considered. These standards are applied so that the College can obtain the maximum information on a student in order to come to the fairest decision. However, the special circumstances of an individual student would always be considered. Other suitable pre-university qualifications such as International Baccalaureate are also welcome. It is best to consult with the Admissions Tutor if you are in doubt about the suitability of your qualifications.

Applicants for Veterinary Medicine are expected to have spent some time with a veterinary surgeon to gain some experience of the profession, and to appreciate a practitioner's routine, lifestyle and expertise. 'Hands on' experience with a variety of animals is also to be encouraged. However, prospective students should not spend too much time on 'work experience' and need to balance time spent with vets and with animals with their other interests and with their academic work.

BIOMEDICAL ADMISSIONS TEST (BMAT)

All candidates are required to sit the 2-hour Biomedical Admissions Test (the BMAT) in the November before coming to interview. For pre-A-level candidates this is normally taken within your school/college, and individual arrangements are made for post A-level candidates. We will decide which candidates to invite to interview once we have the results of the BMAT.

NB: All offers of a place on this course (for UK students) will be subject to a satisfactory standard disclosure from the Criminal Records Bureau. You will be sent the relevant forms to complete only if you are offered a place.

Why study Veterinary Medicine at Clare College?

Preclinical veterinary subjects are taught mainly alongside the medics, except for specific veterinary subjects like anatomy or veterinary physiology. In Clare, we take 4 vets and 12 medics, which reflects the ratio in the university as a whole. It is a good group size for positive interactions. Students have close contact with fellows. There are enough vet students to retain a sense of their own identity but with the advantage of having contact with the medics, which prevents a more parochial outlook. Clare has its own teaching fellows in most biomedical subjects taken during the preclinical years, and also others with expertise more widely in the natural sciences.

Historically, we have been very strong in these subjects: David Attenborough, James Watson and Tim Hunt (Nobel Prizes for Medicine and Biochemistry) were all at Clare. A current fellow, Prof Bill Harris, is an FRS in developmental neuroscience and head of the Department of Physiology, Development and Neuroscience (PDN), which delivers about two-thirds of the teaching to first and second year vets and medics. Library facilities for vets are excellent. Geographically, we are positioned half-way between Downing Site (where most of the preclinical lectures and practicals occur) and the vet school (for clinical years). Finally, we have three qualified vets on the fellowship. One teaches anatomy and carries out neurophysiological research in PDN; the Director of Studies for both preclinical and veterinary clinical sciences are vets, working at the vet school - one is an active equine clinician, the other specialises in pathophysiological research with active collaborations in the preclinical departments.

CHALLENGES TO TODAY'S VETERINARY MEDICINE

Today, the veterinary profession is confronted with a different set of problems compared with the middle of last century. Now, veterinarians often have to deal with herds or regions remaining diseased after lengthy disease control campaigns. In addition, it is considered necessary to take into account the economic aspects of disease control through the use of benefit/cost analyses of disease control campaigns. Costly multi-factorial *disease complexes* such as mastitis or cattle lameness have become quite common. In addition, old, emerging or new *diseases* with complex aetiologies pose a difficult challenge for the profession. Veterinarians have to respond to the challenges posed by problems such as BSE, FMD and antimicrobial resistance. All these problems require identification, quantification and intensive examination of multiple, directly or indirectly causal, and often interacting, disease determinants.

Veterinary epidemiology and evidence-based veterinary medicine provide overlapping sets of tools which can be used to approach these new challenges. In clinical practice, there is now a daily need for valid, up-to-date information about diagnosis, therapy and prevention. This situation is complicated by the inadequacy of traditional sources for this type of information, since they may be out-of-date, they are frequently wrong, it may be ineffective (didactic CPD), too overwhelming in volume, or too variable in validity. In addition, the clinician has to deal with the disparity between diagnostic skills and clinical judgement (increasing with experience) on the one hand and up-to-date knowledge and clinical performance (declining with time) on the other. The fact that he/she has insufficient time to examine the animal patient and to practice CPD further complicates the situation.

VETERINARY EPIDEMIOLOGY

Veterinary epidemiology deals with the investigation of diseases, productivity and animal welfare in populations. It is used to describe the frequency of disease occurrence and how disease, productivity and welfare are affected by the interaction of different factors or determinants. This information is then used to manipulate such determinants in order to reduce the frequency of disease occurrence. Veterinary epidemiology is a holistic approach aimed at co-ordinating the use of different scientific disciplines and techniques during an investigation of disease or impaired productivity or welfare. The field of veterinary epidemiology can be divided into different components.

One of its essential foundations is the collection of data, which then has to be analysed using qualitative or quantitative approaches in order to formulate causal hypotheses. As part of the quantitative approach to epidemiological analysis, epidemiological investigations involving field studies or surveys are being conducted and models of epidemiological problems can be developed.

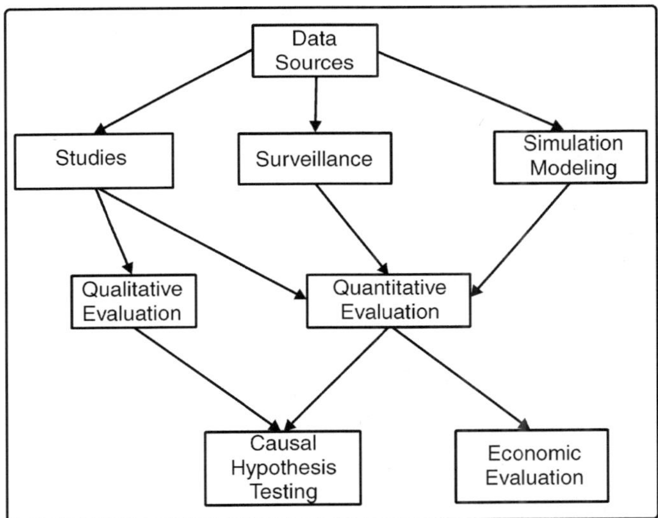

Fig. Components of Veterinary Epidemiology

The ultimate goal is to control a disease problem, reduce productivity losses and improve animal welfare.

MEASUREMENT OF DISEASE FREQUENCY AND PRODUCTION

One of the most fundamental tasks in epidemiological research is the quantification of the disease occurrence. This can be done simply on the basis of *counts* of individuals which are infected, diseased, or dead. This information will be useful for estimating workload, cost, or size of facilities to provide health care. More commonly, *counts* are expressed as a *fraction* of the number of animals capable of experiencing infection, disease or death.

These types of quantities are used by epidemiologists to express the *probability* of becoming infected, diseased or dying for populations with different numbers of individuals (= populations at risk).

From a mathematical perspective, frequency of disease occurrence can be expressed through *static* or *dynamic* measures. *Static measures* include proportions and ratios. A *proportion* is a fraction in which the numerator is included within the denominator.

It is dimensionless, ranging from 0 to 1 and is often expressed as a percentage (x 100). The *ratio* is a fraction in which the numerator is not included in the denominator and it can be with or without dimension.

Dynamic measures include *rates* which represent the instantaneous change in one quantity per unit change in another quantity (usually time). They are not dimensionless and do not have a finite upper bound. Measures of disease frequency can be based only on new (=incident) cases of disease or do not differentiate between old and new disease.

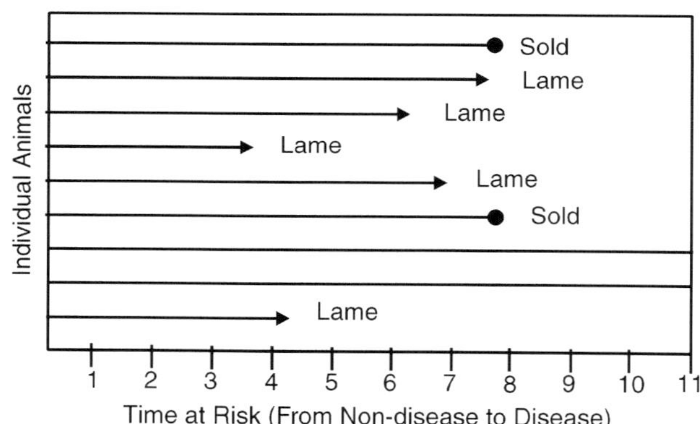

Fig. Incidence of Disease

Figure shows the principles behind incidence measures. They are derived from data for animals which did not have the disease at the beginning of the study period. These animals are followed over time until they develop the disease (eg become lame) or until the observation period finishes (eg sold or end of study period).

CUMULATIVE INCIDENCE

The risk of new disease occurrence is quantified using *cumulative incidence,* also called *incidence risk*. It is defined as the proportion of disease-free individuals developing a given disease over a specified time, conditional on that individual's not dying from any other disease during the period.

Note that animals have to be disease free at the beginning of the observation period to be included in the enumerator or denominator of this calculation. It is interpreted as an individual's risk of contracting disease within the risk period. The quantity is dimensionless, ranges from 0 to 1 and always requires a period referent. As an example, last year a herd of 121 cattle were tested using the tuberculin test and all tested negative. This year, the same 121 cattle were tested again and 25 tested positive. The cumulative incidence over a period of 12 months would then be calculated as 25/121 which amounts to 0.21. Hence, an individual animal within this herd had a 21% chance of becoming infected over the 12 month period.

MISCELLANEOUS MEASURES OF DISEASE OCCURRENCE

Other measures of disease frequency include the *attack rate* which is defined as the number of new cases divided by the initial population at risk. As it is based on the same calculation as cumulative incidence it really is a subtype of cumulative incidence. It is confusing though that despite its name it is in fact a probability and not a rate. The attack rate is used when the period at risk is short. *Mortality rates* are applied using a number of different interpretations, and often do not represent a true rate. The *crude mortality rate* has death as the outcome of interest and is calculated analogous to incidence density. The *cause-specific mortality rate* is estimated for specific causes of death and also calculated analogous to incidence density. *Case fatality rate* represents the proportion of animals with a specific disease that die from it. It is a risk measure, not a rate, and is used to describe the impact of epidemics or the severity of acute disease.

Time to the occurrence of an event such as death or onset of clinical disease can be estimated for many epidemiological data sets describing repeated observations on the same sample of animals. This type of data can be summarised using for example mean survival time. This particular method has the disadvantage that the estimate will depend on the length of the time period over which data was collected. If the interval is too short, survival time is likely to be estimated incorrectly, as only individuals who experienced the event of interest can be included in the calculation.

at which the event occurs is constant throughout the period of study. The most appropriate technique for this data is based on the *survivor* and *hazard function*. The survivor function (=cumulative survival probability) is a functional representation of the proportion of individuals not dying or becoming diseased beyond a given time at risk. It can be interpreted as the probability of remaining alive for a specific length of time. The survival function is often summarized using the *median survival time* which is the time at which 50% of individuals at risk have failed (died or became diseased).

The *hazard function* (=instantaneous failure rate, force of mortality, conditional mortality rate, age specific failure rate) is calculated by dividing the conditional probability of an individual dying or becoming diseased during a specific time interval provided it has not died or become diseased prior to that time divided by the specified *time interval*. This parameter does represent a rate expressing the potential of failing at time *t* per unit time given survival up until time *t*. In the context of survival data, *censoring* is an extremely important concept. In the case of *right censoring*, individuals are lost to follow-up or are not dead/diseased at the end of the follow-up period.

This particular type of censoring can be easily accounted for in survival analysis by excluding them from the denominators of the calculations following their departure from the population at risk. With *left censoring*, beginning of the time at risk is not known, and the commonly used analysis techniques cannot take account of this type of censoring. An example calculation for survival data is presented in Figure Animal A survived for 4 months, animal B survived the whole period of 12 months and animal C was removed from the population after 7 months. The number of survivors is based on the actual number of animals still alive after a given time period. The value for the cohort is used as the denominator for calculation of cumulative survival. The number is adjusted for censored observations. The failures represents the number of deaths during a particular time interval. And the hazard rate is the probability of death per unit time (one month in this case).

STANDARDISATION OF RISK

A crude risk estimate summarises the effects of the specific risk and the subgroup distribution. But in the presence of a confounding factor a crude risk estimate may distort the true pattern. In such a situation, patterns of disease should be described using host-attribute specific risk estimates (e.g. age, sex).

For each level of the attribute a separate stratum is formed and stratum-specific risk estimates are calculated. Summary figures can be produced using *standardised* or *adjusted risk* estimates. The two main methods available to perform these calculations are *direct* and *indirect standardisation*.

DIRECT STANDARDIZATION

Direct standardization involves weighting a set of observed category specific risk estimates according to a *standard* distribution. First, stratum-specific risk rates are calculated. Then a *standard* population distribution is estimated and the proportion of the standard population in each stratum calculated. The direct adjusted risk rate estimate is obtained as the sum of the products across the strata between the proportion of the *standard* population in stratum *i* and the observed risk rate estimate in stratum *i* in the *study* population. As an example, the mortality in humans in 1963 was compared between Sweden and Panama. In this particular year, Sweden had a population size of 7.496.000 and 73.555 deaths resulting in a *mortality rate* of 0.0098 per year. Panama had a population size of 1.075.000 with 7871 deaths giving a *mortality rate* of 0.0073 per year. Based on these figures it appeared that life in Sweden was more risky than in Panama. It becomes apparent that in his comparison the confounding factor was the difference in age structure between the two populations. Sweden had a much lower mortality in young people, but because it had a large proportion of old people this effect did not come through in the aggregated analysis. After adjustment for differences in age structure it turns out that mortality was higher in Panama with 0.0162 per year than it was in Sweden with 0.015 per year.

INDIRECT STANDARDISATION

An alternative approach to standardisation of risk estimates is called *indirect standardisation*. In this case, a *standard* population does not supply the weighting distribution, but a set of stratum-specific risk estimates which are then weighted to the distribution of the *study* population. This technique is used if stratum-specific risk estimates are not available.

But in order to be able to use the method, stratum-specific risk estimates for the *standard* population and the frequency of the adjusting factor in the *study* population have to be available.

As a first step, the expected number of cases is calculated on the basis of the sum of the products between stratum-specific rates for the *standard* population and the total number of individuals in each stratum in the *study* population. The standardised morbidity or mortality ratio (SMR) is calculated using the number of observed cases divided by the number of expected cases, and the indirect adjusted risk is obtained from multiplying the overall observed risk in the *study* population with the SMR.

PREVENTIVE MEDICINE FOR ANIMALS

It is important for veterinary surgeons not only to deal with disease and injury, as they occur, but also to try to prevent disease and injury wherever and whenever possible, whether through education, management advice, nutrition or medical intervention. This is an important route to enhanced animal welfare, in line with holistic thinking, and is a major part of the AVMC's mission.

In the modern veterinary world, the notion of preventive medicine for infectious diseases is all too often left to vaccination, with insufficient emphasis on good nutrition, holistic management and education. While it has been proven that vaccination has achieved a positive impact on disease incidence, in the case of viral or bacterial diseases, it is also widely known that vaccines bring their own risks. Homeopathic methods have not been widely explored by the veterinary profession, to the loss of the animal community that the profession serves. Nosodes are a massively under-utilised resource for preventive medicine and some clinical trials demonstrate their benefit. The use of nosodes is a form ofhomeoprophylaxis and many animal 'owners' use them as an alternative to vaccination, apparently without penalty.

There is no match for a healthy diet (attuned to the evolutionary and biological needs of the species), a healthy environment and a healthy mind (*i.e.* not stressed or distressed) as a means of prevention of disease and to nurture a healthy immune system. A species-relevant natural diet is essential to maintain a healthy mouth and healthy digestive system, as the cost of feeding unsuitable manufactured feeds shows very eloquently, let alone its implications for general constitutional health. Farm or home management should allow optimal welfare, to reduce stress and to allow normal behaviours, to encourage a sound mind and body. In the case of horses, feeding, saddling, shoeing, grazing and stabling all require close attention, to optimise the health and welfare of the animal. We cannot, as holistic vets, leave correctible problems unattended (*e.g.* ill-fitting saddle, bad shoeing etc.), as these can significantly impede the healing process and potentially lead to problems further down the line. Avoidable problems should be avoided.

In the case of farm animals, a great deal of 'preventive medicine' can be achieved via good nutrition. At the AVMC, we encourage all these management issues, whatever the situation or species and offer advice to clients on the best ways to achieve and to maintain the health of their animal charges. Wherever possible, we try to ensure that lifestyle and diet enhance welfare and health, without reliance on medication. Medication is only used where necessary.

ANIMAL HEALTH MONITORING AND REPORTING

VETERINARY ROUNDS

All animals in RAR's facilities are observed daily by an animal care staff. Each area of the facility is also assigned a veterinary technician and an Area Veterinarian. The veterinary staff make regular rounds through the facility to observe the animals, their housing conditions and husbandry procedures.

REPORTING ANIMAL HEALTH PROBLEMS

RAR laboratory animal care staff can report animal health problems to the veterinary staff through an "Animal Health Report" card system. Animal health problems may also be reported to the RAR office at 624-9100. If the phone is not picked up a message can be left, or the on-duty veterinarian can be paged at the Emergency Veterinary Pager, and this number is posted by the phones in all housing areas.

Animal health problems may also be reported to the RAR Veterinary Services office. A message may be left there. Alternatively, the emergency veterinarian can be paged. The numbers for the Veterinary Services Office and the Emergency Veterinary pager are posted next to the phones in all housing areas. Any type of serious animal health problem should be treated as an emergency. Any health problem noted on a weekend or at the end of the day should be treated as an emergency. Animal health problems should not be reported by leaving a voice mail message or e-mail with a veterinary technician or veterinarian. These messages may not be picked up soon enough to respond appropriately.

RESOLVING PROBLEMS: DIAGNOSIS, TREATMENT AND EUTHANASIA

When an animal is experiencing a health problem, the resolution involves a team effort. The area veterinarian or veterinary technician will contact the investigator or their research staff to discuss the problem. Thus it is very important that labs maintain current emergency contact information for RAR veterinary staff to use when there is an animal issue.

This information may be part of the cage card, listed as contact name/phone #/e-mail, or it may be provided to the Area RAR staff to post and/or maintain. Since health problems may be discovered any day of the week, labs are encouraged to provide contact information for one or more people who are willing to be contacted on weekends and holidays.

If an animal health problem arises and the research staff cannot be contacted (and no other instructions have been provided), RAR veterinarians are required to use professional judgement on how to proceed. This may involve initiating treatment, palliative care, or euthanasia depending on the situation.

Mouse breeding programmes sometimes result in situations where there are newborn pups whose dam has died. If the research staff cannot be contacted and have not left instructions on whether to proceed with an attempt at cross-fostering, RAR will euthanize the newborn litter in those situations..

If a problem is expected as part of the experimental procedure the nature of the problem must be documented in the Animal Care and Use Protocol form. The experimental endpoint and clinical or other criteria for euthanasia of the animal must also be indicated. There must be a scientific justification for allowing an animal to experience unrelieved pain or distress. The veterinary staff will review the Animal Usage Form whenever a new problem is seen.

If a problem occurs that is unexpected the veterinarian will assist in developing a diagnosis and prognosis for the problem:

- Veterinary examinations and consultations are not charged to investigators
- Diagnostic testing can be performed on a fee-for-service basis
- A sick animal may be selected for euthanasia and necropsy to assist in the diagnosis

The veterinarian will discuss treatment options with the investigator. Normally any animal health problem must be treated or monitored until the animal meets criteria requiring euthanasia.

- Investigators may provide their own drugs and perform their own treatments under the direction of RAR. RAR can provide the names of suppliers for common drugs and supplies.
- Drugs can be purchased through RAR.
- RAR can perform treatments.

- RAR will monitor the progress of all animals and maintain a medical record of its observations and any treatments it performs.
- If an animal is not responding to treatment the treatment plan will be re-assessed. Euthanasia may be requested.
- Treatment can be directed towards correcting the primary problem, or it may involve providing supportive care or analgesia until the animal recovers, is euthanized or reaches the experimental endpoint.
- An animal should never be allowed to reach a moribund state or die spontaneously unless it is an approved part of the experiment.

LIVESTOCK MEDICINES ON THE DAIRY FARM

The use of livestock medicines on the dairy farm by producers and veterinarians is important for disease prevention and control. Management practices which prevent disease will reduce the need for drug treatment. Planned animal health and production programmes commit the milk producer, the veterinarian and other herd advisors to the implementation of herd management policies which optimize health and production. However, when needed, medicines must be used responsibly. This factsheet provides recommendations on dairy cattle treatment, product label interpretation, treatment recording and antibiotic residue testing of milk. Information about the storage and handling of livestock medicines can be found on the OMAFRA web site.

LABELING

It is essential to read and understand drug labels to use medications safely and effectively. All livestock medicines bear labels which describe product information, indications for use, dosage, route of administration, warnings and storage instructions.

Product information includes:

- The product name ("brand name")
- The name of the manufacturer or distributor
- The drug identification number (D.I.N.)
- The manufacturers lot number
- The active ingredient in the product, and
- The concentration of active ingredient

Information provided by the label on product usage includes:

- The indications for medicine use, such as:
- The species (cattle, horses, swine)
- The class of livestock (lactating cows, non-lactatingcows,calves)
- The disease conditions (mastitis, foot rot, metritis)
- The directions for medicine use, such as
- The dosage (how much, how often and for how long)
- The method of administration
- Intramuscular - into the muscle

- Subcutaneous - under the skin
- Oral - by mouth
- Intramammary - into the udder through the teat end
- Intrauterine - into the uterus
- Storage requirements such as refrigeration, and
- The expiry date, the date past which the product should not be used.

All licensed products carry labels with warnings, cautions or precautions about the use of the product. For example, when an antibiotic product is recommended for use in cattle the label may include a warning statement "Warning: Not for use in lactating animals". This means that the product is for use only in non-lactating cattle such as dry cows and heifers. Products licensed for use in lactating cattle will indicate a with-holding time for milk following the last treatment. Products recommended for use in cattle will have a pre-slaughter withholding time on the label. With-holding times for milk and meat will only be valid if the product is used according to label instructions.

Labels may also provide information about disease management or product safety under the "Caution(s)" section. For example, a product recommended for intramuscular administration under directions for usage, may carry a caution that it is "not to be given intravenously" if the product is not safely given by that route. For further interpretation of the cautions, precautions or warnings on a product label consult your veterinarian.

Inserts included with many products provide additional information such as side effects which may occur following product use in some animals. The inserts may contain scientific and medical terms which require interpretation by a veterinarian. Carefully read and understand all insert information before using the product.

Veterinarians must meet the same labelling requirements when drugs are dispensed in non-original containers. Information must be provided which identifies the product, the species and class of animals on which the product is to be used, directions for use and with-holding times. As well, the label must carry the name of the veterinary clinic and the veterinarian prescribing the product. Drug labels are only useful to those who read them. Make a habit of reading the label before every use of a livestock medicine.

EXTRA-LABEL DRUG USE

"Extra-label" drug use is the use of a drug in any manner other than that listed on the label.

Examples of extra-label use include:

- Using a product to treat a lactating cow when the label does not list lactating dairy cattle
- Using a product at a higher dosage than that listed on the label,
- Using a product labelled for intramuscular injection as a subcutaneous injection, and

- Using a drug to treat mastitis when the label recommends it only for use in the treatment of respiratory disease.

Extra-label drug use is permitted only under the supervision of a veterinarian. The with-holding time given on the medicine label does not apply when a drug is used in an extra-label manner. The veterinarian advising extra-label use of a livestock medicine is responsible for recommending a proper with-holding time for milk and meat.

THERAPY

Livestock medicines are an important tool in the treatment and prevention of disease. Correct treatment methods assure the safety of food products and insure an effective response to treatment. Consider the following points before treating dairy cattle.

Selection of Cases: Medication is not always the best option for controlling animal disease. Treat animals based on the diagnosis, the expected response to therapy and the economic benefit expected. For example, viral infections do not respond to antibiotic therapy while those caused by bacteria will. Treating subclinical mastitis at dry off is effective and economical while treating cows with subclinical mastitis during lactation may not be. Select suitable cases to treat with the help and advice of the veterinary practitioner.

Medicine selection: Select the correct therapy. Consult your veterinarian for advice on the correct medication, the route of treatment, the treatment dosage, the time between treatments and the number of treatments. Veterinarians should leave clear written instructions with the herd owner identifying the treated animal and giving information on the treatment protocol. The veterinarian also plays an important role in monitoring the response to treatment.

Treatment Method: Treatment must be given correctly to be effective and to prevent complications. Use the following guidelines to develop good treatment habits.

- Wash your hands before and after handling livestock medicines.
- Use proper equipment: Choose the correct syringe and needle size for the animal size, the dosage and the type of injection to be given.
- For intramuscular injection use a 11/2 in., 16 or 18 gauge needle to insure the drug goes in the muscle and not under the skin. Before injecting, pull back on the plunger to insure the needle tip is not in a blood vessel. Select appropriate injection sites with the help of your veterinarian. Read the label for the maximum amount to be injected in one site.
- For subcutaneous injection use a 1/2" to 1", 16 or 18 gauge needle. Check that the needle tip is moveable. Inject a small amount of drug to see if a "bleb" of skin starts to rise in the area of the needle tip. This will verify that the needle is under the skin and not in the muscle. Inject only in sites recommended by your veterinarian.

- Inject only in clean body sites.
- Use clean equipment. Single use, sterile, disposable needles and syringes are preferred.
- Give repeated injections in different body sites.
- Before infusing antibiotics into the udder, wash and dry your hands. Wash and dry the teat with single use paper towels. Disinfect the teat end with the alcohol swab provided in the medication package. Avoid touching the infusion canula at the end of the treatment tube. Use only single dose infusion products in disposable syringes. Teat dip the teat after infusion of medication.

Dosage Calculation: To calculate the correct dosage you must know the weight of the animal and the dosage rate. For example, to treat a 600 kg cow with procaine penicillin at the label dosage of 2.5 mL per 100 kg of body weight once daily, inject: 600 kg/100 x 2.5 mL = 15 mL.

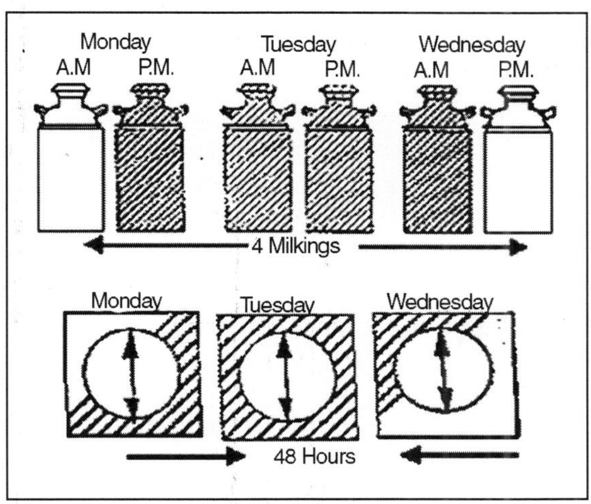

Fig. Diagrams Illustrating how a 48 hour Milk discard time should be Calculated. One shows the number of Milkings to be Discarded and the other the Discard time in Hours.

One millilitre (ml) and one cubic centimetre (cc) represent the same volume and are interchangeable in calculating drug dosages. *Repeat Treatments:* Determine the number of treatments to be given from the product label or as recommended by the veterinarian. The duration of treatment should result in a cure without risk of relapse, yet be short enough to insure withholding times are not extended. *Withholding Times:* Withholding times for milk and meat are given on product labels. A withdrawal day is a full 24 hours starting after the time of treatment. A 48 hour withdrawal time for milk is illustrated in Figure above.

Errors in calculating withdrawal times of only a few hours could result in a residue violation. Label withdrawals are not accurate if products are used in an extra-label fashion, if drugs are used in combination (for example intramammary and intramuscular treatments for mastitis given at the same time), or if the treated animal is severely sick and unable to clear the drug from its body at normal rates. In these cases you must test the milk before addition to the bulk tank to insure it is residue free.

Prevent Residues: Simple management practises will prevent contamination of milk or meat.

To prevent residues:

- Record all treatments given;
- Visibly mark all treated cows;
- Inform all people involved in milking of treated cows;
- Milk treated cows last or use separate "bypass" equipment to insure that no contaminated milk enters the milk supply;
- Discard milk from all quarters of treated cows;
- Discard milk from all cows calving within 30 or 42 days of dry treatment according to label directions;
- Discard milk from fresh cows for the required period if dry treatment was used;
- Use antibiotic test kits as needed; and follow label directions for all medications used. These include feed additives, medicated feeds such as calf starter, topical preparations, as well as injectable and infusion products.

TREATMENT RECORDS

Many antibiotic residue violations result from failure to: identify treated cows, maintain treatment records, and use proper milk withholding times. The record system must make all staff involved in milking aware of treated cows and the period for withholding milk from sale. Identify treated cows in a manner clearly visible to the person milking.

Some methods used are:

- Leg bands,
- Coloured tape or fluorescent hockey tape around the legs or tail, or
- Paint markings on the cow's flank, rump or legs.

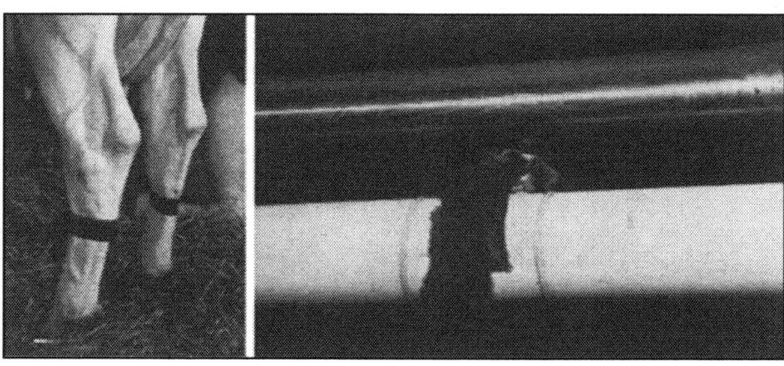

Fig. Clearly Visible Identification of treated Animals such as leg Bands (left) or Tags on the Pipeline (right).

Bibliography

V A Sapre and N P Dakshinkar: *A Handbook for Veterinary Physician* , International Book Dist, 2007, pbk

S N Khosla: *Digestive System and Liver Ailments*, Peacock Books, 2006

Suman Kumari Joshi, Manish Kr. Singh and Srinivas Sathapathy: *A Textbook on Zoonotic Disease*:, Satish Serial Publishing House, 2015.

H. Rahman, Rajeswari Shome and M. Nagalingam: *Brucellosis : A Zoonotic Disease,* Biotech Books, 2015.

S. Nandi: *Zoonotic Diseases* : , New India Publishing Agency, 2014.

Ashok Kumar: *Encyclopaedia of Animal Diseases (5 Vols-Set)* , Discovery, 2007.

Arvind N. Shukla and Rajiv Tyagi: *Encyclopaedia of Animal Diseases (6 Vols-Set)* , Anmol, 2001.

Subrata Bhattacharjee: *Handbook of Animal Diseases*, Dominant, 2001.

Makarand Madhukar Gore,: *Anatomy and Physiology of Yogic Practices : Understanding of the Yogic Concepts and Physiological Mechanism of the Yogic Practices* , Motilal Banarsidass, 20142014 .

S. Sathapathjy, M.K. Singh and S.K. Joshi: *A Handbook on Anatomy and Physiology of Domestic Animals and Birds*, Satish Serial Publishing House, 2015.

Ram Mohun Mojumdar: *Anatomy and Physiology*, Sports Pub, 2009.

Ashok Kumar Sharma: *Anatomy and Physiology Insects*, Oxford Book Company, 2012.

Clark: *Anatomy And Physiology: Understanding The Human Body*, Jones and Bartlett Publishers, 2010.

Vaidyaratnam P.S. Varier: *Astangasariram : Concise and Complete Text Book of Human Anatomy and Physiology in Sanskrit with Commentary and Illustrations Compiled for the Use of Ayurveda Colleges* , Chowkhamba Sanskrit Series, 2005.

Piyush Jain: *Basic Anatomy and Physiology of Exercise*, Khel Sahitya Kendra, 2006.

B K Sheshadri: *Human Anatomy and Physiology in Pharmacy*, Sonali Pub, 2007.

Aslam Khan: *Plant Anatomy and Physiology*, Kalpaz, 2001.

Rajaram Choyal: *Plant Anatomy and Physiology* , Sonali Publications, 2012.

S. Mariappan, N. Deepa Devi, V. Premalakshmi, S. Manisegaran and V. Swaminathan: *A Text Book on Greens and Salad Vegetables*, Jaya Publishing House, 2014.

Gautam Murthy: *India: Bilateral and Regional Economic Co-operation*: , New Century Publications, 2015 .

Makarand Madhukar Gore: *Anatomy and Physiology of Yogic Practices : Understanding of the Yogic Concepts and Physiological Mechanism of the Yogic Practices* , Motilal Banarsidass, 2014.

Rudrajeet Desai: *Breaking Out and Making Big : A No Nonsense Book on Start-Ups and Entrepreneurship*: HarperCollins, 2014.

K. B. Saxena: *Contemporary Practices of Mahatma Gandhi National Rural Employment Guarantee Scheme: Insights from Districts*, Sage, 2015.

Neelima Gupta and D.K. Gupta: *Environment and Biodiversity*, Narendra Publishing House, 2014.

Kulwant Singh Phull: *Foreign Institutional Investors FIIs and Capital Market In India*, New Century Publications, 2014.

Philip Stevens and Debashis Chakraborty: *Free Trade and Markets in Healthcare: Lessons from Asian Countries*, Synergy Books India, 2013.

Josukutty C.A: *India-U.S. Relations and Asian Rebalancing*, New Century Publications, 2015.

Index